Endophthalmitis

Endophthalmitis
Diagnosis and Management

Gholam A Peyman MD
Professor of Ophthalmology
Tulane University Health Sciences Center School of Medicine
New Orleans, LA, USA

Paul J Lee MD
Assistant Professor of Ophthalmology
State University of New York, Buffalo, NY, and
Retina Consultants of Western New York
531 Farber Lakes Drive
Williamsville, NY, USA

David V Seal MD FRCOphth FRCPath DipBact MIBiol
Visiting Professor
Applied Vision Research Centre, City University
Northampton Square
London, UK

With the assistance of

Trisha Chiasson
Editorial Consultant

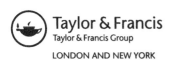
Taylor & Francis
Taylor & Francis Group
LONDON AND NEW YORK
A MARTIN DUNITZ BOOK

© 2004 Taylor & Francis, an imprint of the Taylor & Francis Group

Transferred to Digital Printing 2005

First published in the United Kingdom in 2004
by Taylor & Francis, an imprint of the Taylor & Francis Group,
2 Park Square, Milton Park, Abingdon, Oxfordshire, OX14 4RN

Tel.:   +44 (0) 1235 828600
Fax.:   +44 (0) 1235 829000
E-mail: info@dunitz.co.uk
Website: http://www.dunitz.co.uk

A CIP record for this book is available from the British Library.

Library of Congress Cataloging-in-Publication Data

Data available on application

ISBN 1 84184 278 8

Distributed in North and South America by

Taylor & Francis
2000 NW Corporate Blvd
Boca Raton, FL 33431, USA

Within Continental USA
Tel.: 800 272 7737; Fax.: 800 374 3401
Outside Continental USA
Tel.: 561 994 0555; Fax.: 561 361 6018
E-mail: orders@crcpress.com

Distributed in the rest of the world by
Thomson Publishing Services
Cheriton House
North Way
Andover, Hampshire SP10 5BE, UK
Tel.: +44 (0)1264 332424
E-mail: salesorder.tandf@thomsonpublishingservices.co.uk

Composition by Scribe Design, Ashford, Kent, Great Britain

Dedication

This book is dedicated to those members of the ASCRS (American Society of Cataract and Refractive Surgeons) and the ESCRS (European Society of Cataract and Refractive Surgeons) who have given their time and energy toward studying the best ways to prevent postoperative endophthalmitis after cataract surgery by both surgical and chemotherapeutic approaches. Their aim is to prevent and treat postoperative endophthalmitis to make intraocular procedures as safe as possible.

Contents

Preface

The rapid advance of our knowledge base and development of surgical techniques have culminated in a new era of ophthalmic care. Yet, new developments only broaden the horizon. For this we thank the pioneers as well as the innovators. They have led the paradigmatic shift from the 'appropriate method' of parenteral antibiotic delivery to the delineation of intravitreal techniques and the range of 'appropriate' antibiotics that we enjoy today.

Many forthright investigators have been vilified for going against dogma. Yet, it is this spirit of challenging the 'truth' that has driven our field to its heights. The change of perspective of treating endophthalmitis with parenteral antibiotics in the 1960s to the current milieu of intravitreal injections has been challenging. Our collective psyche in approaching endophthalmitis as a feared condition to a manageable state is still evolution in the making.

Our goal has been to summarize comprehensively the work that has been put into endophthalmitis. As in any body of knowledge, there have been many unacknowledged investigators who had planted the seeds which bore fruit. We are indebted to all whose effort contributed to the present state of understanding and management of endophthalmitis. With time, our knowledge will change, but our practice of knowledge will survive. The accuracy of our current position can only be determined retrospectively in the future.

Gholam A Peyman
Paul J Lee
David V Seal

Acknowledgments

We acknowledge with much gratitude the considerable assistance given by our colleagues below in helping us to produce this book. We are grateful to them for their contributions as follows:

Jorge Abreu MD and Luis Cordoves MD University Hospital of the Canary Islands, Tenerife, Spain, for advice and Figures 6.1 A–D, 6.17 A–C and 6.20 A&B.

Peter Barry, Dublin, Ireland, for advice.

Delmar R Caldwell MD Professor and Chairman, Department of Ophthalmology, Tulane University Health Sciences Center, New Orleans, Louisiana; and Morton F Goldberg MD former Chairman, Department of Ophthalmology, Johns Hopkins University, Baltimore, Maryland, for their support and encouragement.

Mandi D. Conway MD Professor of Ophthalmology, Tulane University Health Sciences Center, New Orleans, Louisiana, for her significant contribution to Chapter 8 on the surgical management of endophthalmitis.

Robert Cooling, Moorfields Eye Hospital, London, England, for Figure 7.4C.

John Dart, Moorfields Eye Hospital, London, England, for Figure 6.21.

Consuelo Ferrer PhD and Jorge Alio MD Instituto Oftalmológico de Alicante, Alicante, Spain for their major contribution of the entire molecular biology section of Chapter 3 and Figures 3.17, 3.18, 3.19, 3.20, 3.21, 3.22, 6.14A, 6.15 A&B and 7.6A–C.

Richard Fiscella RPh MPH Chicago, Illinois, for his contribution towards Chapter 11.

Suzanne Gardner PhD formerly of Emory University, Atlanta, Georgia for her joint authorship of Chapter 5 on pharmacokinetics.

Klaus Geldsetzer PhD Santen Gmbh, Munich, Germany, for the graph on tear levofloxacin levels in Chapter 5 and other advice on quinolone drugs.

Suleyman Kaynak MD Retina Goz Merkezi, Izmir, Turkey, for Figures 6.2, 6.3 A–E, 6.4 A&B, 6.5, 6.6, 7.4 A&B, 7.11, 9.1, 9.2 G–I and 9.3.

Manus C Kraff, MD, Kraff Eye Institute, Chicago, Illinois; and Norman Jaffe MD Miami, Florida, for their encouragement and advice over many years.

Susan Lightman, Moorfields Eye Hospital, London, England, for Figures 10.2(B–D) and 10.7(A-E).

Mary Moore PhD St Thomas' Hospital, London, England for Figures 3.12 A, 3.13, 3.14, 3.15 A&B and 6.12C.

Jerry Niederkorn PhD University of Texas Southwestern Medical Center, Dallas, Texas for advice on immunology.

Joel Schulman MD Associate Professor of Ophthalmology, Louisiana State University Medical School, Shreveport, Louisiana, for contributions towards Chapters 6 and 7.

Thomas Spoor MD Professor of Ophthalmology and Neurosurgery, Kresge Eye Institute, Wayne State University, Detroit, Michigan, for Figures 7.3, 7.8 A&B, 7.9 A&B, 7.10 A&B and 9.2F.

Philip Thomas MD Joseph Eye Hospital, Tiruchirapalli, India for contributing the fungus section and tables in Chapter 3 – Microbiology, for Table 11.4 and for other advice on fungi and antifungal drugs as well as Figures 3.12B&C and 6.12A&B.

Kirk Wilhelmus MD Cullen Eye Institute Baylor College of Medicine, Houston, Texas for advice and Figure 6.7 on Acremonium endophthalmitis.

Our medical students, residents, and fellows for their contributions.

Alan Burgess, Senior Publisher, Martin Dunitz & Parthenon Publishing, London, for his support and patience in bringing our book to press.

Giovanna Ceroni, Senior Production Editor, Martin Dunitz & Parthenon Publishing, for overseeing this project through to completion.

Trisha Chiasson BA Editor, Department of Ophthalmology, Tulane University Health Sciences Center, New Orleans, Louisiana, for editing this work.

Mike Meakin, Yorkshire, UK, formerly of Martin Dunitz Ltd, for his freelance work as a proofreader on this project and his in-house editorial work on an earlier project.

1

Inflammation

Introduction

Inflammation is a biological, chemical, and physical response that the body mounts in response to injury. This response is mediated through vascular, cellular, and humoral pathways and modified by the stimulus and the host's ability to elicit a response. Furthermore, both the nature of the stimulus and the extent of local tissue injury determine the type of inflammatory response. Resolution results in a combination of destruction and repair of the pre-existing tissues.

An inflammatory response occurs in four different phases:

- Recognition that normal tissue equilibrium has been disturbed
- Rapid response involving vascular and cellular events leading to exudation
- A variable phase dependent on the causative agent and the host's response
- Resolution to preinjury state or development of granulation tissue and scarring.

Host damage is a culmination of three factors:

- Etiology. Bacteria generally invoke a polymorphonuclear cell response while most viruses typically elicit only a lymphocyte response.
- Host immune system. Intrinsic enzymes such as collagenase, complement components, and clotting mechanism may have primary damaging consequences.
- Physical/chemical host mechanisms modulate the inflammatory process.

Immunodeficient patients (e.g. patients with human immunodeficiency virus [HIV]) may not be able to mount a robust inflammatory response.

Ocular immune privilege

Resolution of inflammation results in destruction and repair of the preexisting tissues. In the eye, even a mild inflammation and subsequent repair can cause significant vision loss by disrupting the precise collagen fibril organization that is needed for transparency. Immune privilege refers to a protective mechanism in highly specialized organs such as the eye in which sequelae of inflammation would cause severe disruption of function. Immune privilege limits the inflammatory response and allows extended antigen survival within its milieu, thereby sparing inflammation-induced injury. In the eye, this phenomenon is called anterior chamber-associated immune deviation (ACAID). Experimentally, it was noted that antigens such as allografts prepared from a variety of tissues (skin, thyroid, islets of Langerhans, cornea, and retina) experienced prolonged and even indefinite survival when placed in the anterior chamber. *The same immune deviation (ACAID) occurs in the vitreous cavity and subretinal space, but not within the choroid.*

ACAID limits inflammation-induced damage and the repair process in order to maintain the fine organization of tissues required for visual clarity. Specifically, immunosuppressive factors secreted by parenchymal cells in the iris and ciliary body selectively suppress the T cells (delayed hypersensitivity reactions) and complement-fixing antibodies (see Chapter 2).

In sympathetic ophthalmia, ocular penetrating trauma causes uveitis in the fellow eye directed at retinal autoantigens; the implication is that these antigens were released in the traumatic eye and sensitized the systemic immune system. This condition occurs in only a small portion of patients. It has been hypothesized that antigen released by the trauma induces ACAID in the same eye but not in the fellow eye.

Given the recent evidence linking inflammation with diabetes,[1] glaucoma, and age-related macular degeneration (ARMD), deducing the molecular basis for ocular immune privilege may enable novel approaches to these problematic disorders. Experimental studies conducted in mice showed that newborn neural retinal grafts implanted in the subretinal space and vitreous cavity experienced immune privilege. Furthermore, Fas ligand, a component of the Fas/FasL interaction that modulates peripheral tolerance and induction of immune privilege, has also been identified in the eye.[2] Immune tolerance/deviation will likely play a significant role in the treatment of ocular diseases.

Fibrin membrane formation

If immune deviation fails and significant inflammation occurs in the eye, a fibrin membrane will form. Fibrin is the end-product of the coagulation cascade (fibrinogen and thrombin) and comprises the major component of clotted blood. The fibrinolytic system is activated simultaneously with the coagulation pathway, resulting in the conversion of plasminogen into plasmin, which lyses fibrin. Complex autoregulatory mechanisms exist between the coagulation and fibrinolytic systems.

The balance between plasminogen activator and plasminogen activator inhibitor (PAI) determines the level of fibrin formation. The eye may be favored toward coagulation because of the deficiency of plasminogen activator relative to its inhibitor.

Under normal circumstances, the blood–ocular barrier blocks fibrinogen from entering the eye. However, severe inflammation (i.e. endophthalmitis) results in extensive blood–ocular barrier breakdown. Migration of fibrinogen, plasminogen, and leukocytes into the eye occurs and a cascade of reactions is initiated leading to fibrin membrane formation (Figure 1.1, Box 1.1). Leukocytes produce PAI-2 which diminishes the normal fibrinolytic mechanisms and results in severe fibrin formation. Bacterial products such as endotoxins also stimulate its production.

Under normal circumstances, plasminogen activator promotes fibrinolysis by cleaving

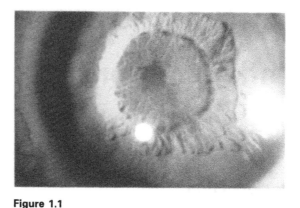

Figure 1.1

Fibrinous deposition in the vitreous after endophthalmitis.

Box 1.1 Ocular sequelae of fibrin and fibrinogen-derived peptides

Retinal pigment epithelium migration
Leukocyte influx
Microvascular permeability
Corneal endothelium damage
Recurrent tractional and rhegmatogenous retinal detachments
Pupillary block and glaucoma

plasminogen into plasmin which lyses fibrin in the process. A balance between plasminogen activators and PAI regulates fibrinolysis. In the eye, the balance may already be tilted toward a procoagulant state. In the aqueous fluid, plasminogen activator concentration is 0.5 ng/ml to 0.9 ng/ml, which is an order of magnitude less than its plasma concentration but PAI-1, its principal antagonist, is absent. Only PAI-2, which is a far less effective antagonist, is present. Therefore, the presence of the plasminogen activator in low levels albeit without its primary inhibitor suggests a profibrinolytic state in the aqueous without inflammation present.

Clinically, patients with diabetes are known to be at increased risk of developing fibrin membrane after surgery. These patients demonstrate both enhanced coagulation and depressed fibrinolysis. Elevated fibrinogen levels and abnormal antithrombin III (AT III) metabolism are among proposed mechanisms. AT III inhibits procoagulant proteases and its activity is enhanced by heparin and endogenous mucopolysaccharides. The end result is that deficient AT III enhances the breakdown of fibrinogen into fibrin. In diabetes, AT III metabolism may be decreased due to:

- Renal loss of AT III as a result of proteinuria.
- Glycosylation of AT III which results in diminished activity.

Other mechanisms accounting for a procoagulant state among patients with diabetes include:

- Depression of fibrinolysis.
- Glycosylation reducing the susceptibility of fibrin to plasmin.
- PAI activities that are elevated in diabetes.

In this state of increased fibrin formation and decreased fibrinolysis, the net result of a significant ocular insult may be fibrin membrane formation.

A similar imbalance between coagulation and fibrinolysis may be responsible for fibrin formation in proliferative vitreous retinopathy (PVR) and endophthalmitis. Given that not all patients with PVR or endophthalmitis develop significant fibrin formation, there may be individual variations in the balance between plasminogen activator and PAI. Increased systemic PAI levels have been documented in a variety of conditions, including advanced age, obesity, and connective tissue disease. Furthermore, because ocular PAI-2 is present over a wide physiologic range in human aqueous, individuals with elevated systemic or ocular PAI activity might be predisposed to fibrin formation.

In a series of 194 consecutive vitrectomies, Jaffe's group identified preoperative clinical risk factors for fibrin formation.[3] The risk factors included:

- Severe flare
- Presence of a previously placed scleral buckle
- Hand motion or light perception preoperative visual acuity
- Vitreous-base dissection
- Iris sutures.

There was an increased incidence of fibrin formation among patients with PVR, compared with other preoperative diagnoses. Overall, the incidence of fibrin formation was 32%.

Inflammatory response

Host response

The host response to bacteria is mounted against the types of adhesion structures expressed on the bacteria and the toxins produced by these bacteria.[4] In Gram-positive organisms, these attachment structures are called fibrillae, while Gram-negative organisms use filamentous attachment structures known as fimbriae (pili). Minor changes in protein structure at the tips of pili also enable the bacteria to adhere to different cell receptors and modify the location/nature of inflammation. Host receptors such as integrins and CR3 serve as binding points.

Microorganisms have evolved many mechanisms to combat the host immune response. One method is to inflict maximal host damage using toxins. Gram-positive organisms use exotoxins and Gram-negative organisms use endotoxins. The exotoxins of clostridia and *Corynebacterium diphtheriae* are particularly potent and typically invoke an acute inflammatory response. Endotoxins are insoluble lipopolysaccharides (LPS) that form integral cell wall components of Gram-negative bacteria. Intravascular exposure may cause intravascular coagulation, peripheral vascular collapse, and shock. Endotoxins elicit an acute inflammatory response through cytokines, the complement system (alternate pathway), and the contact-coagulation system. Polyclonal B lymphocytes are also activated and amplify the inflammatory response.

Microorganisms also combat the immune system by evading it completely. Bacteria such as pneumococci and some *Haemophilus* strains produce capsules while others proliferate within mononuclear phagocytic cells and inhibit microbial killing in phagolysosomes. Examples include *Toxoplasma gondii*, tuberculosis, leprosy, typhoid, tularemia, brucellosis, and listeriosis. Once the immune system determines that the intruders cannot be eradicated, a granuloma forms to physically isolate the organisms. Granulomatous inflammation is discussed in Chapter 10.

Viral particles are able to incorporate into the host genetic DNA or RNA and sometimes avoid detection this way. The immune response is generally virus-dependent and consists of a combination of antibody-mediated and/or lymphocyte-dependent responses. Some viruses exhibit extremely long incubation periods. Some of these organisms show evidence of the immune response directed against virus particles contained in cells and can be responsible in part for the expression of the disease. However, others are able to evade detection and avoid inflammation altogether. Such organisms show no evidence of inflammatory response or ultrastructural evidence of virus. These organisms are called slow viruses and can be transmitted by ultrafiltrates of infected tissue. Subacute sclerosing panencephalitis is an example of the former.

Fungi typically produce a wide variety of inflammatory responses from hypersensitivity reaction to a chronic suppurative or granulomatous inflammation in immunosuppressed individuals. Proteolytic enzymes allow these organisms to gain access to tissues. Live helminths at times do not cause an inflammatory reaction; response occurs only with the death of the organism. Fungi, certain bacteria, protozoa, and helminths can usually be identified in tissues by diligent examination or by using special stains.

Acute inflammatory response

The classic signs of acute inflammation are rubor (redness), calor (heat), tumor (swelling), dolor (pain), and functio laesa (loss of function). These signs can be correlated to microscopic changes causing vascular changes, exudation, and leukocyte emigration. Initial mechanical vascular damage causes flush, which is followed by arteriolar dilation causing increased blood flow, resulting in flare. Next, a wheal is formed by serous or exudative fluid accumulation in the extracellular spaces resulting from vascular permeability.

Several cytokines play key roles in mediating acute inflammatory reactions, namely interleukin (IL)-1, tumor necrosis factor-alpha (TNF-α), IL-6, IL-11, IL-8, G-colony stimulating factor (CSF), and granulocyte-macrophage (GM-CSF) (Table 1.1).[5] Of these, IL-1 and TNF are extremely potent inflammatory molecules that primarily mediate

Table 1.1 Cytokines active in acute inflammation		
IL-1	IL-6	IL-11
Tumor necrosis factor (TNF)	IL-8	IL-16
IL-17	Eotaxin	Colony stimulating factors (CSF)

IL, interleukin.

acute inflammation induced in animals by intradermal injection of bacterial LPS.

Vascular events

Vascular flow

The acute vascular inflammatory response is a combination of two seemingly opposing processes. On one hand, vasodilation and platelet aggregation inhibition promote migration of the body's defense to the site of damage. But a slightly delayed vasoconstriction and platelet aggregation eventually prevail and promote containment of the antigen. An army of lymphokines and cytokines working in concert orchestrates these events.

The initial events in acute inflammation are vasodilation, increase in blood flow, and prevention of platelet aggregation (Table 1.2).[6–8] Prostacyclin (PGI2) and nitric oxide primarily mediate these events. In mild ocular inflammation, a relative increase in blood flow can persist throughout the period of the inflammatory response. In more severe infections, simultaneous intravascular events occur, causing vasoconstriction and blood flow stasis. In response to the early vasodilation and increased blood flow, platelets become activated and release thromboxane A2, serotonins, and platelet-activating factor (PAF). Endothelial cells release endothelin. Subsequently, circulation slows down and increased vascular permeability and leukocyte extravasation into the injured site occur. Severe ocular inflammation eventually results in vasculitis with subsequent thrombus formation in vessels with consequent decrease of blood flow in the area.

Table 1.2 Factors affecting vascular reaction in acute inflammation

Prostacyclin (PGl2)	Vasodilation, inhibition of platelet aggregation
Nitric oxide	Vasodilation
Thromboxane A2	Platelet aggregation
Serotonins	Vasoconstriction
Platelet-activating factor	Progression activation
Endothelin	Vasoconstriction

Vascular permeability and exudation

Increased vascular permeability also develops as a result of direct endothelial injury and vaso-active mediators. In direct endothelial injury, vascular changes occur both in capillaries and venules, whereas the vasoactive mediators act only on the postcapillary venules. Plasma extravasation and continuing activation of plasma components cause coagulation and fibrin formation. This results in diffuse edema in the interstitial tissues and body cavities.

Exudation is the passage of protein-rich fluid through the now increasingly permeable vasculature. This phase responds to the wheal phase in Lewis's triple response. Functionally, fluid increase results in dilution of toxins and allows fibrin deposition, which helps to limit bacterial spread. Two types of exudate exist – cellular and fluid.

Different patterns of vascular leakage have been identified by Albert:[9]

- Immediate transient leakage, located entirely in the venules, that is produced by mediators.
- Immediate prolonged leakage, which is in part due to mediators such as cytokines and in part as the result of direct damage to vessels.
- Delayed, prolonged leakage that does not become manifest for several hours, resulting primarily from mild direct injury.

Of interest, delayed and prolonged leakage has been associated with phospholipase enzymes released from *Clostridium* species. Furthermore, mild acute anterior uveitis can be produced experimentally by the intravenous injection of bacterial endotoxin. This response is caused by increased permeability in the vessels of the ciliary process and correlated with fibrin deposition and platelet aggregation. These clotting events increase the vascular damage.

All components of plasma, including fibrinogen, kinins, the complement system, and immunoglobulins, are present in the fluid exudate. Fibrinogen is important in clot formation and the prevention of further loss of blood. Fibrin is the building block on which further repair occurs. The coagulation pathway reaction must be balanced to limit collateral damage to surrounding undamaged tissue. Fibrinolysis controls the ultimate clearing of the clots. The kinins system produces bradykinin. The complement cascade is responsible for the ultimate destruction of the invading microorganism. Immunoglobulins may act to facilitate phagocytosis or may participate in antibody-dependent cell-mediated cytotoxicity.

Cellular exudate is formed during the acute and chronic cellular response. Neutrophils predominate in the acute phase, whereas mononuclear cells (macrophages and lymphocytes) become predominant in the later chronic phase. The type of inflamed tissue and factors triggering the inflammatory process also determine the cellular make-up of the exudate. Neutrophils dominate when a pyogenic bacterial infection or local deposition of immune complexes containing IgG causes the inflammation. Mononuclear cells (monocytes) dominate in the subacute and chronic phases of inflammatory reactions, and parasitizing microorganisms. Eosinophils and basophils are predominant when inflammation has been initiated by immediate allergic reactions or by parasites.

Cellular events

The net effect of the vascular alterations is to promote accumulation of appropriate immune elements. In this process, various factors are released from the endothelium and blood components (platelets, monocytes, and neutrophils). These factors upregulate the expression of mechanisms that allow the migration and accumulation of the inflammatory cells.

The cellular events of acute inflammation begin soon after the vascular response is initiated. The sequence of events is margination of leukocytes in the blood vessels, migration of the

Table 1.3 Adhesion molecules

Selectins Family of transmembrane molecules expressed on the surface of leukocytes and activated endothelial cells	• E-selectin (activated endothelium) • P-selectin (activated platelets and endothelium) • L-selectin (leukocytes)
Integrins Transmembrane glycoproteins that attach cells to extracellular matrix proteins of the basement membrane or to ligands on other cells	• Very late activation (antigen)-4 (VLA-4) • VLA-4 is chiefly responsible for lymphocyte adhesion to vascular endothelium and leukocyte recruitment to the inflamed area
Immunoglobulin superfamily	

leukocytes into the injured tissue (directed by chemotaxis), attachment of the phagocytes to the antigens, and the ingestion and degradation of these particles.

Margination

In this phase, leukocytes appear to line up along the endothelium. Through a variety of chemotactic mechanisms, leukocytes accumulate intravascularly at the site of inflammation. The different proposed mechanisms are:

*   Alteration in the relative negative charge of cell surfaces of both leukocytes and endothelial cells, allowing closer attachment.
*   The balance of procoagulant factors and fibrinolytic factors (plasminogen) affecting leukocyte accumulation. For instance, the peptide that results when fibrinolysis splits fibrin is a leukocyte chemoattractant.
*   The expression of adhesion molecules by leukocytes and endothelial cells, allowing margination and eventual emigration of leukocytes through the endothelial cells and eventually the vascular wall.

There are at least three adhesion molecules involved in acute inflammation: selectins, integrins, and members of the immunoglobulin superfamily (Table 1.3). Selectin molecules are expressed on the surfaces of endothelium and leukocytes, and a firm adhesion is established. P-selectin is stored in platelet granules and in Weibel–Palade bodies in endothelial cells. The surface expression of this molecule is initiated by

thrombin, histamine, and PAF among others. The expression of E-selectin is induced by the cytokines IL-1, TNF-α, and LPS. E-selectin and P-selectin bind neutrophils and monocytes. L-selectin binds endothelial cells.

Integrin proteins bind to adhesion molecules found on endothelial cells. Their expression on the leukocyte surface is initiated by products of the complement C5a, arachidonic acid metabolism (leukotriene B4), bacteria (formyl peptides), and cytokines (IL-8). Other cytokines (IL-1, TNF-α, and interferon-gamma [IFN-γ]) and LPS from bacteria induce intercellular adhesion molecule-1 expression on endothelial cells. The end result is a firm adherence between the integrin on leukocytes and the endothelial surface.

Migration and chemotaxis

In this phase, the marginated leukocytes migrate through the interendothelial junctions into the extravascular space. As endothelial cells are drawn apart or injured, the leukocytes also become adherent to the exposed basement membrane. Specifically, the activated leukocytes form adhesions to fibronectin and laminin.

Leukocyte migration is mediated via chemotaxis (directed locomotion), in which injured tissue elaborates specific mediators and attracts leukocytes to a particular location. These chemotactic mediators (C5a, LTB4, IL-8, and formyl peptides) activate intracellular signals and induce myofilament assembly, contraction, and subsequent leukocyte migration. The intracellular signals involve membrane phospholipids, intracellular calcium, and protein kinases. This cellular activation requires an orchestrated release of mediators from neutrophils, monocytes, mast cells, or basophils and platelets acting together. Acute inflammation can be viewed as a concerted event involving plasma components, endothelium, neutrophils, platelets or basophils, and monocytes.

Phagocytosis

Macrophages are able to destroy antigens through phagocytosis and subsequent degradation. Antigen recognition is enhanced by opsonins (plasma antibodies), for which both neutrophils and macrophages have specific Fc receptors. After a phagocyte attaches to the surface of the antigen, the particle is ingested by cytoplasmic engulfment. Granules and vesicles converge on the resulting phagosome (engulfed antigen) and discharge their contents to degrade the antigen. Ingestion is an energy-dependent activity, and is a continuation of the leukocyte activation process beginning with receptor induction and proceeding to chemotaxis.

Chronic inflammation

Chronic inflammation is a prolonged inflammatory response occurring:

* As a progression from persistent acute inflammation
* As a result of repeated episodes of acute inflammation
* As a primary event if the antigen produces only a mild acute response.

Granulomatous inflammation is a form of chronic inflammation histologically characterized by the presence of granulomas which are collections of activated macrophages with epithelioid morphology, macrophage-derived giant cells, and surrounding infiltrate of lymphocytes, plasma cells, and granulocytes. Because this type of inflammatory response can be seen in relatively few disease processes, identification of granulomas in tissue has important diagnostic implications.

Causes of granulomatous inflammation

During this phase of inflammation, cytokine interactions result in monocyte chemotaxis to the site of inflammation. Macrophage-activating factors (MAF), such as IFN-γ, membrane cofactor protein (MCP-1), and other molecules then activate the macrophages while migration inhibition factors (MIF), such as GM-CSF and IFN-γ, retain them at the inflammatory site. The macrophages contribute to the inflammatory process by chronically elaborating low levels of IL-1 and TNF.

Chemical mediators of inflammation

Chemical mediators released from cells

GM-colony stimulating factor (GM-CSF) enhances the survival and activates the immunological functions of granulocytes and macrophages (Table 1.4).

Cytokines are peptides produced from other cells that help to regulate the immune response. Each cytokine can have contradictory functions: at times proinflammatory and at times anti-inflammatory. The cytokine network is analogous to a code that orchestrates the inflammatory response in initiating, curtailing, and sustaining complex biologic responses (Table 1.5).

Histamine, which is stored in mast cells, basophil and eosinophil leukocytes, and platelets, causes vasodilation and an increase in vascular

Table 1.4 Chemical mediators released from cells

Granulocyte-macrophage colony stimulating factor (GM-CSF)	Tumor necrosis factor-alpha (TNF-α)
Platelet-derived growth factor (PDGF)	

Table 1.5 Cytokines		
Cytokines primarily involved in the *humoral* inflammatory response		
IL-3	IL-7	IL-13
IL-4	IL-9	IL-14
IL-5	IL-10	TGF-β
Cytokines involved primarily in the *cellular* inflammatory response		
IL-2	Interferon	
IL-12	IFN-γ inducting factor	
IL-15		
IL, interleukin; IFN, interferon.		

Box 1.2 Nomenclature of prostaglandins

PGE₂: PG means prostaglandin, E means that the cyclopentane ring has a carbonyl group at position 9 and a hydroxyl group at position 11 (E is because the prostaglandin is ether-soluble) and 2 means that there are 2 double bonds.

PGF₂ is a prostaglandin with hydrophilic hydroxyl groups at both positions 9 and 11 (so it is soluble in phosphate buffer), the hydroxyl in the 9 position is in the beta configuration and there are 2 double bonds.

permeability. Histamine release is stimulated by complement components C3a and C5a and by lysosomal proteins released from neutrophils.

Lysosomal compounds are released from neutrophils and include cationic proteins, which may increase vascular permeability, and neutral proteases, which may activate the complement system.

Platelet-derived growth factor (PDGF), which induces proliferation of fibroblasts, microglia, and smooth muscle, is stored in platelet granules and is released following platelet aggregation. PDGF also serves as a chemotactic agent for inflammatory cells.

Prostaglandins are long-chain fatty acids (Box 1.2) derived from arachidonic acid and synthesized by many cell types. Some prostaglandins potentiate the increase in vascular permeability caused by other compounds. Others include platelet aggregation (prostaglandin 1 is inhibitory while prostaglandin A2 is stimulatory). Part of the antiinflammatory activity of drugs such as aspirin and the nonsteroidal antiinflammatory drugs (NSAIDS) is attributable to inhibition of one of the enzymes involved in prostaglandin synthesis.

Leukotrienes are also synthesized from arachidonic acid, especially in neutrophils, and appear to have vasoactive properties. SRS-A (slow-reacting substance of anaphylaxis), involved in type I hypersensitivity, is a mixture of leukotrienes.

5–Hydroxytryptamine (serotonin) is a vasoconstrictor found in high concentrations in mast cells and platelets as well as in the central nervous system.

Lymphokine is a generic term for molecules produced by lymphocytes other than antibodies which are involved in cellular signaling in the immune system. Lymphokines play a major role in type IV hypersensitivity as well as displaying vasoactive and chemotactic properties.

TNF-α is a proinflammatory cytokine that can force cells to undergo apoptosis. It is essential in the control of many intracellular infectious agents in humans.[10]

If TNF-α is inhibited with drug antagonists, such as Infliximab or Etanercept®, in conditions such as rheumatoid arthritis or Crohn's disease, then the incidence of severe sepsis increases with only a few signs to alert the clinician[11,12] – this can be due to reactivation of latent granulomatous infections such as tuberculosis, histoplamosis and candidiasis.

TNF-α has also been implicated as a key agent in tumor regression initiated by some physiological conditions and also in such pathological states as septic shock and cachexia.

Factors released from plasma

Three major interrelated systems are involved with the release of chemical mediators from plasma: the kinin, clotting, and complement systems. Kinin activation, coagulation, and fibrinolytic systems are closely related, sharing several factors. The complement system is a separate system that also has points of interaction.

Complement system

The complement system was first described by Jules Bordet in 1895. It is a component of the immune response system which culminates in lysis of antigens and onset of local inflammatory reaction. It comprises more than 25 plasma and membrane-bound interacting proteins and functions to:

- Bind foreign cells and destroy their membranes (complement fixation)
- Recruit phagocytic cells to sites of infection and effect phagocytosis (opsonization)
- Trigger inflammatory reactions that attract phagocytes to 'wall off the area.'

Because of its lethal consequences, the complement system is tightly regulated to prevent unnecessary collateral damage. Two antibody-independent activation pathways (alternative and lectin-mediated) found in mammals are remnants of a prevertebrate origin. The classical pathway was added with the appearance of antibodies in primitive vertebrates and complement became involved in orchestrating lymphoid responses.

The classical pathway is activated by the binding of an antibody to an antigen. Specifically, it is activated by the formation of C1 esterase by immune complexes (the Fc portion of immunoglobulin G [IgG] and IgM). It is antibody-dependent and lacks the ability to recognize antigen and initiate inflammation that the alternate pathway possesses. In this pathway, the proteins sequentially form the recognition unit, the activation unit, and the membrane attack complex (MAC) to cause cell lysis. The MAC is a complex formed from five complement proteins which puncture the plasma membrane of the infected cell. One MAC can be sufficient to kill an infected cell.

The alternate pathway is directly activated by antigens and plays a major role in the immune response against infectious agents. Specifically, this pathway is activated by bacterial endotoxins, cell membranes, and aggregated gamma globulin. This pathway is antibody-independent. Six proteins, C3, B, D, H, P, and I, cause initiation, recognition, and activation of this pathway. Formation of activator-bound C3/C5 convertase is the end result.

Both activation pathways contain an initial enzyme that catalyzes the formation of the target cell-bound C3 convertase which in turn generates the C5 convertase (see Figure 2.1). This activity results in the cleavage and activation of C5 and, therefore, in the assembly of the MAC. The MAC is assembled from five hydrophilic precursor proteins: C5, C6, C7, C8, and C9. Activation of the MAC is a consequence of the activity of either the classical or the alternative pathway on the surface of a cell.

Complement components also regulate the immune response and stimulate release of interleukins, PAF, and eicosanoids.

- C3a and C5a cause vasodilation by releasing histamines from mast cells and basophils, causing increased vascular permeability.
- All three are also leukocyte chemoattractants.
- C5a enhances phagocytosis and superoxide ion production in neutrophils.
- C3b makes leukocytes adhere and induces phagocytosis (opsonization).

Plasmin or fibrinolysin is a pivotal point because of its ability to activate the Hageman factor, cleave C3 into fragments, and digest fibrin.

Arachidonic acid metabolism

Prostaglandins are a group of unsaturated fatty acids that belong to the eicosanoid family (compounds having 20 carbon molecules). Other members of the eicosanoids include thromboxanes, leukotrienes, and lipoxins. Eicosanoids have paracrine effects and have been implicated in the immune system, coagulation system, smooth muscle, and as hypothalamic releasing factors. Although considered lipid-soluble hormones that normally enter the cells, these molecules function more as peptide hormones by binding to receptors on the plasma membrane.

Activation of a phospholipase A2 by an extracellular molecule such as thrombin, hormone, or damage to the cell causes the release of arachidonic acid. Next, cyclooxygenase catalyzes the formation of a five-membered carbon ring and bridging endoperoxide, and addition of an –OOH group to carbon resulting in PGG. PGH is formed next and serves as the precursor of the other prostaglandins and thromboxanes (see Figure 2.4). Cyclooxygenase exists in two forms, COX-1 and COX-2. COX-1 exists and functions in normal physiologic states in a variety of locations; COX-2 becomes active under inflammatory conditions. Several medications have been developed recently that specifically inhibit COX-2 (Chapter 2).

Physically, a 'tunnel' extends into the enzyme from the fatty acid tail part of the membrane. Arachidonic acid presumably enters this tunnel, where it is converted to PGH. Aspirin (acetylsalicylate) functions by preventing arachidonic acid from entering the tunnel in an irreversible fashion. Other NSAIDs such as ibuprofen and indomethacin also inhibit cyclooxygenase, but by simply competing with arachidonic acid for entry into the tunnel; therefore, this inhibition is reversible. Recent studies have shown that some prostaglandins such as PGF may act to resolve inflammation. Therefore, while cyclooxygenase inhibitors may inhibit inflammation, they may also slow recovery.

Leukotrienes and lipoxins

Lipoxygenase adds a peroxide group to the 5 position of arachidonic acid to form 5–hydroperoxyeicosatetraenoic acid (5–HPETE). Subsequent forms of leukotriene (A, C, D, and E) are formed through further reaction. Lipoxygenase is inhibited by nordihydroguaiaretic acid but not by aspirin or NSAIDS. Leukotriene E is associated with bronchoconstriction with asthma. Leukotriene C4 may act as a hypothalamic-releasing hormone that regulates luteinizing hormone secretion. Lipoxins contain four conjugated double bonds and three hydroxyl groups that also exert regulatory effects on the immune system, the vascular system, and smooth muscle.

Steroid antiinflammatory drugs activate the synthesis of a protein that inhibits phospholipase A2 and also inhibits the synthesis of phospholipase A2 itself. These compounds intervene in the release of arachidonic acid by phospholipase A2.

Coagulation cascade

The coagulation cascade is composed of two pathways: intrinsic and extrinsic. The intrinsic pathway is activated by physical/chemical activation and the extrinsic pathway is activated by tissue factors released from damaged cells. Both pathways are thought to be activated simultaneously to initiate and sustain clot formation. At the same time, platelets are also activated.

Intrinsic pathway. Trauma to the blood vessel, exposure of blood to collagen in a damaged vascular wall, or exposure of blood to a surface such as glass activates this pathway. First, Factor XII (Hageman factor) is activated from its inactive form (zymogen). Next, platelets are activated. Activated Factor XII is a protease and activates Factor XI. This reaction requires the presence of high molecular weight kininogen and prekallekrein. Activated Factor XI is also a protease which activates Factor IX. Activated Factor IX then converts Factor X to Factor Xa which is accelerated by Factor VIIIa. Deficiencies in either Factor VIII or Factor IX lead to hemophilia A and B.

Extrinsic pathway. Damage to the vessel wall or extravascular tissue exposes the plasma to tissue factor found in nonvascular tissue cells as an integral membrane protein. In this process, Factor VII is activated to Factor VIIa which, in the presence of Ca^{2+} and phospholipids, activates Factor X to Factor Xa. The remainder of the cascade is similar to the intrinsic pathway.

Combined pathway. Activated Factor X functions as a protease to convert prothrombin to the active thrombin; this conversion requires the presence of Factor Va. Thrombin then cleaves fibrinogen to fibrin, which then polymerizes to form fibrin strands. Thrombin is a powerful procoagulant. It catalyzes conversion of Factors V and VIII to their activated forms through a positive feedback mechanism and converts more prothrombin to thrombin. The end result is acceleration and amplification of the entire cascade.

The kinin system

The kallikrein-kinin system is one of the first inflammatory pathways activated after tissue damage; it produces one of its most potent inflammatory mediators, bradykinin. The kinin system is activated by coagulation Factor XII (Hageman factor). Activated Hageman factor activates prekallikrein via a series of prekallikrein activators, resulting in the production of kallikrein. The generation of kallikrein triggers kinin production, including bradykinin, which is responsible for inducing pain, increasing vascular permeability, and causing vasodilation. Kallikrein also activates the fibrinolytic pathway, leading to the removal of blood clots.

References

1. Hinkelmann L, Struck HG, Lautenschlager C. Inflammatory reaction of the anterior eye segment: cataract extraction in patients with and without diabetes mellitus, *Ophthalmologe* (1998) **95**:213–18.

2. Gregory MS, Repp AC, Hohlbaum AM et al. Membrane Fas ligand activates innate immunity and terminates ocular immune privilege, *J Immunol* (2002) **169**:2727–35.

3. Jaffe GJ, Schwartz D, Han DP et al. Risk factors for postvitrectomy fibrin formation, *Am J Ophthalmol* (1990) **109**:661–7.

4. Spencer WH. Inflammation. In: *Ophthalmic Pathology: An Atlas and Textbook*, 4th edn (WB Saunders: Philadelphia, 1996) 56–67.

5. Feghali CA, Wright TM. Cytokines in acute and chronic inflammation, *Front Biosci* (1997) **2**:12–26.

6. Fantone JC, Ward PA. In: Rubin E, Farber JL, eds. *Pathology* (JB Lippincott: Philadelphia, 1994) 32–67.

7. Lentsch AB, Ward PA. Regulation of inflammatory vascular damage. *J Pathol* (2000) **190**:343–8.

8. Ward PA, Lentsch AB. Endogenous regulation of the acute inflammatory response. *Mol Cell Biochem* (2002) **234-5**:225–8.

9. Albert DM. Principles of pathology. In: Albert DM, Jakobiec FA, eds. *Principles and Practice of Ophthalmology: Clinical Practice* (Saunders: Philadelphia, 1994) 2101–26.

10. Beutler B, Grau GE. Tumor necrosis factor in the pathogenesis of infectious diseases, *Crit Care Med* (1993) **21**(Suppl 10):S423–35.

11. Kroesen S, Widmer AF, Tyndall A et al. Serious bacterial infections in patients with rheumatoid arthritis under anti-TNF-alpha therapy. *Rheumatol (Oxford)* (2003) **42**:617–21.

12. Wallis RS, Broder MS, Wong JY et al. Granulomatous infectious diseases associated with tumor necrosis factor antagonists. *Clin Infect Dis* (2004) **38**:1261–5.

2

Immunology

Ocular immune privilege

Ocular immune privilege has five primary features:[1]

- The blood–ocular barriers, considered in Chapter 5 (pharmacokinetics)
- The absence of lymphatic drainage
- Soluble immunomodulatory factors in the aqueous humor
- Immunomodulatory ligands on the surface of ocular parenchymal cells
- Tolerogenic antigen-presenting cells (APCs) in the anterior and posterior chambers.

Immune-privileged sites such as the eye have evolved with these mechanisms to prevent the induction of inflammation. Only recently have neuropeptides, constitutively present in ocular tissue, been recognized as part of the immune privilege mechanism.[2]

Local corneal surface immunity consists of immunoglobulin M (IgM), C1 complement, and Langerhans' (dendritic) cells (LC); until recently, these cells were thought to be found only in the peripheral corneal epithelial sheet in the normal noninflamed eye.[3] Irritation of the central cornea, such as with herpetic infection, can result in centripetal migration of these dendritic cells to promote an immunoinflammatory response. Dekaris et al suggested that interleukin (IL)-1 induction of the dendritic cell migration, first observed 15 years ago, was mediated by tumor necrosis factor (TNF) receptor function rather than TNF-α which had an independent stimulatory role.[4] They also found that p55 and p75 signaling pathways were important in mediating dendritic cell migration.

The normal cornea has large numbers of dendritic cells in the epithelium which are important for antigen recognition and processing, with monocytes (APCs) in the stroma.[5] In addition, conjunctival macrophages can function as APCs and have been shown to be important in the control of an invasion of *Acanthamoeba* sp., by phagocytosis,[6] as well as to have a role in corneal graft rejection.[7,8] The dendrite is the only corneal cell to express the major histocompatibility class (MHC) II molecules without prior inducement by cytokines. Class II MHC molecules are responsible for presenting processed peptides from exogenous antigens to receptors on CD4+ T helper lymphocytes. A recent advance has been the discovery of the CIITA protein which is a nonDNA binding activator of transcription that is a master control gene for class II gene expression;[9] current research is focused on understanding situations where class II gene expression occurs in a CIITA-independent pathway and the molecular basis for this expression.

Hamrah et al[10,11] have studied the phenotype and distribution of dendritic cells in the periphery and central zone of normal and inflamed corneas. They have shown that in the periphery nearly one half of the dendritic cells expressed MHC class II positive (CD80+CD86+) molecules; the central cornea contained immature and precursor dendritic cells which were uniformly MHC class II negative (CD80–CD86–). These authors have also found immature monocyte APCs in the stroma of the central cornea. After 24 hours of inflammation, Hazlett and associates found an increased number of dendritic cells in the central cornea with up-regulation of expression of MHC class II receptors with co-stimulatory molecules CD80 and CD86; in addition, a CD11c-CD11b positive population of macrophages (monocytes) was found exclusively in the posterior stroma.

Hazlett et al[12] have investigated the B7/CD28 co-stimulatory pathway for LC migration and activation in the central cornea. These findings mean that the concept of the cornea being immune privileged from a lack of resident lymphoreticular cells needs revision because the cornea is capable of diverse cellular mechanisms for antigen presentation.[11]

The dendritic cell takes up antigen by pinocytosis. Upon exposure to antigen, the dendritic or other APC undergoes functional maturation and gains the ability to present the antigen to CD4 T helper cells attracted to the area by cytokine production.[3] The APCs take up antigens intracellularly and express them on their surface as antigenic peptides bound to MHC class II molecules; during antigen processing, partial degradation of oligopeptides occurs with unfolding of the secondary structure.

Corneal epithelial cells or nonactivated macrophages in the anterior and posterior chambers can produce IL-1, activating macrophages which then express MHC class II molecules and become APCs. These cells will then process antigenic peptides in a binary complex with MHC class II molecules similarly to dendritic cells. Macrophages can process particulate antigens including whole bacteria such as staphylococci and propionibacteria, but can more effectively process soluble antigens, e.g. protein A, internalized in endocytic vesicles.

T lymphocytes exert their local effector function by secreting cytokines in tissue for direct interaction with target cells. Interferon-gamma (IFN-γ) induces expression of MHC class II molecules by keratinocytes, epithelial cells, endothelial cells, and fibroblasts, which can all vary in their capacity to serve as APCs. These cells can process and present immunogenic peptides complexed with MHC class II molecules. However, they differ in their capacity to produce co-stimulatory signals and do not stimulate resting T cells, which require IL-2 to become activated.

Diamond et al[13,14] demonstrated an antimicrobial effect in rabbit aqueous humor, finding a 90% drop (1 $\log_{10}$) in viable colony count for *Staphylococcus aureus* and *Pseudomonas aeruginosa* compared with controls in rabbit serum. They found that rabbit aqueous humor could be bactericidal for *S. aureus* and *Ps. aeruginosa* but not for micrococcus, *Escherichia coli* or *Streptococcus pneumoniae*. Defensins are naturally occurring antimicrobial peptides.[15] Reverse transcription-polymerase chain reaction (RT-PCR) was performed on human postmortem ciliary body samples for beta defensin-1 (HBD-1) and beta defensin-2 (HBD-2), and alpha defensins 5

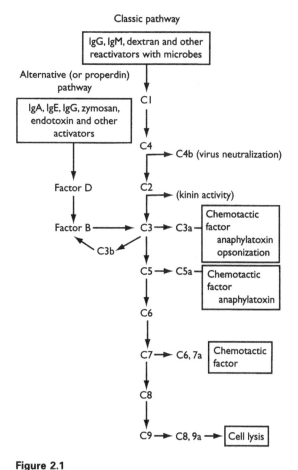

Figure 2.1

Classic and alternate complement pathways. (Adapted from Foster CS[16].)

and 6. This study demonstrated that HBD-1 is constitutively present in the aqueous and vitreous, probably at sub-bactericidal concentrations. HBD-2 was absent from aqueous, but cytokine stimulation studies suggested that it may be generated in response to inflammatory cytokines during infections. HBD-2 has a wider antibacterial spectrum, is 10–fold more potent, and may play a more significant role in antimicrobial defense than HBD-1.[15] Caution is required for the use of defensins therapeutically because they also promote cell proliferation and fibrin formation, two key elements in ocular scarring processes such as proliferative vitreoretinopathy.

Immune complex activation occurs by stimulation of either the C1 complement component, with a resulting cascade to C5a which acts chemotactically for polymorphonuclear leukocytes (PMNs) and causes release of cytokines, or the alternative pathway (Chapter 1 and Figure 2.1).[16] Aqueous humor contains three complement regulatory proteins, membrane cofactor protein (MCP), decay-accelerating factor (DAF) and CD59, and a cell surface regulator of complement (Crry) that inhibit complement activation.[17–19] These proteins have been found in normal human aqueous humor and vitreous as well as in Lewis rats; the results of these experiments suggest that the complement system is continuously active at a low level in the normal eye but is tightly regulated. Severe inflammation developed if these regulatory proteins were blocked with monoclonal antibodies or otherwise inactivated. The cornea, choroid, and retina are particularly susceptible to autoimmune-mediated, immune-complex disease; however, the vitreous and the subretinal space are not. The expression of ICAM-1–β2 integrin is needed to attract neutrophils to the site, as part of the inflammatory process, and will attract activated Th1 lymphocytes as well.

Delayed-type hypersensitivity from cell-mediated immunity

Delayed-type hypersensitivity (DTH) from cell-mediated immunity (CMI) has been proposed in humans[20] for recurrent episodes of chronic blepharitis caused by S. aureus, leading to local conjunctival enhancement of CMI, expressed as DTH, to cell wall antigens of S. aureus, especially protein A. S. aureus repeatedly colonizes the lids of both normals (approximately 10%) and atopes (approximately 50%) from other sites of human carriage, as well as causing chronic folliculitis in patients with blepharitis. DTH is also the mechanism that is suppressed in anterior chamber-associated immune deviation (ACAID) and posterior chamber-associated immune deviation (POCAID) (Figure 2.2). Johnson et al[21] first showed in rabbits that had been immunized subcutaneously with a whole-cell vaccine to develop systemic enhancement (CMI/DTH) to S. aureus, that there was tolerance instead of DTH in the anterior chamber. This situation applies

similarly to most other organisms able to induce a systemic DTH reaction.

The CD4 T helper cell (Th) is responsible for most DTH reactions.[22] The Th1 subtype mediates DTH, not given by the Th2 subtype, based on an array of cytokines produced by T cell clones including IL-2, IFN-γ, and TNF-α. The Th2 subtype stimulates B lymphocytes with IL-4, IL-5, IL-10, and IL-13 cytokines to produce an antibody response (see Figure 2.2). Other cytokines not characterized as either Th1 or Th2 include IL-12, which promotes IFN-γ and TNF-α production and hence a Th1 response, and IL-18. Polymorphonuclear (PMN) cells, macrophages, and dendritic cells can produce both Th1 and Th2 cytokines but ocular APCs cannot produce the Th1–inducing cytokine IL-12. DTH is thought to be responsible for the underlying mechanisms for the pathogenesis of trachoma, herpes simplex virus (HSV) stromal keratitis, and some forms of idiopathic uveitis. DTH is recognized as the primary cause of experimental autoimmune uveitis (EAU) in rodents. ACAID is believed to be a mechanism that prevents trivial activation of the DTH arm of the immune response as a method for sustaining immunohomeostasis in the eye.

Macrophages produce IL-1, stimulating other macrophages to become APCs and to present antigen to Th1 lymphocytes. IL-1 also regulates macrophage inflammatory protein-2 (MIP-2)[23] which acts as a chemoattractant for PMN influx and may be susceptible to 'down-regulation' to reduce the inflammatory response.[24]

Th1 produces IL-2 and IFN-γ, responsible in part for the induration response of the DTH reaction. Th1 and Th2 each cross-regulate the activities of the other via cytokine production with one inhibiting production by the other; e.g. IFN-γ inhibits the effect of IL-4 on B lymphocytes. This may be the mechanism for the in vivo observation of a strong DTH response with weak antibody production and vice versa so that preferential 'up-regulating' of the Th1 response down-regulates the Th2 response. The roles of Th1 and Th2 responses in cross-regulating each other and thereby maintaining a balance in the immune response are responsible for the adaptive immunity to various pathogens, e.g. Th1 protects against intracellular pathogens while Th2 protects against helminths. Several novel therapeutic strategies hold promise for modulating the alloimmune response to corneal allografts by either promoting antigen-specific tolerance or redirecting the host's response from a Th1 pathway toward a Th2 pathway to reduce immune rejection.[8]

The activated CD4 Th cell secretes IFN-γ at the site of antigen entry, inducing class II expression on 'non-professional' APCs, which activates them.

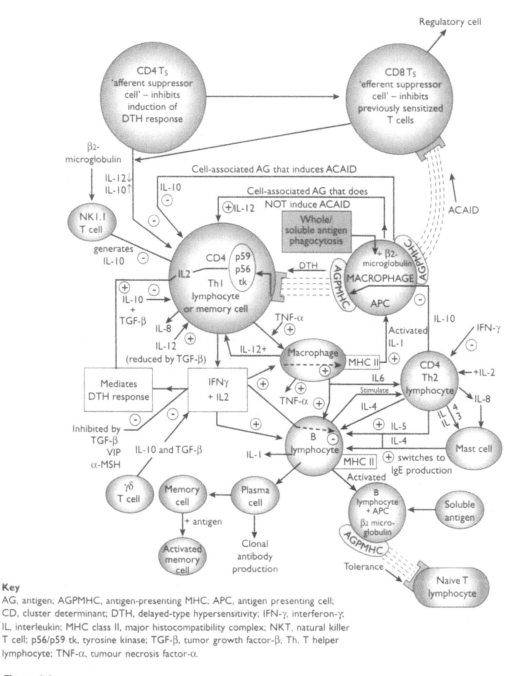

Key

AG, antigen; AGPMHC, antigen-presenting MHC; APC, antigen presenting cell; CD, cluster determinant; DTH, delayed-type hypersensitivity; IFN-γ, interferon-γ, IL, interleukin; MHC class II, major histocompatibility complex; NKT, natural killer T cell; p56/p59 tk, tyrosine kinase; TGF-β, tumor growth factor-β; Th, T helper lymphocyte; TNF-α, tumour necrosis factor-α.

Figure 2.2

Delayed-type hypersensitivity (DTH) and POCAID.

The recognition of the MHC-peptide complex of the APC by a T cell receptor initiates an intracellular signal transduction pathway within the cell. The molecules that are then produced increase binding of Th cells to the APC and are called adhesion molecules (ADM); for CD4 cells, this includes the 55 kd monomeric transmembrane glycoprotein belonging to the Ig gene superfamily and, for CD8 cells, two 34 kd alpha chain molecules.

The cellular response is regulated by expression of ADMs on inflammatory cells and the vascular endothelium, which in turn is controlled by cytokines that can also act as chemotactic factors for PMN cells. These ADMs cause an adhesion cascade of PMNs and lymphocytes via the nearby vascular endothelium when they bind to it and migrate to the site of activated lymphocytes. Memory Th lymphocytes will also migrate to this site if the patient has previously induced systemic enhancement to cell wall antigens such as *S. aureus*, hence the need for 'tolerance' (ACAID/POCAID) within the eye.

The expression of integrins ($\beta1$, $\beta2$, $\beta3$) attracts these activated Th cells to the inflammatory site. The expression of $\beta1$ is up-regulated on the surface of activated memory cells which bind to the counter receptor on the vascular endothelium (VLA-4, a member of the Ig superfamily) which results in extravasation to the site of the processed antigen.

The cell–cell interaction between the APC and the Th lymphocyte combination of CD3–TCR, recognizing the MHC/oligopeptide antigen expressed, and the complex of CD4 and CD5 receptors, activates p59 and p56 tyrosine kinases by dephosphorylation as an 'activity cascade.' Synthesis of IL-2 and its receptor expression are induced to give proliferation of selected antigenic specificity, resulting in the inflammatory DTH reaction.

Anterior chamber- and posterior chamber-associated immune deviation

ACAID- and POCAID-associated immune deviation (Figure 2.3) exist to protect the single cell-layered corneal endothelium, the anterior chamber, and the subretinal space and vitreous from immune-mediated damage by cell-mediated immunity or DTH.[25,26] This POCAID effect is not present in the retina or choroid. Immune deviation is achieved by avoidance of CD8 cytotoxic T lymphocyte (CTL)-mediated cytolysis and inhibition of CD4 Th1 lymphocyte response in the AC.[7,8,25] These aims are achieved by an absence of class I MHC expression on endothelial and lens cells, avoiding lysis by class I restricted CTLs similarly to the brain. The problem with this mechanism for the anterior chamber endothelium is the inability to prevent persistent viral infection; this problem also applies to the immunoprivileged retinal pigment epithelium (RPE) in which cytomegalovirus (CMV) can persist.

Recent evidence has found that CMV immediate early (IE) gene expression in RPE cells deviates ocular antiviral inflammation via FasL (FasLigand, see Figure 2.3).[27] TNF-α and IFN-γ, found elevated in patients with acquired immunodeficiency syndrome (AIDS) with retinitis, sensitize RPE cells to FasL-mediated cytolysis, contributing to retinal destruction rather than inflammation. One explanation that has been proposed for the normally reduced immune response is engagement of the pro-apoptotic molecule Fas by its ligand (FasL), which leads to apoptosis and consequently limits an inflammatory response.[28]

The prevention of a DTH (cell-mediated) immune reaction is gained by the camero-splenic axis (see Figure 2.3). Microbial antigen in the AC is discharged in the aqueous to the venous blood flow, often phagocytosed within 'tolerogenic' APCs, and so to the spleen instead of to the lymphatics. However, there is experimental evidence that up to 25% of antigens in the anterior chamber reach T cells in the submandibular lymph nodes of an anterior chamber-injected mouse via the uveal/scleral pathway. However, because of the inability of ocular APCs to produce IL-12 and hence to stimulate a Th1 reaction, the responding T cells fail to differentiate into functioning Th1 cells.[7,8] Within the spleen, T suppressor (T_s) lymphocytes are produced that migrate back to the anterior chamber to inhibit Th1 lymphocytes. These T_s cells also suppress a DTH response acting systemically to the specific antigen. This systemic protection is lost with the removal of the spleen, which is the source of the T_s cells. A functioning spleen has been proven essential for developing and maintaining ACAID.

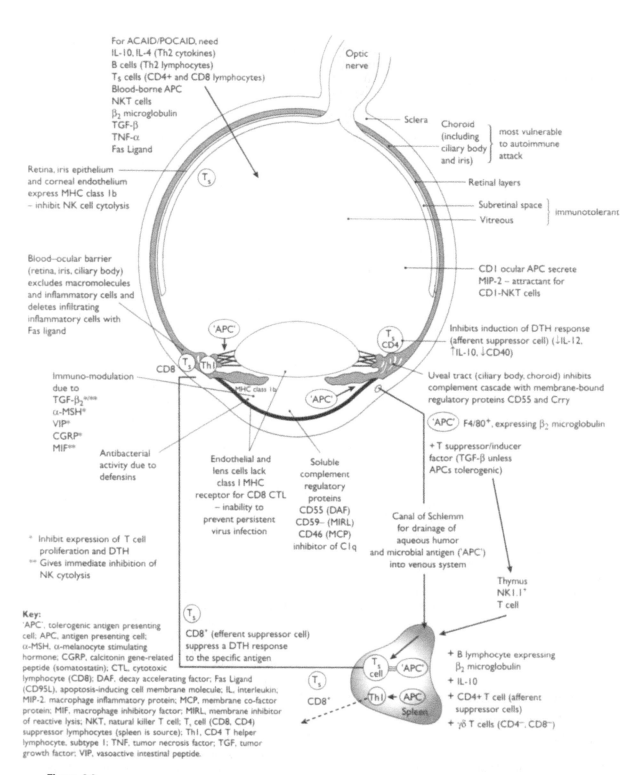

For ACAID/POCAID, need
IL-10, IL-4 (Th2 cytokines)
B cells (Th2 lymphocytes)
T_s cells (CD4+ and CD8 lymphocytes)
Blood-borne APC
NKT cells
β_2 microglobulin
TGF-β
TNF-α
Fas Ligand

Optic nerve

Sclera

Choroid (including ciliary body and iris) } most vulnerable to autoimmune attack

Retina, iris epithelium and corneal endothelium express MHC class Ib – inhibit NK cell cytolysis

Retinal layers

Subretinal space } immunotolerant
Vitreous

Blood–ocular barrier (retina, iris, ciliary body) excludes macromolecules and inflammatory cells and deletes infiltrating inflammatory cells with Fas ligand

CD1 ocular APC secrete MIP-2 – attractant for CD1-NKT cells

Inhibits induction of DTH response (afferent suppressor cell) ($\downarrow$IL-12, $\uparrow$IL-10, $\downarrow$CD40)

Uveal tract (ciliary body, choroid) inhibits complement cascade with membrane-bound regulatory proteins CD55 and Crry

'APC' F4/80$^+$, expressing β_2 microglobulin

Immuno-modulation due to
TGF-β_2*/**
α-MSH*
VIP*
CGRP*
MIF**

+ T suppressor/inducer factor (TGF-β unless APCs tolerogenic)

Antibacterial activity due to defensins

Endothelial and lens cells lack class I MHC receptor for CD8 CTL – inability to prevent persistent virus infection

Soluble complement regulatory proteins
CD55 (DAF)
CD59– (MIRL)
CD46 (MCP) inhibitor of C1q

Canal of Schlemm for drainage of aqueous humor and microbial antigen ('APC') into venous system

* Inhibit expression of T cell proliferation and DTH
** Gives immediate inhibition of NK cytolysis

Thymus
NK1.1$^+$
T cell

Key:
'APC', tolerogenic antigen presenting cell; APC, antigen presenting cell; α-MSH, α-melanocyte stimulating hormone; CGRP, calcitonin gene-related peptide (somatostatin); CTL, cytotoxic lymphocyte (CD8); DAF, decay accelerating factor; Fas Ligand (CD95L), apoptosis-inducing cell membrane molecule; IL, interleukin; MIP-2, macrophage inflammatory protein; MCP, membrane co-factor protein; MIF, macrophage inhibitory factor; MIRL, membrane inhibitor of reactive lysis; NKT, natural killer T cell; T_s cell (CD8, CD4) suppressor lymphocytes (spleen is source); Th1, CD4 T helper lymphocyte, subtype 1; TNF, tumor necrosis factor; TGF, tumor growth factor; VIP, vasoactive intestinal peptide.

T_s
CD8$^+$ (efferent suppressor cell) suppress a DTH response to the specific antigen

+ B lymphocyte expressing β_2 microglobulin
+ IL-10
+ CD4+ T cell (afferent suppressor cells)
+ $\gamma\delta$ T cells (CD4$^-$, CD8$^-$)

Figure 2.3

Anterior (ACAID)- and posterior (POCAID)-associated immune deviation.

An afferent (CD4 T_s) and efferent (CD8 T_s) mechanism is able to achieve this suppression or immune tolerance (see Figures 2.2 and 2.3). The afferent CD4 T_s lymphocyte, generated in the spleen, inhibits induction of the DTH response within the anterior chamber and subretinal space. The CD4 T_s cells go to the spleen via the aqueous humor/venous system with the tolerogenic APC that has captured eye-derived antigens. A multi-cellular interaction occurs within the spleen with natural killer (NK) T cells, splenic B lymphocytes expressing β_2 microglobulin, IL-10, and γδ T cells (CD4–, CD8–), which creates an antigen-presentation environment that leads to CD4+ and CD8+ alpha/beta T cells which suppress induction of Th1 and Th2 immune expression.[1] The spleen releases CD8 T_s efferent suppressor lymphocytes which can suppress a DTH response to a specific antigen and which return to the eye via the arterial blood flow. Splenic production of T_s lymphocytes can also be observed with intravenous (IV) injection of antigens, but while the classic model of IV antigen-induced immune deviation shares many characteristics with ACAID including down-regulation of DTH, there are also major differences.[7,8] In particular, IL-4 is required for IV-induced immune deviation but not for ACAID, while IL-10, B cells, blood-borne APCs, IV NKT cells, and β_2 microglobulin are not required for IV-induced immune deviation but are for ACAID.[7,8]

TNF-α and the Th2 cytokine IL-10 within the anterior chamber have to induce an ACAID response to an antigen. The anterior chamber also contains TGF (tumor or transforming growth factor)-β which renders local APCs 'tolerogenic' and is another necessary part of ACAID, particularly if the host has DTH systemically enhanced to the specific antigen. Such tolerance within the anterior chamber was first shown for *S. aureus* in rabbits with specific systemic DTH enhancement.[21] Another associated mechanism is FasL-induced apoptosis (see Figure 2.3) when infiltrating cells are apoptopically killed within the blood–ocular barrier (retina, iris, and ciliary body).[28,29]

Not all antigens produce ACAID or POCAID; notable exceptions are purified protein derivative of *Mycobacterium tuberculosis*, large simian virus-40 T antigens, and some experimental tumor allografts.[25] The reasons and mechanism for such antigen selection remain unclear.

Macrophages within the anterior chamber are not always able to kill bacteria such as *Propionibacterium acnes* and coagulase-negative staphylococci (CNS). This finding is well illustrated in chronic 'saccular' or granulomatous endophthalmitis resulting from *P. acnes* and, less frequently, CNS.[30–32] Macrophages phagocytose *P. acnes* and CNS within the capsule fragment (Chapter 6) but are unable to kill the bacteria due to the lack of a functioning cell-mediated immune system with cytokine expression, so that these bacteria are able to multiply within them. The macrophages within the anterior chamber function as 'tolerogenic' APCs rather than as 'scavenger' cells. A chronic inflammatory reaction is recognized clinically as 'saccular', plaque, or granulomatous endophthalmitis with white plaque in the capsular bag (Chapter 6). The anterior chamber tap is often culture-negative because the bacteria are intracellular only; however, a PCR test can be positive (Chapter 3). When released from the macrophages the bacteria may be killed by the antibacterial effect within the aqueous humor.

Our hypothesis suggests that the continued intracellular replication of the bacteria may allow the macrophage to express MHC class II molecules and to give a limited Th1 response that is susceptible to suppression with corticosteroids. This explains why the inflammation returns when corticosteroid therapy is withdrawn and why the capsule fragment often has to be removed surgically, after which there are no recurrences of chronic inflammation. The most useful antibiotic to use is clarithromycin, by the oral or intravitreal route, which penetrates into the anterior chamber and is concentrated up to 200 times intracellularly within macrophages to kill intracellular bacteria (Chapters 5, 6, and 11). Therapeutic success has been reported with clarithromycin oral therapy of 500 mg b.i.d.[33–35] without the need for surgical removal of the capsule and intraocular lens. Clarithromycin can be injected intravitreally with a nontoxic dose of up to, but not more than, 1.0 mg in 0.1 ml.[36]

Specific production of antibodies within the vitreous and posterior chamber during endophthalmitis has been investigated by Ravindranath et al.[37] Using a rat model of *Staphylococcus epidermidis* endophthalmitis, the authors found that IgG and IgM but not IgA antibodies against glycerol teichoic acid (GTA) of the staphylococcal cell wall were present in the vitreous from day 1 onward and declined by day 7. Plasma cells were seen in the vitreous between days 1 and 3, and B lymphocytes (CD45+, CD3−) were present in pooled vitreous humor. In contrast, serum anti-GTA IgM antibodies were raised for 1 week. These vitreous antibodies may be involved in neutrophil-mediated opsonophagocytosis leading to spontaneous sterility within their rat model. Recent work by Meek et al[38] investigated the specificity of intraocularly produced antibodies, demonstrating that antibodies recognizing the same antigen in both serum and intraocular fluid differ in the epitopes that are recognized. This finding demonstrates that the intraocular compartment determines its own antibody profile against intraocular pathogens. The authors presented several models for how an exclusive intraocular B cell lymphocyte repertoire may function.

In the conjunctiva, Th2 lymphocytes play a key role in immediate hypersensitivity reactions, producing IL-4 and IL-5 to stimulate B cells and expression of IgE receptors; IL-4 induces mast cell proliferation. This explains why adult patients with severe allergic keratoconjunctivitis, who have very high systemic IgE antibodies associated with IL-5 induction of eosinophils, have lids colonized by S. aureus but lack DTH to S. aureus protein A.[39] Th2 cells are found in the conjunctiva of children with vernal disease. Recent experimental models have demonstrated that inhibition of Th2 cells and their secreted cytokines could be a therapeutic target for inhibiting chronic allergic inflammation on the ocular surface.[40]

Immunopathogenesis

Considerable work by Hazlett et al explored the role of Langerhans' dendritic cells, cytokines, and subsets of T lymphocytes in the pathogenesis of Ps. aeruginosa infection of the cornea in a mouse model.[41–43] The authors have demonstrated that dendritic cells are crucial in the innate immune response.[41] In B6 mice, which produce a Th1 type response to a challenge of Ps. aeruginosa and ulcerate,[44] the early induction of dendritic cells made no difference. However, in BALB/c mice, which give a Th2 response, early induction of dendritic cells was disastrous: instead of the infection resolving and healing, the cornea perforated.[41] Hazlett and associates compared this

model with human extended-wear contact lens wearers (EWCLWs), in whom chronic irritation leads to centripetal migration of dendritic cells into the central cornea[45]; such EWCLWs may therefore be at greater risk of corneal ulceration caused by Ps. aeruginosa (Chapter 6).

Hazlett and co-workers, exploring the differing pathogenesis between Th1 and Th2 responses in their mouse model, found the presence of IL-12 to be important in stimulating production of IFN-γ and TNF-α and therefore in giving a Th1 response.[42,43] If IL-12 was absent, there was unchecked bacterial growth; however, if IL-12 was present, the bacterial growth was stopped, although the cornea ulcerated. They found that differing genetic strains of mice would either produce a Th1 response (B6, BL10) or a Th2 response (BALB/c).[46]

This important work begins to explain how the immune response to a bacterial challenge, such as contamination of the anterior chamber with phacoemulsification surgery, influences the outcome in association with numbers and virulence of the organism. The combination of the type of immune response (Th1 or Th2 with relevant cytokines) together with the bacterial virulence factors and toxins, if any, will determine whether there is an acute or chronic inflammatory response or, when the immune response is satisfactory, there is no inflammatory effect at all. A high bacterial count can also influence the outcome, overcoming the host immune response to lead to infection.

Others have made important contributions in studying the role of DTH, Th1 cells, and latency for the immunopathogenesis of herpes virus infections.[47] Khanna et al have challenged the concept that HSV-1 latency represents a silent infection that is ignored by the host immune system; they suggested that antigen-directed retention of memory CD8(+) T cells specific for the immunodominant gB (498–505) HSV-1 epitope are selectively retained in the ophthalmic branch of the latently infected trigeminal ganglion.[48] They concluded that CD8(+) T cells provide active surveillance of HSV-1 gene expression in latently infected sensory neurons.

Immune suppression

The drug cyclosporine can cause immunomodulation, which suppresses the activity of the p56 and p59 tyrosine kinases in the Th1 lymphocytes when the DTH activity cascade is blocked. This drug also acts on calcineurin-blocking T cell activation. Cyclosporine acts specifically and reversibly on lymphocytes, does not depress hemopoiesis, and has no effect on the function of PMNs. It is a potent immunosuppressive drug and prolongs survival of allogeneic transplants involving heart, kidney, pancreas, bone marrow, lung, and the cornea. Cyclosporine prevents and treats rejection and graft-versus-host disease; it has also been found beneficial in psoriasis, atopic dermatitis, rheumatoid arthritis, uveitis, and Sjögren's syndrome, all conditions considered to have an immunologic pathogenesis. Cyclosporine inhibits the development of cell-mediated reactions. It blocks the lymphocytes in the early phase of their cycle, as described above, and inhibits lymphokine production and release including IL-2 (T cell growth factor).

Fucidin (fusidic acid) is an antistaphylococcal antibiotic, for which there is a topical preparation (Fucithalmic), and also has an immunosuppressive action similar to cyclosporine. These factors may explain its beneficial effect for treating the blepharitis of rosacea, usually associated with both S. aureus colonization of the lids and systemically enhanced DTH to its antigens.[49] In the future, there may be potential for therapeutic application of ACAID mechanisms to prevent progression of ocular immunoinflammatory disease.[26]

Corticosteroids act by affecting the functions of cell populations and their distribution. They have a specific role, inhibiting phospholipase conversion of membrane phospholipids to arachidonic acid (Figure 2.4).

Corticosteroids have both antiinflammatory and immunosuppressive effects. The antiinflammatory effects are nonspecific to the cause of the

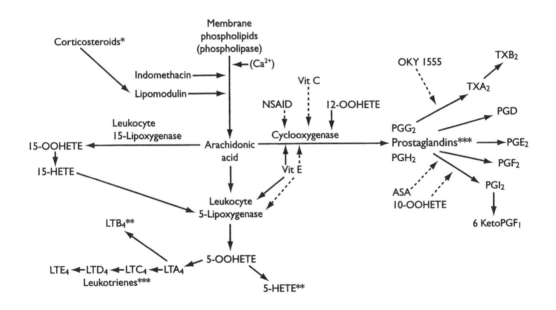

NSAID =   nonsteroidal antiinflammatory drug, includes salicylate, diflusinol, indomethacin, naproxon, ibuprofen, sulindac, and piroxicam
5-HETE   (hydroxy-5,8,10,14-eicosatetraenoic acid)
*   corticosteroids inhibit phospholipase converting membrane phospholipids to arachidonic acid
**   neutrophil attractant
***   give massive amplification of the inflammatory reaction

Figure 2.4

Arachidonic acid metabolic pathways. (Adapted from Foster CS[16].)

disease process and will inhibit the inflammatory reaction to nearly any type of stimulus.

Antiinflammatory effects include:

- Inhibition of increased capillary permeability caused by the acute inflammatory reaction and suppression of vasodilation.
- Inhibition of degranulation of neutrophils, mast cells, and basophils with monocytopenia and eosinopenia.
- Reduction of prostaglandin synthesis by inhibiting phospholipase (see Figure 2.4).
- Temporary neutrophil leuokocytosis 4–6 hours after administration but with reduced adherence to vascular endothelium.

Immunosuppressive effects include:

- Induction of lymphocytopenia: T lymphocytes are more susceptible than B lymphocytes; therefore antibody production is not reduced while DTH/CMI reactions are modified at low concentrations.
- Inhibition of migration of macrophages and neutrophils.
- Suppression of lymphocyte proliferation.
- Suppression of action of cytokines.
- Inhibition of DTH/CMI by decreasing recruitment of macrophages.
- Alteration of antigen processing by macrophages.
- Depression of bactericidal activity of monocytes and macrophages.

Corticosteroids reduce the activity of macrophages but not necessarily their activation by cytokines. Corticosteroids inhibit cytokine release with additional suppression of PMN activity, explaining the progression of fungal, protozoal, or parasitic infections in their presence; these latter infections especially require macrophages as 'scavenger' cells.

The use of corticosteroid therapy in managing endophthalmitis has continued to be a necessary albeit controversial treatment (Chapter 8).[50,51] Our findings generally correspond to those provided by others in that intravitreal corticosteroid therapy should be used for bacterial and considered for fungal endophthalmitis and should be injected at the same time as the antibiotics. Dosing is considered in Chapter 8 (Management and treatment).

NSAIDS act by inhibiting the conversion of arachidonic acid to prostaglandins by cyclooxygenase (see Figure 2.4). NSAIDS such as flurbiprofen (Froben) may in the future supersede conventional steroid preparations, such as dexamethasone or prednisolone, by removing unwanted side effects, particularly when corticosteroids are introduced systemically for treatment of severe ocular inflammatory disease. Flurbiprofen, given orally, has been found particularly effective for suppressing the acute inflammation of ocular infection, especially keratitis, episcleritis, and limbitis, as well as providing analgesia without interfering with satisfactory chemotherapy. Flurbiprofen is also a mydriatic drug.

References

1. Streilein JW. Ocular immune privilege: the eye takes a dim but practical view of immunity and inflammation, *J Leukoc Biol* (2003) **74**:179–85.
2. Taylor AW. Neuroimmunomodulation and immune privilege: the role of neuropeptides in ocular immunosuppression, *Neuroimmunomodulation* (2002–2003) **10**:189–98.
3. Seal DV, Bron AJ, Hay J. *Ocular Infection – Investigation and Treatment in Practice* (Martin Dunitz: London, 1998) 1–275.
4. Dekaris I, Zhu SN, Dana MR. TNF-alpha regulates corneal Langerhans cell migration, *J Immunol* (1999) **162**:4235–9.
5. Brissette-Storkus CS, Reynolds SM, Lepisto AJ et al. Identification of a novel macrophage population in the normal mouse corneal stroma, *Invest Ophthalmol Vis Sci* (2002) **43**:2264–71.
6. Hurt M, Proy V, Niederkorn JY et al. The interaction of *Acanthamoeba castellanii* cysts with macrophages and neutrophils, *J Parasitol* (2003) **89**:565–72.
7. Niederkorn J. Immune privilege in the anterior chamber of the eye, *Crit Rev Immunol* (2002) **22**:13–46.
8. Niederkorn JY. Immunology and immunomodulation of corneal transplantation, *Int Rev Immunol* (2002) **21**:173–96.
9. Radosevich M, Ono SJ. Novel mechanisms of class II major histocompatibility complex gene regulation, *Immunol Res* (2003) **27**:85–106.
10. Hamrah P, Liu Y, Zhang Q et al. Alterations in corneal stromal dendritic cell phenotype and distribution in inflammation, *Arch Ophthalmol* (2003) **121**:1132–40. [erratum appears in *Arch Ophthalmol* (2003) **121**:1555]

11. Hamrah P, Huq SO, Liu Y et al. Corneal immunity is mediated by heterogeneous population of antigen presenting cells, *J Leukoc Biol* (2003) **74**:172–8.

12. Hazlett LD, McClellan S, Barrett R et al. B7/CD28 costimulation is critical in susceptibility to *Pseudomonas aeruginosa* corneal infection: a comparative study using monoclonal antibody blockade and CD28-deficient mice, *J Immunol* (2001) **166**:1292–9.

13. Diamond JP, Leeming JP, Smart AD et al. An antimicrobial effect associated with rabbit primary aqueous humour, *Br J Ophthalmol* (1994) **78**: 142–8.

14. Diamond JP, Moule K, Leeming JP et al. Purification of an antimicrobial peptide from rabbit aqueous humour, *Curr Eye Res* (1998) **17**:783–7.

15. Haynes RJ, McElveen JE, Dua HS et al. Expression of human beta-defensins in intraocular tissues, *Invest Ophthalmol Vis Sci* (2000) **41**:3026–31.

16. Foster CS. Nonsteroidal anti-inflammatory and immunosuppressive agents. In: Lamberts DW, Potter DE, eds. *Clinical Ophthalmic Pharmacology* (Little Brown: Boston/Toronto, 1987) 173–92.

17. Sohn JH, Kaplan HJ, Suk HJ et al. Chronic low level complement activation within the eye is controlled by intraocular complement regulatory proteins, *Invest Ophthalmol Vis Sci* (2000) **41**:3492–502.

18. Sohn JH, Kaplan HJ, Suk HJ et al. Complement regulatory activity of normal human intraocular fluid is mediated by MCP, DAF, and CD59, *Invest Ophthalmol Vis Sci* (2000) **41**: 4195–202.

19. Bardenstein DS, Cheyer CJ, Lee C et al. Blockage of complement regulators in the conjunctiva and within the eye leads to massive inflammation and iritis, *Immunology* (2001) **104**:423–30.

20. Ficker L, Ramakrishnan M, Seal D et al. Role of cell-mediated immunity to staphylococci in blepharitis, *Am J Ophthalmol* (1991) **111**:473–9.

21. Johnson JE, Cluff LE, Goshi K. Studies on the pathogenesis of Staphylococcal infection, *J Exp Med* (1960) **113**:235–47.

22. Hendricks RL, Tang Q. Cellular immunity and the eye. In: Pepose GS, Holland G, Wilhelmus K, eds. *Ocular Infection and Immunity* (Mosby Year Book: Chicago, 1996) 71–95.

23. Rudner XL, Kernacki KA, Barrett RP et al. Prolonged elevation of IL-1 in *Pseudomonas aeruginosa* ocular infection regulates macrophage-inflammatory protein-2 production, polymorphonuclear neutrophil persistence, and corneal perforation, *J Immunol* (2000) **164**:6576–82.

24. Kernacki KA, Barrett RP, Hobden JA et al. Macrophage inflammatory protein-2 is a mediator of polymorphonuclear neutrophil influx in ocular bacterial infection, *J Immunol* (2000) **164**: 1037–45.

25. Niederkorn JY, Ferguson TA. Anterior chamber associated immune deviation. In: Pepose GS, Holland G, Wilhelmus K, eds. *Ocular Infection and Immunity*. (Mosby Year Book: Chicago, 1996) 96–103.

26. Stein-Streilein J, Streilein JW. Anterior chamber associated immune deviation (ACAID): regulation, biological relevance, and implications for therapy, *Int Rev Immunol* (2002) **21**:123–52.

27. Scholz M, Doer HW, Cinatl J. Human cyto-megalovirus retinitis: pathogenicity, immune evasion and persistence, *Trends Microbiol* (2003) **11**:171–8.

28. Green DR, Ferguson TA. The role of Fas ligand in immune privilege, *Nat Rev Mol Cell Biol* (2001) **2**:917–24.

29. Feltkamp TE, Ringrose JH. Acute anterior uveitis and spondyloarthropathies, *Curr Opin Rheumatol* (1998) **10**:314–18.

30. Abreu JA, Cordoves L, Mesa CG et al. Chronic pseudophakic endophthalmitis versus saccular endophthalmitis, *J Cataract Refract Surg* (1997) **23**:1122–5.

31. Warheker PT, Gupta SR, Mansfield DC et al. Post-operative saccular endophthalmitis caused by macrophage-associated staphylococci, *Eye* (1998) **12**:1019–21.

32. Kresloff MS, Castellarin AA, Zarbin MA. Endophthalmitis, *Surv Ophthalmol* (1998) **43**: 193–224.

33. Warheker PT, Gupta SR, Mansfield DC et al. Successful treatment of saccular endophthalmitis with clarithromycin, *Eye* (1998) **12**:1017–19.

34. Okhravi N, Guest S, Matheson MM et al. Assessment of the effect of oral clarithromycin on visual outcome following presumed bacterial endophthalmitis, *Curr Eye Res* (2000) **21**:691–702.

35. Karia N, Aylward GW. Postoperative *Propionibacterium acnes* endophthalmitis, *Ophthalmology* (2001) **108**:634–5.

36. Unal M, Peyman GA, Liang C et al. Ocular toxicity of intravitreal clarithromycin, *Retina* (1999) **19**: 442–6.

37. Ravindranath RM, Hasan SA, Mondino BJ. Immunopathologic features of *Staphylococcus epidermidis*-induced endophthalmitis in the rat, *Curr Eye Res* (1997) **16**:1036–43.

38. Meek B, Speijer D, de Jong PTVM et al. The ocular humoral immune response in health and disease, *Prog Retin Eye Res* (2003) **22**:391–415.

39. Tuft SJ, Ramakrishnan M, Seal D et al. Role of *Staphylococcus aureus* in chronic allergic conjunctivitis, *Ophthalmology* (1992) **99**:180–4.

40. Calonge M, Siemasko KF, Stern ME. Animal models of ocular allergy and their clinical correlations, *Curr Allergy Asthma Rep* (2003) **3**:345–51.

41. Hazlett LD, McClellan SA, Rudner XL et al. The role of Langerhans cells in *Pseudomonas aeruginosa* infection, *Invest Ophthalmol Vis Sci* (2002) **43**: 189–97.

42. Hazlett LD, Rudner XL, McClellan SA et al. Role of IL-12 and IFN-γ in *Pseudomonas aeruginosa* corneal infection, *Invest Ophthalmol Vis Sci* (2002) **43**:419–24.

43. Hazlett LD, Houang X, McClellan SA et al. Further studies on the role of IL-12 in *Pseudomonas aeruginosa* corneal infection, *Eye* (2003) **17**: 863–71.

44. Huang X, Hazlett LD. Analysis of *Pseudomonas aeruginosa* corneal infection using an oligonucleotide microarray, *Invest Ophthalmol Vis Sci* 2003; **44**:3409–16.

45. Hazlett LD, McClellan SM, Hume EB et al. Extended wear contact lens usage induces Langerhans cell migration into cornea, *Exp Eye Res* (1999) **69**:575–7.

46. Hazlett LD, McClellan S, Kwon B et al. Increased severity of *Pseudomonas aeruginosa* corneal infec-tion in strains of mice designated as Th1 versus Th2 responsive, *Invest Ophthalmol Vis Sci* (2000) **41**:805–10.

47. Hendricks RL. Immunopathogenesis of viral ocular infections, *Chem Immunol* (1999) **73**:120–36.

48. Khanna KM, Bonneau RH, Kinchington PR et al. Herpes simplex virus-specific memory CD8+ T cells are selectively activated and retained in latently infected sensory ganglia, *Immunity* (2003) **18**:593–603.

49. Seal D, Wright P, Ficker L et al. Placebo-controlled trial of fusidic acid gel and oxytetracycline for recurrent blepharitis and rosacea, *Br J Ophthalmol* (1995) **79**:42–5.

50. Coats ML, Peyman GA. Intravitreal corticosteroids in the treatment of exogenous fungal endoph-thalmitis, *Retina* (1992) **12**:46–51.

51. Schulman JA, Peyman GA. Intravitreal corticos-teroids as an adjunct in the treatment of bacterial and fungal endophthalmitis: a review, *Retina* (1992) **12**:340–66.

3

Microbiology and molecular biology

MICROBIOLOGY

Invasion and virulence

A microbe has to penetrate the eye to cause infection; penetration can occur as the result of trauma or surgery, either into the cornea or anterior chamber or directly into the posterior segment, where endophthalmitis can develop. Trauma often involves an accident with hammering on dirty metal involving the penetration of a metallic chip contaminated with *Bacillus* species, considered in detail in Chapter 7. The trauma may also be relatively minor, caused by wearing contaminated soft contact lenses, or may be associated with an epithelial defect from dry eye (Sjögren's syndrome) or other external disease. Surgical complications include cataract surgery, extracapsular cataract extraction (ECCE) or phacoemulsification, and penetrating keratoplasty, which are reviewed in Chapter 6. The blood-borne route must always be considered for endophthalmitis when there is no history of accidental or surgical trauma, particularly the possibility of endocarditis or a previous, possibly contaminated blood transfusion; intravenous drug abusers are also more likely to develop endophthalmitis, particularly with *Candida albicans* (Chapter 9).

To gain entry superficially, the organism needs to adhere to the epithelium and to invade through the epithelial sheet into the corneal stroma. *Pseudomonas aeruginosa* is particularly adept at invading from a superficial source, often from contaminated contact lenses or eye drops.[1] *Ps. aeruginosa* has been shown experimentally to be able to adhere to the corneal epithelium in mice and invade the stroma within 1 hour because of the toxins and proteases that this pathogen produces.[2–9] The immunopathogenesis of invasion by *Ps. aeruginosa*, including molecular identification of involved cytokines, is considered in Chapter 2.

Penetration alone by an organism is not sufficient to cause infection. Proliferation is required for the establishment of sufficient numbers of cells to be able to overcome the host defenses aimed at its eradication. Studies found that up to 35% of anterior chamber irrigation samples contained bacteria following cataract surgery[10–13] compared with an expected rate of postoperative endophthalmitis of between 0.02% and 0.5%.[14–17] In most cases, the bacterial inoculum is too low to establish multiplication, because the cells are inactivated by the innate immune system, such as phagocytic cells, and by antibacterial substances such as defensins (Chapter 2). However, in a few patients, bacterial proliferation occurs, resulting in devastating endophthalmitis.

A prospective, randomized, placebo-controlled multi-center clinical trial is needed to establish whether antibiotics used at the time of surgery, either topically or by intracameral injection, are effective in reducing the chances of such proliferation, causing postoperative endophthalmitis. The European Society of Cataract and Refractive Surgeons (ESCRS) is currently conducting such a trial for a 2-year period (January 2004 to December 2005) with a Fisher 2×2 factorial design in 30,000 patients, comparing the use of topical 0.5% levofloxacin (Chapter 5) versus saline, with or without an intracameral injection of 1 mg of cefuroxime[17] during phacoemulsification cataract surgery and placement of an intraocular lens. Additionally, all patients receive preoperative prophylaxis with 5% povidone iodine for a minimum of 3 minutes and, starting 18 hours postoperatively, 6 days of 0.5% levofloxacin given topically every 6 hours (Chapters 5 and 6).

The virulence of the organism also dictates the outcome in the patient and is usually related to the production of lethal toxins by the bacterium that are quickly effective at causing tissue necrosis. *Streptococcus pyogenes* and *Bacillus cereus* are highly virulent for the eye, needing a very small inoculum, possibly as low as 10 cells, to cause a fulminant endophthalmitis within 24 hours. While this situation applies to all the tissues of the body, it is different for *Ps. aeruginosa*, which is highly pathogenic for the eye but not for the skin or other organs, except in the immunocompromised host. The eye is unique with the cornea and vitreous having no direct vascular supply to provide an immediate vascular and immunological reaction to trauma, hence *Pseudomonas* can establish a fulminant necrotic infection in the first 24 hours which does not occur similarly at other sites in the body. The posterior segment is a sterile site and therefore more vulnerable to bacterial multiplication whether small numbers reach it by the blood-borne, surgical, or traumatic routes.

Bacteriology

Cell wall

Bacteria are divided into Gram-positive and Gram-negative groups based on their cell wall structure (Box 3.1). The bacterial cell wall is a rigid structure surrounding a flexible cell membrane. The cell wall maintains the shape of the cell: its rigid wall compensates for the innate flexibility of the phospholipid membrane and also maintains the cellular integrity when the intracellular osmotic gradient is unfavorable. The wall is also responsible for attachment: teichoic acids attached to the outer surface of the wall serve as attachment sites for bacteriophages. Flagella, fimbriae, and pili all come from the wall.

The composition of the Gram-positive cell wall is 90% peptidoglycan polymer that is made of alternating sequences of N-acetylglucosamine (NAG) and N-acetyl-muramic acid (NAMA) with each layer cross-linked by an amino acid bridge. The peptidoglycan polymer imparts thickness to the Gram-positive cell wall. In contrast, peptidoglycan makes up only 20% of the Gram-negative cell wall. Periplasmic space and an outer membrane also differentiate the Gram-negative organism and contain proteins that destroy potentially

dangerous foreign matter. The outer membrane, composed of lipid, protein, and lipopolysaccharide (LPS), is porous because porin proteins allow free passage of small molecules. The lipid portion of LPS also contains lipid A, a toxic substance, which imparts the pathogenic virulence associated with some Gram-negative bacteria.

The Gram stain was the innovation of Hans Christian Joaquim Gram, a Danish physicist, who sought to distinguish bacterial organisms based on their different cell wall structures. The crystal violet primary stain in Gram stain preferentially binds peptidoglycan. Because the cell wall of Gram-negative bacteria is low in peptidoglycan content and high in lipid content, the primary

---

Box 3.1 Gram-positive and Gram-negative bacteria

- Gram-positive bacteria
  - Cocci
    - *Staphylococcus* species
    - *Streptococcus* species
  - Rods
    - *Bacillus* species
    - *Listeria* species
    - *Lactobacillus* species
    - *Erysipelothrix* species
    - *Corynebacterium* species
    - *Actinomyces* species
    - *Propionibacterium* species
    - *Clostridium* species
- Gram-negative bacteria
  - Rods
    - Enterobacteriaceae
      Escherichia coli
      Klebsiella species
      Proteus species
      Serratia species
      Providencia species
      Salmonella species
      Shigella species
      Citrobacter species
      Morganella species
    - Pleomorphic group
      - *Haemophilus* species
      - *Brucella* species
      - *Pasteurella* species
      - *Legionella* species
    - Nonfermenters
      - *Pseudomonas* species
    - Others
      - *Vibrio* species
      - *Campylobacter* species
      - *Helicobacter* species
  - Coccobacilli
    - *Haemophilus influenzae*
    - *Neisseria*

crystal violet stain is washed out when the decolorizer (acetone) is added. Instead, the Gram-negative organism incorporates the safranin counterstain that stains red.

Methylene blue is a simple stain that is taken up by all bacteria and can be used to show if bacteria are present or not. Other useful stains include acridine orange (all bacteria, fungi, and

---

Box 3.2 Biochemical tests

Tests for distinguishing Gram-positive organisms
Catalase test
This test distinguishes *Staphylococcus* organisms, which are catalase-positive, from *Streptococcus* species, which are catalase-negative. Catalase is a self-defense enzyme employed by certain Gram-positive bacteria to neutralize hydrogen peroxide, which is toxic to the bacteria.

$2H_2O_2$ catalase $2H_2O + O_2$

Gas that is produced as O_2 can be seen as a white froth after adding a few drops of 3% H_2O_2.
Coagulase test
Along with mannitol salt agar medium, the coagulase test is another method for differentiating *S. aureus*, which is coagulase-positive, from the other strains of staphylococci, which are coagulase-negative. Bacteria that produce coagulase use it as a defense mechanism by clotting the areas of plasma around them, enabling the organisms to resist phagocytosis by the host's immune system. The sample is inoculated into 0.5 ml of rabbit plasma and incubated at 37°C for 1–4 hours. Clot formation in the test tube indicates a positive test.
Christie, Atkins, and Munch-Petersen (CAMP) test
This test is used to differentiate *Streptococcus agalactiae*. *S. aureus* beta toxin binds to bovine erythrocytes and this sensitizes it to the lytic activity of the *Strep. agalactiae* ceramide-binding factor. A positive test produces a complete hemolysis and is seen as an arrowhead-shaped clearing on the blood agar plate.
Bile-esculin test
This test differentiates group D streptococci from other *Streptococcus* organisms. Group D organisms are positive for bile-esculin hydrolysis. In the presence of bile or bile salts, group D streptococci hydrolyze the esculin with the by-products reacting with the iron salts in the medium, causing it to blacken.
Optochin test
The optochin test is a presumptive test that is used to distinguish *Strep. pneumoniae* from the other alpha-hemolytic streptococci. Optochin (ethyl hydrocupreine) disks are placed on inoculated blood agar plates kept overnight in a CO_2 incubator. Because *Strep. pneumoniae* is sensitive to optochin, a zone of clearing will develop around the disk where the *Strep. pneumoniae* have been lysed.

Tests for distinguishing Gram-negative bacteria
Citrate test
The citrate test is used to determine the ability of a bacterium to use citrate as its only source of carbon. Ammonia is released if the bacterium grows and a pH indicator in the medium detects the presence of this compound and turns blue (a positive test). This is a part of the indole, methyl red, Voges–Proskauer, and citrate test (IMViC) used for differentiating the Enterobacteriaceae. For instance, *Enterobacter cloacae* tests positive while *Escherichia coli* tests negative. *Klebsiella pneumoniae* also tests positive.
Indole test
The indole test is part of the IMViC test. *Proteus* species and *E. coli* are prototype indole-positive organisms. Some bacteria are able to break down the amino acid tryptophan, releasing indole; its presence can be detected through the use of Kovacs' reagent, which turns red.
Oxidase test
This test is used to identify bacteria containing cytochrome oxidase. It is useful in differentiating the oxidase-negative Enterobacteriaceae from the oxidase-positive Pseudomonadaceae. *Neisseria* organisms also test positive. The presence of cytochrome oxidase can be detected through the use of an oxidase disk which acts as an electron donor to cytochrome oxidase. If the bacteria oxidize the disk (remove electrons), the disk will turn purple, indicating a positive test. Unchanging color indicates a negative test.
Urease test
This test is used to distinguish *Proteus* organisms, which produce urea, from other enteric bacteria. When urea is broken down and ammonia is released, the pH of the medium becomes more alkaline, causing the pH indicator to turn pink.
Other tests
Automated identification systems are now widely used based on 10 or 23 differentiating media-impregnated well 'strips' (API) that cost approximately $1 each.

protozoa), modified Ziehl-Neelsen (*Nocardia* species), full Ziehl–Neelsen (mycobacteria), lactophenol blue (wet preparation for fungi), immunofluorescent stains, and fluorescein-labeled molecular probe stains.

Organisms

Even within the broad rubric of the Gram reaction, many different taxonomy schemes are used to group various bacteria. For instance, they are further subdivided by their physical morphology (coccus or rod), metabolic pathway (aerobe, anaerobe, or facultative anaerobe), and survival function (spore-forming). In this section, these organisms have been grouped in the simplest way possible (Box 3.1).

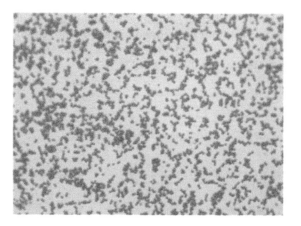

Figure 3.1

Gram-positive cocci – staphylococci in clusters.

Gram-positive cocci

The Gram-positive cocci are grouped together based on their Gram stain reaction, thick cell wall structure, and spherical shape. *Staphylococcus, Streptococcus*, and *Enterococcus* species are members of this group with medical importance. *Enterococcus* organisms are a part of the group D streptococci that were designated a new genus. Various biochemical tests are employed to differentiate these species. For instance, staphylococcal organisms are catalase-positive, whereas streptococci and *Enterococcus* species are catalase-negative. These tests are listed in Box 3.2.

Staphylococcus organisms

There are 23 recognized staphylococcal species; three of them, *S. aureus, S. epidermidis,* and *S. saprophyticus* are recognized as being the most clinically significant. The *Staphylococcus* genus appears as Gram-positive cocci in grape-like clusters (Figure 3.1). Staphylococci are classified into *S. aureus* and non-*aureus* organisms by the coagulase test. The former is coagulase-positive while the latter are all coagulase-negative, hence known collectively as coagulase-negative staphylococci (CNS).

The pathogenic effects of staphylococci are mainly produced by a variety of toxins. For instance, enterotoxin causes food poisoning and

exfoliative toxins cause scalded skin syndrome. A more thorough listing of toxins associated with staphylococci is found in Table 3.1. *S. aureus,* the pyogenic and virulent organism, is almost always resistant to penicillin because of beta-lactamase production, but is usually susceptible to the beta-lactamase-stable penicillins (e.g. methicillin, nafcillin, oxacillin, [di]cloxacillin), but may become resistant on the basis of altered penicillin-binding proteins. Methicillin-resistant *S. aureus* (MRSA) has become a major concern within hospitals, as part of hospital-acquired infection. *S. aureus* has a propensity for invasion of the vascular system, leading to bacteremia, and is distinguished from other bacteria by its ability to establish metastatic sites of pyogenic infection throughout the body, including endophthalmitis.

Table 3.1 Staphylococcal toxins

Staphylococcal toxin	Pathogenic effect
Enterotoxin	Food poisoning
Exfoliative toxin	Scalded skin syndrome
Toxic shock syndrome toxin	Toxic shock syndrome
Leukocidin	Formation of pus and acne
Others: coagulase, hemolysin, protein A	

Systemically, *S. aureus* is the most pathogenic of this group of organisms and is also associated with endophthalmitis, pneumonia, meningitis, boils, arthritis, and osteomyelitis. *S. epidermidis* is a CNS which is part of normal skin flora. Infection with *S. epidermidis* usually occurs in the presence of a foreign body such as an intraocular lens, catheter, prosthetic device; surgery; or trauma. *S. saprophyticus* is a common cause of infection of the urinary tract, both upper (i.e. kidney – pyelonephritis) and lower (i.e. bladder – cystitis) segments, in sexually active young women. This bacterium may possess adhesin for urothelial cell adhesion.

Intraocularly, involvement of staphylococcal organisms with postoperative endophthalmitis has been well documented. *S. epidermidis* was the most frequent organism isolated in the Endophthalmitis Vitrectomy Study (EVS),[18] although bias in recruitment explains this finding (Chapter 8). *S. aureus* is associated with a severe form of acute postoperative endophthalmitis while CNS cause both subacute and chronic postoperative endophthalmitis. In a Finnish study, 23% of post-cataract extraction endophthalmitis was caused by *S. saprophyticus*.[19]

Streptococcus species

The *Streptococcus* genus consists of Gram-positive cocci in chains or clusters (Figure 3.2).

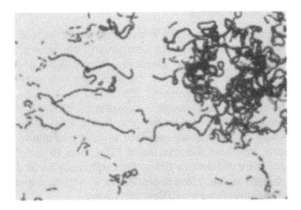

Figure 3.2

Microaerophilic streptococci in long chains. Gram stain.

Several classifications have been proposed for this genus. Hemolytic activity has been used as a preliminary criterion for classifying some streptococci.

- Alpha-'hemolysis' – incomplete lysis causing 'greening' around colonies on blood agar – viridans group and *S. pneumoniae*.
- Beta-hemolysis – complete lysis (contains most of the major human pathogens) – *S. pyogenes*.
- Gamma-'hemolysis' completely nonhemolytic.

Rebecca Lancefield devised a scheme of classification based on the antigenic characteristics of a cell wall carbohydrate called the C substance. Group A was named *Streptococcus pyogenes*; more than 90% of streptococcal disease in humans is caused by beta-hemolytic group A streptococcus which is extremely virulent although it also colonizes the throats of 10% of the population. Group A streptococcal diseases are divided into suppurative (primary) and nonsuppurative (sequelae) diseases. Suppurative diseases include impetigo, erysipelas, puerperal fever, cellulitis, and necrotizing fasciitis. Group A streptococcus also causes a highly virulent and purulent acute postoperative endophthalmitis. Subsequent nonsuppurative complications include scarlet fever, rheumatic fever, glomerulonephritis, and erythema nodosum. Streptococci perpetuate their pathology via elaborated toxins including erythrogenic toxins, cardiohepatic toxins, nephrotoxins, hemolysins, and spreading factors.

Lancefield group B streptococcus is called *Strep. agalactiae* and is found in the oral cavity, intestinal tract, and vagina. It is not beta-hemolytic. In the USA, it is the most frequent cause of life-threatening disease in newborns including meningitis and the occasional case of endophthalmitis. Adult diseases include meningitis, endocarditis, and pneumonia.

Lancefield groups C and G streptococci are beta-hemolytic and cause pyogenic infections, including endophthalmitis in the elderly and compromised individuals.

Lancefield group D is divided into enterococcal and nonenterococcal organisms. Enterococcal members such as *Strep. faecalis, Strep. faecium*, and *Strep. durans* have been assigned the genus name *Enterococcus* and thus are referred to as *E. faecalis, E. faecium*, and *E. durans*, respectively.

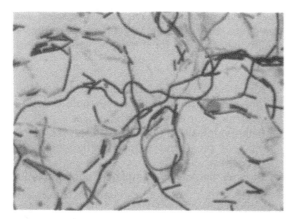

Figure 3.3

Long chains of *Bacillus* species in culture; may form spores in human tissue, which does not occur with *Clostridium perfringens*.

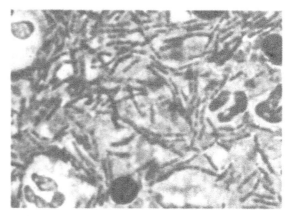

Figure 3.4

Methylene blue stain of *Bacillus anthracis*.

Enterococcal organisms have long been known to cause infective endocarditis, but have also been recognized to cause nosocomial infection and 'superinfection' in patients receiving antimicrobial agents.[20] Further, *Enterococcus* species are now receiving increased attention because of their resistance to multiple antimicrobial drugs, probably contributing to their prominence in nosocomial infections.[21,22] The most common enterococci-associated nosocomial infections are those of the urinary tract, followed by surgical wound infections and bacteremia. Other enterococcal infections include meningitis and bacteremia in ill neonates; central nervous system infections in adults, typically with a history of central nervous system surgery or intrathecal chemotherapy; and rarely, osteomyelitis and pulmonary infections. Enterococci frequently arise from colonization of indwelling drainage tubes, causing liver or biliary infection in liver transplant patients. Enterococci have been recognized as a cause of endophthalmitis post-cataract surgery, particularly in women over 80 years of age.[17] It is not particularly virulent and reasonable vision is retained.

Viridans streptococci are mostly alpha-hemolytic bacteria that do not fit into the Lancefield rubric; they are responsible for subacute bacterial endocarditis but occasionally possess a selection of substance antigens. Patients with a history of rheumatic fever or congenital heart disease are susceptible to seeding of these displaced organisms on the heart valves or other vital systems.

Gram-positive rods (spore-forming)

The Gram-positive rods are ubiquitous organisms divided into three groups based upon their ability to produce endospores and their morphological appearance.

Bacillus species

Bacilli are ubiquitous organisms found in soil, water, airborne dust, and even the human intestines. *Bacillus* (aerobic, Figure 3.3) and *Clostridium* (anaerobic) bacteria are the only spore-forming organisms. On blood agar plates, bacilli produce large, spreading, gray-white colonies with irregular margins. In the spore state, these organisms are resistant to heat and chemicals; however, autoclaving at 120°C and 15 lbs of pressure will destroy them. Although most *Bacillus* species are harmless saprophytes, *B. anthracis* and *B. cereus* cause significant pathology.

B. anthracis, the organism that causes anthrax, primarily affects herbivorous animals. The bacterium is transmitted to humans through

Table 3.2 Gram-positive rod classification

Aerobic bacteria	Anaerobic bacteria		Toxin	Disease
Endospore-forming organisms	Endospore-forming organisms			
Bacillus species	Clostridium species			
Nonendospore-forming organisms				
Corynebacterium species	Cl. difficile		Exotoxins	Pseudomembranous colitis
Erysipelothrix species	C. septicum		–	Wound infection
Lactobacillus species	C. sporogenes		–	Wound infection
Listeria species	Cl. perfringens		Enterotoxin	Myonecrosis/intestinal necrosis, food poisoning, diarrhea, gas gangrene
	Cl. tetani		Neurotoxin	Tetanus
	Cl. botulinum		Neurotoxin	Botulism

inhalation of endospores or direct contact with animal products. In order to be fully potent, *B. anthracis* must produce a capsule and a protein exotoxin. Under the microscope, these organisms are nonmotile and appear to have square ends and to be attached by a joint to other cells (Figure 3.4). Sources of infection are usually industrial or agricultural. Unfortunately, recent events have added terrorism as another cause. The infection is classified as one of three types:

* Cutaneous infection (95% of human cases)
* Inhalation anthrax (rare)
* Gastrointestinal anthrax (very rare).

Although extraocular and eye surface complications have been reported,[1] no intraocular complications have been noted. Cutaneous anthrax leading to corneal scarring from cicatricial ectropion[23] has been reported, as well as preseptal cellulitis.[24]

B. cereus

Unlike *B. anthracis*, *B. cereus* is a motile bacterium that can cause toxin-mediated food poisoning. Its association with traumatic endophthalmitis has been documented in detail in the literature (Chapter 7). *B. cereus* has also been associated with endogenous endophthalmitis, especially in immunocompromised hosts. *B. cereus* produces beta-lactamases and is resistant to beta-lactams, including third-generation cephalosporins. It is also found in different foods, including stew, cereal, fried rice, and milk. The toxin is produced after the infected foods are cooked and causes symptoms similar to those of staphylococcal food poisoning.

Clostridium species

Clostridium species are Gram-positive, anaerobic spore-forming, motile rods found ubiquitously in organisms inhabiting water, soil, vegetation, and the human bowel. These organisms are especially fond of soil. Under the microscope, they resemble long drumsticks with a bulge located at their terminal ends.

Extremely durable *Clostridium* spores are produced when the environment becomes unfavorable. In the active form, potent exotoxins are produced which are responsible for tetanus, botulism, and gas gangrene. The six clinically important *Clostridium* species are listed in Table 3.2.

Endophthalmitis cases related to *Clostridium* organisms have been reported following trauma (Chapter 7) and in one case, after cataract surgery.[25] Coinfection with *Cl. tetani* and *Bacillus* species was noted in one particular traumatic case, the source being contamination with mud.[26] Endogenous endophthalmitis secondary to metastasis of *Clostridium* organisms from the biliary tract has also been reported.[27] In one case of panophthalmitis secondary to *Cl. septicum*, the patient presented with spontaneous gas gangrene panophthalmitis and a gas bubble was present in the anterior chamber.[28] Gram stains of clostridia from cases of gas gangrene show Gram-positive bacilli with no spores, as the bacterium does not produce spores when causing active infection; it does so when exposed to air or when the laboratory cultures are a few days old.

Gram-positive bacilli (nonspore-forming)

Listeria monocytogenes causes listeriosis. Neonates experience granulomatosis infantisepticum. It can also be spread by undercooked meat. Seventeen cases of endophthalmitis associated with *Listeria* species have been reported in the literature since 1977. Most occur as endogenous endophthalmitis in immunocompromised hosts, typically with elevated intraocular pressure, pigment dispersion, and dark hypopyon.[29]

Erysipelothrix rhusiopathiae is usually found in decomposing nitrogenous material; swine are major reservoirs. Most human infections are due to occupational exposure. Systemic infection can cause endocarditis. No cases of endophthalmitis have yet been reported with this organism.

Corynebacterium diphtheriae is found in upper respiratory lesions and skin. Humans are the only natural host of this bacterium that causes respiratory and cutaneous diphtheria. Along with CNS, *Corynebacterium* species are a frequent cause of subacute endophthalmitis following cataract surgery.[12–14] They also comprise the majority of positive cultures after cataract surgery in patients without evidence of endophthalmitis, implying contamination at the time of surgery.[12,30]

Lactobacillus organisms are normal flora in the vagina. One case of posttraumatic endophthalmitis caused by *Lactobacillus* species has been reported in the literature.[31]

Gram-negative organisms

Gram-negative bacteria are deficient in peptidoglycans. They loosely bind the crystal violet primary stain, which is removed on exposure to acetone for 5 seconds (Gram-positive bacteria retain the stain). Therefore, they are stained with the secondary safranin stain, which imparts its red hue. The LPS layer is primarily responsible for endotoxin production. These bacteria are found in the gastrointestinal tract and are a common cause of urinary tract infection.

Gram-negative diplococci

Neisseria species are pathogens as well as normal flora in humans. They are aerobic and facultative anaerobic, Gram-negative diplococci requiring a moist environment and warm temperatures for optimum growth. Where the diplococci abut, they are flat-sided, so each member of the pair presents a bean-shaped configuration. They are found within polymorphs. These organisms grow well on chocolate agar containing antibiotics that inhibit growth of Gram-negative bacteria. The two most clinically significant *Neisseria* species are *N. gonorrhoeae* and *N. meningitidis*.

N. meningitidis (meningococcus)

Humans are the only natural hosts for *N. meningitidis* and transmission is through nasal droplets. Meningococcal diseases can be divided into nasopharyngitis, septicemia, meningitis, arthritis, conjunctivitis, and occasionally bilateral endogenous endophthalmitis. Different strains of *N. meningitidis* are classified by their capsular polysaccharides. This bacterium is the second leading cause of meningitis in the USA. Both exogenous and endogenous endophthalmitis cases related to *N. meningitidis* have been reported.[32,33] Meningococcal endophthalmitis has been reported as both a preceding event and sequela of septicemia (Chapter 9).[34,35]

N. gonorrhoeae

Among the *Neisseria* species, only *N. gonorrhoeae* strains are always pathogenic. This organism colonizes mucosal surfaces of the cervix, urethra, rectum, oropharynx, and nasopharynx, causing the correlating symptoms. Ocular surface sequelae of gonococcal ophthalmia have been well documented; however, intraocular manifestations have not been reported.

Enterobacteriaceae species

The Enterobacteriaceae are a family of large Gram-negative rods (Box 3.3) that are usually associated with intestinal infections but are found in almost all natural habitats. These are among the most pathogenic and frequently encountered organisms in clinical microbiology. Systemically, they have also been known to cause meningitis, pneumonia, bacillary dysentery, typhoid, and food poisoning.

In general, Gram-negative organisms account for 16–18.5% of all cases of culture-proven post-surgical endophthalmitis and up to 30% of post-traumatic cases in rural areas. Among Enterobacteriaceae organisms are the *Proteus* species, *Serratia marcescens*, *Morganella morganii*, *Citrobacter* species, *Escherichia coli*, and *Klebsiella pneumoniae*. This list includes non Enterobacteriaceae organisms such as *Pseudomonas* species and *Haemophilus influenzae*. Enterobacteriaceae organisms have been associated with both endogenous and exogenous endophthalmitis, especially in immunocompromised hosts. However, no cases of endophthalmitis caused by *Shigella*, *Edwardsiella*, or *Providencia* species have been reported.

Ocular sequelae can include central artery occlusion resulting from septic thrombi. *Klebsiella* and *Serratia* species appear to be among the organisms within this group most likely to cause endophthalmitis. Sixty-one percent of the 44 patients with *Klebsiella* endophthalmitis reported in the literature from 1981 to 1994 had diabetes, 68% had suppurative liver disease, and 16% had a urinary tract infection.[36] Although most cases of endogenous endophthalmitis result from metastasis in immunocompromised hosts, a case of exogenous endophthalmitis caused by *Serratia* organisms after an injury with a wood fragment has been reported.[37] Among the less frequent causes of endophthalmitis, *Proteus* species were found in a diabetic patient who underwent a triple procedure (penetrating keratoplasty, cataract extraction, and posterior chamber intraocular lens implantation) as a result of contamination from the donor cornea.[38] *Morganella* organisms have

also been isolated from a postoperative cataract patient.[39] In a case of endophthalmitis induced by *Salmonella* organisms, the use of snake powder as a food seasoning was suspected as the cause. *Salmonella* has also been isolated from a case of endophthalmitis following pneumopexy.

Other Gram-negative rods

Haemophilus species
Haemophilus organisms comprise a significant portion of the indigenous flora of the upper respiratory tract. Given their ubiquity, most of the population are carriers for one or more *Haemophilus* species; they represent a large group of Gram-negative rods with an affinity for growing in blood. The blood medium provides two factors that *Haemophilus* species require for growth: X factor (hemin) and V factor (nicotinamide dinucleotide). *Haemophilus* colonies will usually form satellites around *Staphylococcus* colonies because staphylococci can provide the necessary factors required for optimum *Haemophilus* organism growth. Morphologically, *Haemophilus* bacteria usually appear as tiny coccobacilli under the microscope, but can also assume many other shapes. Some classification systems have grouped them into a pleomorphic category. Using methylene blue stain on a smear may aid in identification.

Haemophilus species are classified by their capsular properties into six different serological groups (a–f). Species that possess the type b capsule are the most clinically significant because of their virulent properties.

H. influenzae
Infection with *H. influenzae* occurs following inhalation of infected droplets. Most invasive upper respiratory infections are caused by type b capsulate strains (HIB). Systemic sequelae can occur after hematogenous spread and can cause meningitis, epiglottitis, cellulitis, septic arthritis, pneumonia, and endophthalmitis. HIB is the major cause of meningitis in children under 4 years of age who have yet to form protective antibodies. This species may exist with or without a pathogenic polysaccharide capsule. Strains that lack the capsule usually cause mild localized infections (otitis media, sinusitis), as opposed to HIB, which can cause several serious infections.

H. influenzae has been well documented as a major cause of bleb-associated endophthalmitis. There have also been cases following strabismus surgery[40] and trauma.[41] *H. aegyptius* and *H. paraphrophilus* have also been reported as causing endophthalmitis. *H. ducreyi* causes chancroid but has not been associated with endophthalmitis.

Brucella species

Brucella species only cause incidental infections in humans; the organism is thought to have been eradicated in many countries, except in agrarian environments. It colonizes the genital tracts of animals and infects the milk. *Brucella abortus* infects cattle and *B. melitensis* infects goats and was the original cause of Malta fever. A case of endophthalmitis caused by *B. melitensis* has been reported in a 17–year-old woman in Saudi Arabia, probably the result of drinking raw goat's milk.[42] Populations avoid brucellosis by pasteurizing milk and producing farm animals from which *Brucella* has been eradicated.

Francisella species

Francisella tularensis causes tularemia from tick bites. This highly infectious disease is carried by rodents, deer, pets, and many other animals. Oculoglandular tularemia has been reported but endophthalmitis has not been noted as a sequela.

Pasteurella multocida infects humans from dog or cat bites. Patients tend to exhibit swelling, cellulitis, and some bloody drainage at the wound site. Infection may also move to nearby joints where it can cause swelling and arthritis. No ocular complications have been noted in the literature.

Legionella pneumophila

L. pneumophila causes legionnaires' disease and Pontiac fever. The first discovery of bacteria from the genus *Legionella* came in 1976 when an outbreak of pneumonia at an American Legion convention led to 29 deaths. Transmission is through respiratory droplets and causes a gradual onset of influenza-like symptoms. Severe pneumonia can develop that is not responsive to penicillins or aminoglycosides but does respond to the quinolones and azithromycin. Legionnaires' disease also has the potential to spread into other organ systems of the body such as the gastrointestinal tract and the central nervous system. No ocular complications have been reported.

Miscellaneous Gram-negative rods

Vibrio species

Vibrio organisms are obligate aerobes with a recognizable curved shape and a single polar flagellum (Figure 3.5). These are waterborne organisms transmitted to humans, especially fishermen, by infected water or through fecal transmission. Thus, in hot countries with poor sewerage or water treatment, cholera is sometimes seen in epidemic proportions.

Ocular involvement usually occurs as a result of trauma involving infected warm seawater, such as the Gulf of Mexico or the South China Sea. In a recent review, Penland et al described 17 cases of eye infections involving *Vibrio* species, in which 11 (65%) involved exposure to seawater or shellfish. Three cases of exogenous endophthalmitis were included in this survey.[43]

Campylobacter species

Campylobacter organisms are microaerophiles that can survive in a low oxygen environment and prefer a relatively high concentration of carbon dioxide, making a suitable growth environment a challenge. Cell motility is achieved through polar flagella that emanate from a curved rod-shaped cell. The unique shapes of the cell and flagella are extremely useful in Gram stain identification. *C.*

Figure 3.5

Gram-negative rod: *Vibrio vulnificus.*

jejuni is an organism that causes gastrointestinal infection. Humans acquire the organisms by eating undercooked chicken or drinking contaminated milk and water. *C. jejuni* causes septicemia but no cases of endophthalmitis have been reported.

Helicobacter species

Helicobacter species are microaerophilic organisms with curved cell bodies. Aside from the well-known association of *H. pylori* with stomach ulcers, *Helicobacter* species have been linked to ocular manifestations of acne rosacea.[44] *H. pylori* has been reported to be found frequently in glaucoma patients.[45] However, no cases of endophthalmitis have been reported.

Pseudomonas species

Pseudomonas species are motile, Gram-negative, aerobic rods that, along with *Xanthomonas* species, comprise a group of bacteria called pseudomonads. These organisms are found commonly in soil and water, as well as on plant and animal surfaces. These bacteria demonstrate significant antibiotic resistance, including innate resistance to many antibiotics, and are capable of surviving in harsh conditions. They also produce a slime layer that is resistant to phagocytosis. *Ps. aeruginosa* is the most common human pathogen and the most frequently isolated nonfermenter in the laboratory. Box 3.4 lists its virulence determi-

nants. Several features distinguish *Ps. aeruginosa* from other *Pseudomonas* species:

- Able to grow at 42°C.
- Produces a bluish pigment (pyocyanin), a greenish pigment (pyoverdin), and a red pigment (pyorubin).
- Characteristic fruity odor.

Upon infection, the LPS layer helps the cell adhere to host tissues and prevents leukocytes from ingesting and lysing the organism. Lipases and exotoxins destroy host cell tissue, leading to the complications associated with infection. *Ps. aeruginosa* prefers moist environments but can survive in a medium as nutritionally deficient as distilled water. It will also grow on most laboratory media.

Pseudomonas species are often encountered in hospital and clinical settings and are a major cause of nosocomial infections. Immunocompromised patients, burn victims, cystic fibrosis patients, and patients on respirators or with indwelling catheters are most susceptible. Infection can occur at many sites and can lead to urinary tract infection, sepsis, endocarditis, pneumonia, pharyngitis, pyoderma, and dermatitis.

Ocular infectious complications can cause devastating vision loss with potential for infection at any location. Both endogenous and exogenous forms of endophthalmitis and panophthalmitis caused by *Pseudomonas* species have been described. The etiologies range from contact lens keratitis to trauma and surgery to an immunocompromised state. These are discussed in further detail in Chapters 6, 7 and 9. *Ps. aeruginosa* is highly virulent for the eye and endophthalmitis caused by it must be managed aggressively with vitrectomy and intravitreal antibiotics (gentamicin or ceftazidime) or the eye will be lost within 48 hours.

Other *Pseudomonas* species include *Ps. cepacia*, which is an opportunistic pathogen of cystic fibrosis patients. *Stenotrophomonas maltophila* (formerly known as *Xanthomonas maltophila*) is very similar to the pseudomonads. This motile bacterium is a cause of nosocomial infections in immunocompromised patients. *S. maltophila* also harbors significant resistance to many antibiotics considered effective for treating infections caused by *Pseudomonas* organisms. However, most strains of the bacterium are susceptible to trimethoprim or sulfamethoxazole.

Box 3.4 Virulence determinants of *Pseudomonas aeruginosa*

Adhesins
Fimbriae, polysaccharide capsule, alginate slime (biofilm)

Invasins
Elastase, alkaline protease, hemolysins, cytotoxin, siderophores and siderophore uptake systems, pyocyanin diffusible pigment

Motility/chemotaxis
Flagella

Toxins
Exoenzyme S, exotoxin A, lipopolysaccharide (LPS)

Acinetobacter species

Acinetobacter species are oxidase-negative, nonmotile bacteria that appear as Gram-negative pairs under the microscope. Identifying the different species of this genus is possible with the use of fluorescence-lactose-denitrification medium that determines the amount of acid produced from metabolizing glucose. Although many *Acinetobacter* species can cause infection, *A. baumannii* is the most frequently encountered species in the clinical laboratory, causing hospital-acquired infections that include skin and wound infections, pneumonia, and meningitis.

Five cases of endophthalmitis caused by *Acinetobacter* species have been reported in the literature; all were exogenous, resulting from either trauma or surgery.[46–50] Some of the postoperative cases presented in a similar fashion to *Propionibacterium acnes*.[46]

Anaerobes

Anaerobic organisms require an oxygen-free environment to grow; strict anaerobes are completely inhibited from growing in the presence of oxygen. Anaerobes represent 5–10% of all clinical infections. Anaerobic infections usually have the following characteristics:

- Foul-smelling discharge
- Proximity to mucosal membrane
- Necrotic tissue
- Gas formation in tissues or discharge
- Infection following a bite.

The significant anaerobes are listed below.

Actinomyces species are Gram-positive, nonspore-forming anaerobic bacilli. They have been described as bacteria that form filamentous branches. They are difficult to culture and thioglycolate fluid medium should be used. They grow as 'bread crumb' colonies at a depth reflecting their ideal microaerophilic environment. Infection usually occurs through trauma with abscess formation at the implantation site. Six cases of chronic postoperative endophthalmitis have been reported in the literature.[51]

Propionibacterium species are among the most commonly isolated Gram-positive anaerobes. They are found as saprophytes in humans, animals, and dairy products. *P. acnes,* among the most commonly isolated nonspore-forming

anaerobic clinical specimens, is found as normal flora on the skin, nasal pharynx, oral cavity, and gastrointestinal and genitourinary tracts. Systemically, *P. acnes* has been associated with acne vulgaris, endocarditis, wound infections, central nervous system shunt infections, and abscesses. Chronic postoperative endophthalmitis, of a granular type involving the capsular bag, is the main ocular complication (Chapter 6). Rarely, optic disk edema with visual defect has been proposed as a possible presenting event.[52] Microscopically, *Propionibacterium* organisms clump and show a tendency to branch. Colonies grow best in an anaerobic or microaerophilic environment using blood agar.

Culturing media

There are two types of culturing medium: selective and differential. A selective medium promotes the growth of desired organisms while inhibiting the undesirable organisms. A differential medium provides a visible indication of a physiologic property, such as the fermentation of a carbohydrate. Routine culture media can be stored in a refrigerator although only fresh plates of media should be used. Media that appears dry in a Petri dish with recessed edges should not be used. Inoculation should be done at room temperature. For most organisms encountered in ophthalmology, blood and chocolate agars (for bacteria), Sabourauds agar (for fungi), and thioglycolate and brain heart infusion broth media (for bacteria and fungi) should be sufficient. Other cultures can be helpful, such as for mycobacteria, depending on specific need and availability.

Blood agar plate

Blood agar consists of a *Brucella* agar base with a peptic digest of animal tissue, dextrose, and yeast extract. It is an enriched, nonselective, general purpose medium able to grow most aerobes (except *Neisseria, Haemophilus*, and *Moraxella* species), anaerobes (with vitamin K, cysteine, and hemin supplementation), and fungi. Using this differentiating medium, the degree of hemolysis caused by hemolysins is assessed to differentiate among Gram-positive cocci.

- Beta-hemolysins completely lyse the red blood cells and hemoglobin, resulting in complete clearing around colonies.
- Alpha-hemolysis refers to the partial lysis of red blood cells and hemoglobin and produces a greenish discoloration of the blood agar around the colonies.
- No hemolysis, sometimes called gamma-hemolysis, results in no change of the medium.
- Hemolysis must be determined before 2 days of incubation as later reactions are nonspecific.

Thioglycolate medium

Thioglycolate medium is a semisolid, nutrient medium that supports the growth of bacteria and fungi of all oxygen requirements: anaerobes, aerobes, and facultative anaerobes. Thioglycolate reaction causes a gradation of oxygen and establishes an anaerobic environment at the bottom of the medium. An oxygen indicator turns the medium pink or blue at the top of the tube. This medium is boiled before use to drive off oxygen, which is less soluble at hot temperatures. The specimen is inoculated after cooling. Obligate aerobes will grow only at the top of the tube of medium, microaerophiles in the middle, while anaerobes grow only at the bottom.

Sabouraud's agar

Sabouraud's agar is a selective medium with low pH which inhibits the growth of most bacteria, making it selective for yeasts and most but not all fungi. It is a rich medium, good for yeasts, but vegetative plant fungi may not grow, preferring a low nutritious medium such as corn meal agar.

Chocolate agar

Chocolate agar comprises heated sheep blood which provides factors X (hemin) and V (nicotinamide adenine dinucleotide) necessary for growth of *Haemophilus* species, *N. gonorrhoeae*, *N. meningitidis*, and *Moraxella* organisms. However, the Thayer–Martin medium containing antimicrobial agents (vancomycin 3.0 mg, colistin 7.5 mg, and nystatin 12.5 units/ml of agar) is used to supplement the chocolate agar when *N. gonorrhoeae* is suspected. These incorporated antimicrobial agents will suppress the growth of other organisms that inhibit the growth of *N. gonorrhoeae*. Thayer–Martin plates are incubated in an atmosphere containing 3–10% CO_2.

MacConkey agar

MacConkey agar, mainly used to differentiate between various Gram-negative rod-shaped organisms, is also used to inhibit growth of Gram-positive organisms; thus it is both differential and selective. Many facultative anaerobes in the intestine are lactose fermenters (*E. coli*). Several well-known pathogens are unable to ferment lactose (*Shigella* and *Salmonella* species). Bacterial colonies that can ferment lactose turn the medium red as a result of the response of the pH indicators to the acidic environment created by the fermentation. Organisms that do not ferment lactose do not cause a color change.

Eosin-methylene blue agar

Eosin-methylene blue (EMB) agar, a differential medium that inhibits the growth of Gram-positive organisms, is used to identify Gram-negative enteric rods. Gram-positive bacteria are inhibited by the dyes eosin and methylene blue which are added to the agar. The medium also allows distinction between lactose-fermenting and nonlactose-fermenting organisms. Two types of coliform colonies are noted:

- Coli-type: very dark colonies but with a green hue in reflected light caused by the precipitation of methylene blue in the medium from the very high amount of acid produced from fermentation. Colonies are composed of methyl red-positive lactose-fermenters such as most strains of *E. coli* and some *Citrobacter* strains.
- Aerogenes-type: less dark colonies with a dark center surrounded by a wide, light-colored, mucoid rim, resulting in a 'fish-eye' appearance. Those organisms which form this type of colony are methyl red-negative lactose-fermenters, including most strains of *Klebsiella* and *Enterobacter* species.

Mannitol salts agar

Mannitol salts agar (MSA) is a common medium used for the isolation of *S. aureus*. This medium contains 7.5% salt, which is inhibitory to most bacteria other than staphylococci. While most *Staphylococcus* species are capable of growing in this high salt concentration, *S. aureus* is also capable of fermenting the carbohydrate mannitol with production of an acid that turns the pH indicator from red to yellow. Nonpathogenic staphylococci can grow on the medium but produce no acid from it.

Bile-esculin agar

Bile-esculin agar is used to identify group D streptococci which are able to grow in the presence of bile, an emulsifying agent produced in the liver. Group D streptococci also have the ability to hydrolyze esculin, which turns the medium black and denotes a positive test. Other bacteria capable of growing in the presence of bile do not turn the medium black. A variation of this medium uses sodium azide to inhibit the growth of all other Gram-positive and Gram-negative bacteria.

Brain-heart infusion broth

This broth is a highly nutritious, buffered liquid used as an adjunct to the solid media. Because the medium is a liquid, material picked up by a swab but not released onto the solid agar thus has an opportunity to grow. Any antibiotics or other inhibitors of bacterial growth will be diluted and have less effect. Inoculation of broth also allows the use of antimicrobial removal devices. However, a fluid medium does not permit confirmation that growth is occurring along an inoculum streak or allow quantification of the amount of growth. This culture medium is useful for enhancing the growth of small numbers of bacteria or fungi.

Löwenstein–Jensen medium

Löwenstein–Jensen medium, commonly used to identify *Mycobacterium* species, is used on initial culture as it will support growth of a very small inoculum. This is an egg-potato-based medium and contains the dye malachite green to inhibit

slow-growing contaminants. The fluid Kirschner medium may also be used for mycobacteria.

Incubation

Agar plates should be incubated for a minimum of 48 hours at 37°C for bacteria and for 4 weeks at 32°C for fungi. Cultures for bacteria should be plated out on two agar plates for both aerobic and anaerobic conditions. If a microaerophilic bacterium is suspected, that growth condition should also be included. Both bacteria and fungi grow better in an atmosphere of 5% carbon dioxide than in air alone. Anaerobic plates should be incubated in an anaerobic cabinet for 7 days or for 14 days if *P. acnes* is suspected. Fluid enrichment media such as BHI or thioglycolate should be incubated for 14 days at 37°C and then subcultured.

Plating and staining

The streak plate technique is the most widely used method of obtaining isolated colonies from a clinical sample or a mix of cultures. This technique dilutes the number of organisms by decreasing the density, allowing individual colonies to be isolated from other colonies. Each colony is considered 'pure,' because theoretically it began with an individual cell.

- Inoculation is begun in the first, or primary, quadrant of the agar plate. A light touch is necessary to avoid penetrating or scraping the agar surface. The plate is covered with a lid.
- The loop is flamed and then allowed to cool.
- An inoculum from quadrant one is chosen and is streaked onto quadrant two.
- The loop is again flamed and allowed to cool. The procedure is repeated for quadrants three and four.

Gram-staining procedure

Before a Gram stain procedure is begun, the specimen must be properly spread onto the glass slide. A smear can be prepared from a clinical sample, such as aqueous humor or vitreous, or a solid agar or broth laboratory medium. The

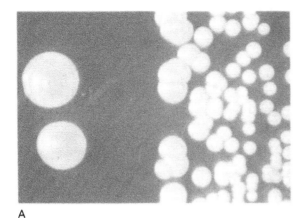

A

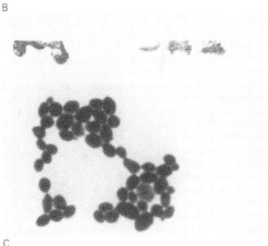

B

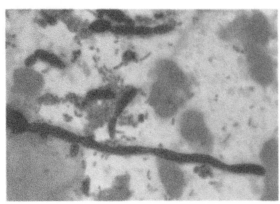

C

Figure 3.6

(A) White colonies of *Candida albicans* on agar. (B) Pseudomycelium of *Candida albicans* (Gram stain). (C) Typical budding yeast cells of *Candida albicans* (Gram stain).

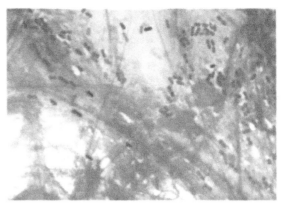

Figure 3.7

Gram-negative rod: *Moraxella* sp.

specimen should be fixed to the slide before starting the procedure. For specimens other than vitreous, the smear can be fixed with heat in a flame. Vitreous specimens must NOT be heat-fixed but allowed to slowly dry in air, which can require up to 45 minutes.

The required reagents are:

- Crystal violet (the primary stain)
- Iodine solution (the mordant)
- Decolorizer (ethanol is a good choice)
- Safranin (the counterstain)
- Water (preferably in a squirt bottle).

STEP 1: The entire slide is flooded with crystal violet. The stain is left on the slide for 60 seconds and then gently washed with water for 5 seconds, taking care not to wash away the specimen, which now appears blue-violet.

STEP 2: The slide is flooded with iodine solution that is allowed to remain for 60 seconds before gentle rinsing with water for 5 seconds. The specimen should still be blue-violet. Step 3 follows immediately.

STEP 3: A decolorizer, ethanol, is added. However, excess application of ethanol will lead to a false Gram-negative result and an insufficient amount will lead to a false Gram-positive result. The ethanol is added drop-wise until the blue-violet color is no longer emitted from the specimen. This takes no longer than 5 seconds. A 5-second gentle rinse with water follows.

STEP 4: The counterstain, safranin, is added. The slide is flooded with safranin which is allowed to remain for 60 seconds to permit the

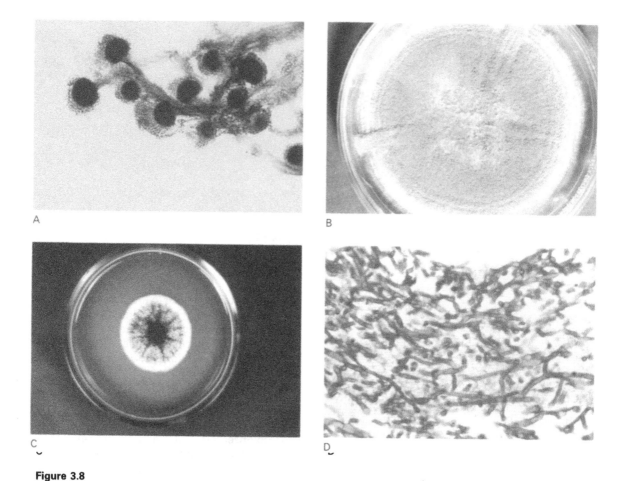

Figure 3.8

(A) *Aspergillus* conidiophore seen in cultures. (B) Aspergillus flavus *(yellow pigment)*. (C) *Aspergillus niger* (black pigment). (D) PAS (periodic acid Schiff) stain of branching mycelium of *Aspergillus* species.

bacteria to incorporate the safranin. Gram-positive cells will incorporate little or no counter-stain and will remain blue-violet in appearance. Gram-negative bacteria, however, will take on a pink color (see Figure 3.7) and are easily distinguishable from the Gram-positive cells. Excess dye is removed with a 5–second water rinse.

The slide is blotted gently or allowed to air dry before viewing under the microscope at ×1,000 with an oil immersion lens.

Mycology

The major causes of intraocular mycoses are species of *Candida*, especially *Candida albicans* (Figure 3.6)*;* *Aspergillus* (Figure 3.8), especially

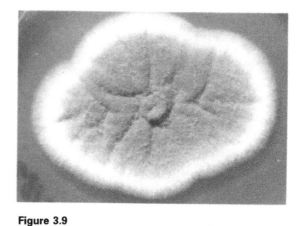

Figure 3.9

Aspergillus fumigatus (green pigment).

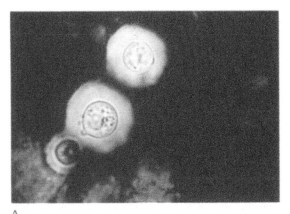

A

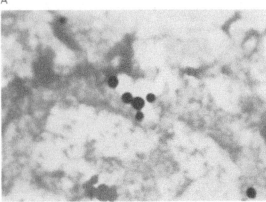

B

Figure 3.10

(A) *Cryptococcus neoformans* and its capsule (wet preparation with indian ink). (B) Budding yeast cells of *Cryptococcus neoformans* (Gram stain).

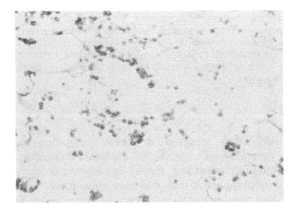

Figure 3.11

Histoplasma capsulatum in tissue.

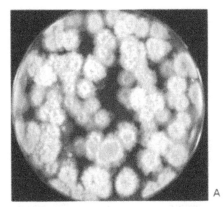

A

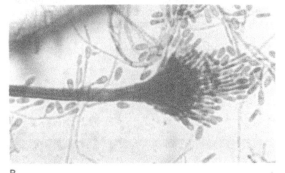

B

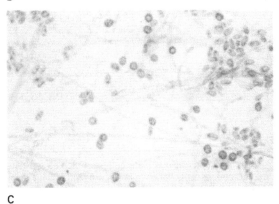

C

Figure 3.12

(A) *Scedosporium apiospermum* plate culture. Colonies are high, flat to dome-shaped and floccose in texture, initially white and later pale smoky-brown in color, and grow rapidly (40 mm/7 days). (B) Microscopy of *Scedosporium apiospermum* (teleomorph *Pseudoallescheria boydii*). Conidia are abundant, yellow to pale-brown in color, oval in shape (6–12 × 3.5–6 μm) with a scar at the base, and are formed from single or branched, long, slender annellides that are sometimes aggregated into bundles of tree-like synnemata (Graphium state). (C) In slide preparations the annellidic tip usually has only a single conidium remaining.

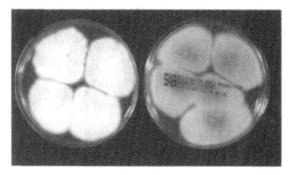

Figure 3.13

Fusarium solani plate culture. Colonies are flat, grayish-white, cream, buff or pinkish-purple in color (reverse is pale cream), floccose in texture, and attain a diameter of 30 mm in 1 week.

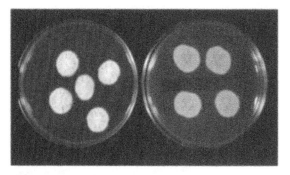

Figure 3.14

Acremonium strictum plate culture. Colonies are flat, smooth, wet or velvety to floccose in texture, rapidly growing (50 mm/7 days), pink to orange in color, with the reverse remaining colorless or turning pink to orange.

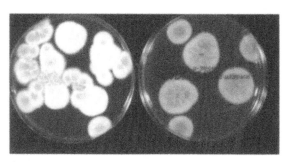

A

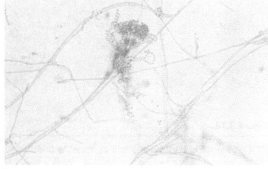

B

Figure 3.15

(A) *Paecilomyces lilacinus* plate culture. Colonies are flat to domed, vinaceous to violet-white in color (reverse is pale or deep purple), densely floccose in texture, and attain a diameter of 30 mm in 1 week. (B) *Paecilomyces lilacinus* microscopy. Conidia (2.5–3 × 2–2.2 µm) are ellipsoidal to fusiform in shape, smooth-walled to slightly roughened in texture, hyaline in color (purple in a mass), arranged in divergent chains; they are borne on irregularly branched heads terminating in long phialides which consist of a swollen basal part, tapering into a thin neck.

Aspergillus fumigatus (Figure 3.9); *Blastomyces dermatitidis*; *Coccidioides immitis*; *Cryptococcus neoformans* (Figure 3.10); *Histoplasma capsulatum* (Figure 3.11); *Scedosporium apiospermum* (*Pseudallescheria boydii*) (Figure 3.12); and *Sporothrix schenckii*.[53] Species of *Fusarium*[54,55] (Figure 3.13), *Acremonium* (Figure 3.14),[56] *Paecilomyces* (Figure 3.15),[57–59] and *Zygomycetes*[60] have also been reported to cause such lesions; *Pneumocystis carinii*[61,62] causes choroiditis. Although most of these organisms produce endophthalmitis, they may also cause focal (localized) chorioretinitis or a granulomatous lesion in the iris or ciliary body.[63]

In the 1970s and 1980s, the incidence of endogenous fungal endophthalmitis in patients with

Table 3.3 Direct microscopic techniques in endophthalmitis

Method and specimens	Features
Potassium hydroxide (KOH) wet mounts 1) KOH only 2) Ink–KOH 3) KOH-dimethyl sulfoxide digestion and counterstaining by periodic acid–Schiff or acridine orange. Used for corneal scrapes, aqueous and vitreous aspirates	Rapid (1–2 steps), inexpensive, easy to perform. KOH ensures good digestion of thick samples. Use of ink, periodic acid–Schiff, or acridine orange as counterstain facilitates detection of fungal structures. *Reported drawbacks:* artifacts common; optimal viewing time for ink–KOH mounts is 12–18 hours; ink–KOH has a short shelf-life (ink precipitates out); fluorescence microscope fitted with appropriate filters needed if acridine orange counterstain is used. If no dye/ink is added, there is no contrast to facilitate detection of usually colorless fungus against a colorless background.
Gram staining Sensitivity: 85%. Used for corneal scrapes, aqueous and vitreous aspirates	Stains yeast cells and fungal hyphae equally well, and bacteria in the preparation can be differentiated. Takes only 5 min to perform. *Reported drawbacks:* fungal hyphae may stain irregularly or not at all; less useful in thick preparations; false-positive artifacts common; crystal violet precipitates may cause confusion.
Giemsa staining Sensitivity: 66–85% in culture-proven mycotic keratitis Used for corneal scrapes, aqueous and vitreous aspirates	Stains yeast cells and fungal hyphae. *Pneumocystis carinii* can be seen. *Reported drawbacks:* staining time of 60 min; staining of nuclei and cytoplasmic granules of tissue cells may cause opacities in smear; false-positive artifacts may occur.
Lactophenol cotton blue (LPCB) staining Sensitivity 75% Used for corneal scrapes, aqueous and vitreous aspirates.	Rapid, simple, inexpensive one-step method which detects all common ocular fungi. Stain commercially available with long shelf-life. *Reported drawbacks:* no tissue digestion, hence thick preparations may pose problems; contrast between fungi and background may be insufficient; unusual fungi may escape detection.
Modified methenamine silver staining Sensitivity: 85%. Used for corneal scrapes, necrotic material, tissue sections	Fungal cell walls and septa clearly delineated against pale green background; *Pneumocystis carinii* can also be detected. *Reported drawbacks:* false positives due to staining of cellular debris and melanin; multi-step procedure requires 60 min; reagents and procedures need standardization.
Calcofluor white Sensitivity: 80–90% Used for corneal scrapes, aqueous and vitreous aspirates	Fungal hyphae and yeast cells clearly delineated against dark background; clearly seen even in thick preparations. *Pneumocystis carinii* also seen. Rapid two-step method. *Reported drawbacks:* fresh reagents needed, otherwise false-positive artifacts occur; fluorescence microscope fitted with appropriate filters needed; reagents and procedures need standardization; viewer should be protected against hazards of ultraviolet light.
Hematoxylin-eosin (H&E) stain Used to detect hyaline and dematiaceous fungi in necrotic material and tissue sections	Host reaction, nuclei of yeast-like cells (especially *Blastomyces dermatitidis*) and hyphae of hematoxylinophilic fungi (aspergilli, zygomycetes) can be visualized. The melanin (brown pigment) of dematiaceous fungi and agents of chromoblastomycosis can be detected. *Drawbacks:* may not be possible to distinguish poorly stained fungi from tissue components; preparation of stained sections requires time and standardization.

candidemia or candidiasis, or both, was reported to range from approximately 10% to 40%. A study in the late 1980s reported that ocular lesions developed within 72 hours of the suspected onset of fungemia in approximately 90% of nontreated, hospitalized patients with candidemia.[64] However, a more recent study estimated the incidence of chorioretinal findings consistent with early endogenous fungal endophthalmitis to be 2.8%.[65] This low incidence was attributed to the fact that 90% of the patients were being treated with systemic antifungal medication (mostly amphotericin B and/or oral fluconazole) at the time of the ophthalmologic consultation. *Candida* endophthalmitis now also appears to be rare in patients with candidemia, with none of 118 adults with candidemia showing evidence of endophthalmitis, only 9.3% exhibiting chorioretinitis, and 20.3% nonspecific fundus lesions.[66] In a study of 30 hospitalized children with suspected or known systemic infections caused by *Candida* species, all of whom had risk factors for disseminated candidiasis (broad-spectrum intravenous antibiotics, chronic debilitation with indwelling catheterization, total parenteral nutrition, immunocompromised state), none were found to have either endophthalmitis or chorioretinitis.[67] The low rate of ocular involvement in both series, compared with earlier reports, was believed to be the result of either earlier treatment with antifungal agents or to the lack of rigorous criteria for endophthalmitis in previous studies.

Direct microscopic techniques to be followed with fresh samples from the aqueous humor or vitreous are listed in Table 3.3.[68] Unfortunately, there are no data pertaining to the sensitivity and specificity of these direct microscopic techniques as aids to the diagnosis of fungal endophthalmitis, unlike the situation in mycotic keratitis. The diagnostic yield from samples of the vitreous is reported to be more than that with samples from the aqueous. Features of the types of fungi causing endophthalmitis are given in Tables 3.4 to 3.8.[68]

Samples for fungus isolation should generally be plated out onto Sabouraud's medium or brain-heart infusion agar. Thioglycolate or brain-heart infusion fluid medium should also be inoculated. Corn meal agar is not generally recommended as a primary isolation medium for filamentous fungi but is used to induce sporulation of a filamentous fungus to facilitate identification, once the fungus has been isolated in the primary isolation medium. Samples should be incubated at 32°C for 4 weeks in 5% CO_2. The plates should be sealed in a plastic box for the agar to remain moist.

Contents of media

Sabouraud's agar (Emmons' modification)

Dextrose 20 g; mycological peptone 10 g; agar 20 g; deionized water 1 liter; final pH 6.8–7.0; chloramphenicol added to a final concentration of 40 mg/l or gentamicin added to a final concentration of 50 mg/l to prevent possible bacterial contamination.

Corn meal agar

Infusion from corn meal (ground yellow corn) 50 g; agar 15 g; deionized water 1 liter; final pH 6.0.

Table 3.4 Yeasts implicated in endophthalmitis

Genus and species	Microscopic morphology in ocular samples	Ophthalmic infections in which implicated
Candida C. albicans, C. parapsilosis, C. guilliermondii	Presence of small 3–4-µm budding yeast cells and pseudohyphae in samples almost diagnostic for *Candida* spp. The bud exhibits an off-axis position and a narrow base at the point of attachment; the yeast cell appears asymmetrical.	Keratitis, endophthalmitis and chorioretinitis. Criteria for diagnosis: growth on multiple media; growth on single medium with positive microscopy.
Cryptococcus C. neoformans var. neoformans, C. laurentii	Typically 2–20 µm in diameter. Presence of tear drop-shaped, narrow-based budding of *C. neoformans* var. *neoformans* is a useful cytologic feature. View characteristic capsule with indian ink.	C. neoformans var. neoformans causes keratitis, chorioretinitis, endophthalmitis, and solitary subretinal lesions. C. laurentii implicated in contact lens-associated keratitis and endophthalmitis.

Table 3.5 Thermally dimorphic fungi (yeast phase in tissue at 37°C, hyphae in culture at 22°C) implicated in endophthalmitis

Fungus and morphology in ocular samples	Ophthalmic lesions in which implicated
Paracoccidioides brasiliensis Spherical, yeast-like cells with multiple buds attached by narrow necks, also called 'steering wheel forms', seen in potassium hydroxide (KOH) mounts of material or in tissue sections	Rarely occurs in absence of lesions elsewhere in body, unless entry is through wound; usually unilateral. Anterior and granulomatous uveitis. Diagnosis by histopathologic examination or direct microscopy of lesions.
Coccidioides immitis Large, multinucleate, thick-walled cells (spherules) filled at maturity with spores; these escape by rupture of cell wall. Spherules usually found within giant cells. Spherules seen on microscopic examination of KOH mounts of pus or necrotic material, or by histopathologic examination of infected ocular tissues.	Anterior segment lesions (phlyctenular conjunctivitis, episcleritis, scleritis, and keratoconjunctivitis) reported in conjunction with underlying pulmonary infection; lid granulomata and inflammation reported in disseminated disease. Diagnostic criteria used unclear. Granulomatous uveitis and iris nodules noted in patients without systemic disease and one patient with previously treated pulmonary disease. Diagnosis established by presence of spherules in various samples and positive cultures.
Blastomyces dermatitidis Spherical, multinucleate yeast-like cells (8–20 μm) with single broad-based bud and refractile double-contoured walls; generally larger than those of cryptococci. Seen in KOH mounts of necrotic material or in tissue sections, and generally extracellularly.	Lesions of eyelids, cornea, conjunctiva, and orbit; intraocular lesions, and endophthalmitis reported. *B. dermatitidis* cultured from orbital lesions and endophthalmitis. Positive immunofluorescence test. Detection of characteristic forms in tissues.
Sporothrix schenckii Small, spherical, oval or elongated 'cigar-shaped' budding yeast cells with irregularly stained cytoplasm, mostly located extracellularly. 'Asteroid bodies', which are central spherical or oval basophilic cells 3–5 μm in diameter surrounded by thick, radiate eosinophilia substance, rarely occur.	Endophthalmitis, scleritis, uveitis, and orbital lesions. In most reports, diagnosis by detection of characteristic forms in affected tissues or by positive culture and histopathology findings.
Histoplasma capsulatum; H. capsulatum var. capsulatum; H. capsulatum var. **duboisii** Organisms may be missed in wet mounts, hence stained smears should be examined. *H. capsulatum* var. *capsulatum*: thin-walled oval yeasts, free or phagocytosed within cells; may be associated infiltrate of lymphocytes and histiocytes. *H. capsulatum* var. *duboisii*: yeast cells larger than those of *H. capsulatum* var. *capsulatum*; cell wall thicker, isthmus and bud scar more prominent.	Endogenous and exogenous endophthalmitis, choroiditis, retinitis, and optic neuritis in patients with AIDS; anterior segment lesions rare.

Thioglycolate broth

Yeast extract 5 g; casitone 15 g; sodium chloride 2.5 g; l-cystine 0.25 g; thioglycolic acid 0.3 ml; agar 0.75 g; methylene blue 0.002 g; deionized water 1 liter; final pH 7.2.

Brain-heart infusion

Infusion from calf brains 200 g; infusion from beef heart 200 g; proteose peptone 10 g; dextrose 2 g; sodium chloride 5 g; disodium phosphate 2.5 g.

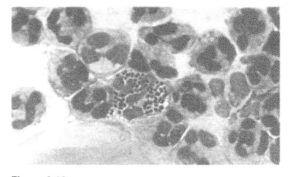

Figure 3.16

Gram stain of *Neisseria meningitidis* in PMNs.

Table 3.6 Hyaline filamentous fungi implicated in endophthalmitis

Genus and species	Microscopic morphology in ocular samples
1. Fusarium F. solani, F. dimerum, F. oxysporum	Septate, hyaline, branching hyphae, 2–4 μm wide, similar to other hyaline filamentous fungi. Adventitious sporulation may be seen; the conidia are larger than those of Paecilomyces spp.
2. Aspergillus A. fumigatus, A. flavus, A. terreus	Septate, hyaline branching hyphae, 3–6 μm wide, which exhibit parallel walls and radiate from a single point in tissues; smaller than hyphae of zygomycetes. Dichotomous (45°) branching may occur; this may not be pathognomonic in ocular infections.
3. Scedosporium S. apiospermum (asexual stage) (teleomorph Pseudallescheria boydii – sexual stage); S. prolificans	Septate, hyaline, branching hyphae, 2–4 μm wide, similar to other hyaline filamentous fungi. Abundant oval conidia formed from single or branched annellides. Conidiophore has long, slender annellides that can be bundled into tree-like synnemata (Graphium state). Conidia are yellow/brown, oval 6–12 × 4–6 μm. Ascocarps sometimes present with black, round and lemon-shaped ascospores. S. prolificans: speciation of isolates reported to be S. prolificans requires confirmation by DNA sequencing.
4. Paecilomyces P. lilacinus, P. variotii	Septate, hyaline, branching hyphae, 2–4 μm wide, similar to other hyaline filamentous fungi. Abundant adventitious sporulation frequently occurs. Adventitious conidia subglobose to very short ellipsoidal.
5. Acremonium A. kiliense, A. potronii	Septate, hyaline, branching hyphae, 2–4 μm wide; adventitious sporulation may occur.
6. Alternaria A. infectosa, A. alternata	Septate, hyaline, branching hyphae, 2–4 μm wide. It is not easy to distinguish between the two species of Alternaria; each is identified based on the characteristics of the conidias; the length of the beak is always one-third larger than the length of the conidium.

Table 3.7 Dematiaceous fungi frequently implicated in endophthalmitis

Fungal genera and species	Morphology	Criteria for diagnosis
Bipolaris (B. spicifera, B. hawaiiensis, B. australiensis)	In tissue: Brown-pigmented , septate, hyphae. In culture: sympodial conidiophore with profuse sporulation. Conidia are oblong, ellipsoidal to fusoid (16-34 x 4–9 μm) with 3–7 pseudosepta	Positive microscopy, culture & PCR
Curvularia (C. lunata, C. geniculata, C. senegalensis)	Erect unbranched conidiophore. Conidia are smooth walled (18–37 x 14–18 μm), olive to brown with 3–4 septa and ovoid or curved.	
Exophiala (E. jeanselmei var. jeanselmei, E. dermatitidis)	Brown cylindrical conidiophore with a narrow apex, that is apical or on the side of hyphae. Conidia single celled, colourless to brown (2–6 x 1–3 μm) and may cluster.	
Exserohilum (E. rostratum, E. longirostratum)	Profuse sporulation. Conidia ellipsoid (30–128 x 9–23 μm), hilum truncate with 7–9 pseudosepta.	
Lecytophora (L. mutabilis, L. hoffmannii)	Condigenous cells that emerge from hyphae. Conidia (5 x 2μm) smooth, thin wall, cylindrical	
Phialophora verrucosa	Conidiophore brown, cylindrical with distinct flared funnel or cup-shaped collarette. Conidia 3–6 x 1–3 μm, pale brown, oval, clusters	
Lasiodiplodia theobromae	Septate, highly bulged, brown-colored hyphae. In culture: Conidia (20–30 μm x 10–15 μm) initially colorless, ellipsoidal, non-septate; later dark-brown and septate, with longitudinal striations and truncate bases.	In culture: rapid growth (90 mm in one week), floccose, grey to brown-black in color; produces macroscopic fruiting bodies (pycnidia).

Table 3.8 Zygomycetes implicated in ophthalmic infections

Genus and species	Microscopic morphology in ocular samples	Ophthalmic infections in which implicated
1. *Rhizopus*: R. arrhizus 2. *Mucor* 3. *Rhizomucor* 4. *Absidia* 5. *Apophysomyces* 6. *Saksenaea* 7. *Cunninghamella* 8. *Syncephalastrum*	Broad, aseptate or sparsely septate hyphae with right-angled 90° branching; these neither possess parallel walls nor radiate from a single point in tissues. Hyphae stain poorly with periodic acid–Schiff, but stain well with hematoxylin-eosin and Gomori methenamine silver stains. Cresyl-fast violet stains zygomycete walls brick red, other fungi blue or purple. Seen in midst of prominent inflammation, necrosis, and invasion of blood vessels	Rhino-orbito-cerebral zygomycosis. Criteria for diagnosis: suggestive clinical features, detection of the characteristic large, broad aseptate hyphae in necrotic material or tissue. Identification of the fungus in culture. *Rhizopus* spp. have been reported as a cause of scleritis but the evidence is not convincing.

MOLECULAR DIAGNOSIS OF ENDOPHTHALMITIS*

Clinical diagnosis of endophthalmitis can be confirmed by numerous techniques based on the microbiologic analysis of ocular samples (aqueous and vitreous). Diagnostic techniques include standard microbiologic tests (culture and stains, as shown in Figure 3.16) and culture-independent diagnostic tests such as those based on methods of molecular biology. The capacity for detection and identification of genomic material in any type of sample was an enormous step in the field of medicine, allowing diagnosis of many genetic or infectious diseases based on the DNA sequence. These molecular techniques have their advantages and disadvantages, offering speed and sensitivity in the detection and identification of pathogens; however, at present they are still not standardized and their cost is high.

The two main determining factors in the microbiologic diagnosis of ocular infections are the scarce quantity of the samples obtained and the possibility that the infecting organism may cause the loss of the eye or vision after a short period, necessitating speedy diagnosis. Molecular biology can resolve these problems because with a minimal quantity of specimen (microliter), it is possible to determine whether the origin of the infection is bacterial or fungal within a few hours. The species can be identified in a matter of hours.

*This section has been contributed by Drs Consuelo Ferrer and Jorge Alio.

Polymerase chain reaction

The polymerase chain reaction (PCR) has surpassed other diagnostic techniques based on the study of nucleic acids, such as Southern blot, because of its simplicity, sensitivity, speed, and specificity. PCR allows amplification of the region of the genome selected for analysis in a minimal

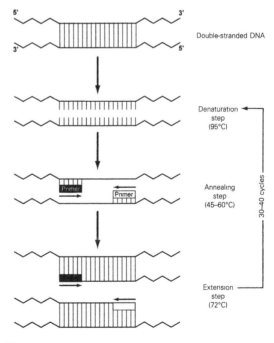

Figure 3.17

Schematic of polymerase chain reaction (PCR).

period of time – approximately 90 minutes. PCR is based on the ability of DNA polymerase to copy a strand of DNA.[69–71] The enzyme initiates elongation at the 3′ end of a short (primer) sequence joined to a longer strand of DNA, known as the target sequence. When two primers bind to a complementary strand of target DNA, the sequence between the two primers' binding sites is amplified exponentially with each cycle of PCR. There are three steps to each cycle: a DNA heat denaturation step (separation of the double strands of the target DNA by heat); a primer-annealing step (primers anneal to their complementary amplification target sequences at a lower temperature); and an extension reaction step (extension of the target sequences between the primers by DNA polymerase). At the end of each cycle, the PCR products are theoretically doubled (Figure 3.17). A thermocycler is used for the procedure. Generally, 30–40 thermal cycles result in detectable amounts of a target sequence originally present in less than 100 copies, and the PCR is theoretically capable of detecting a single copy of DNA.[72,73]

The primers constitute the factor that determines what genome and which part to amplify. These are short sequences of DNA that can vary in size (usually between 10 and 25 nucleotides); the sequences will hybridize specifically with their complementary sequence, permitting elongation of the chain with polymerase. For example, to determine whether there is *P. acnes* in a vitreous sample, a fragment of the *P. acnes* genome (DNA target) flanked by short specific sequences is selected. The primers are bound to these two zones and the amplification of the flanked region is produced. If in the last cycle a product the size of the selected fragment is obtained, it can be determined whether the sample contains *P. acnes* DNA.

Depending on the genome region being amplified, there are DNA ribosomal targets and the nonribosomal targets. Among the nonribosomal targets can be found those that amplify DNA regions codifying certain enzymes (e.g. *Candida* actin gene[74] and cytochrome P450[75]), those that amplify mitochondrial telomere,[76] and methods using arbitrarily primed PCR (AP-PCR).[77]

However, the area of the genome most commonly used as a target to amplify and detect bacterial or fungal DNA is the region within the ribosomal DNA (rDNA) complex. This region is used most frequently because the ribosomal RNA genes have a relatively conserved nucleotide

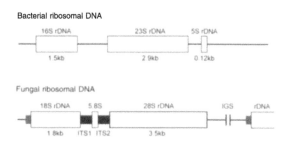

Figure 3.18

Schematic representation of bacterial and fungal ribosomal DNA.

sequence; the genes are present in a high number of copies, achieving the sensitivity of the detection method. The number of copies of 16S rDNA in bacterial pathogens varies between 1 and 10, with *S. epidermidis* having 5, *S. aureus* having 5–6, and *Strep. pneumoniae* 4.[78] In yeast cells, rDNA repeated in tandem number approximately 150.[79]

This bacterial rDNA complex is organized as shown in Figure 3.18: the small subunit 16S rDNA, the longer subunit 23S rDNA, and 5S rDNA. Among the three rRNA molecules (16S, 23S, and 5S rRNA), the 16S rRNA gene has been used most often for bacterial characterization.[80] This sequence contains alternating regions of sequence conservation and heterogeneity.[81] The conserved regions can be used to create PCR amplification primers that anneal to ribosomal targets from all or most bacterial species. The 16S and 23S rRNA molecules consist of variable sequence motifs that reflect their phylogenetic origins. This sequence variability permits the design of probes at different taxonomic levels.

The organization of the fungal rDNA complex includes a sequence coding for the 18S rDNA, an internal transcribed spacer region 1 (ITS1), the 5.8S rDNA coding region, another ITS (ITS2), and the sequence coding for the 28S rDNA (see Figure 3.16). The coding regions of 18S, 5.8S, and 28S nuclear rRNA genes evolved slowly, and are relatively conserved among fungi, providing a molecular basis of establishing phylogenetic relationships.[82] Between these rDNA gene-coding regions are the ITS regions (ITS1 and ITS2), which evolved more rapidly, leading to sequence variability among genera and species of fungi. Early studies in molecular testing used the rDNA

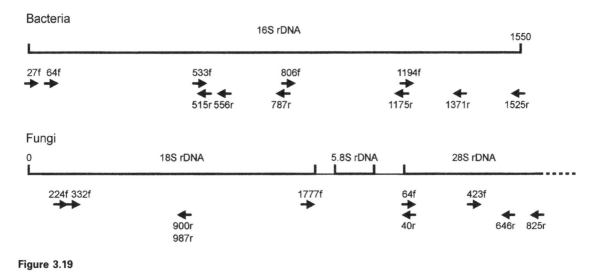

Figure 3.19

Location of broad-range primers used in bacterial endophthalmitis in the 16S rDNA of *E. coli* (see Table 3.9) and broad-range primers used in fungal endophthalmitis in the rDNA complex of *C. albicans* (see Table 3.10).

complex as a target, concentrating on the region of the 18S rDNA. The comparison of nucleotide sequences within this gene region has been successful for the separation of fungal genera and species. However, limited sequence variability within these rDNA, together with a need to compare large sequence regions, has led to a shift to the evaluation of the region between 18S rDNA and 28S rDNA as a target of molecular diagnostic testing. This region includes the shorter spacer regions (ITS1 and ITS2) and the 5.8S rDNA.

Conventional PCR with specific primers and other versions of the PCR are used in the diagnosis of ocular infection. The most frequently used forms of PCR in molecular endophthalmitis diagnosis are described below.

infection. Broad-range rDNA PCR techniques allow rapid and highly specific bacterial identification with a single pair of primers targeting the bacterial small-subunit (16S) rRNA gene. Pan-fungal primers have been designed which may permit the detection and identification of endophthalmitis caused by fungi.

Table 3.9[82–98] shows the primers that have been used thus far for the detection of pathogens in bacterial endophthalmitis by broad-range PCR, their sequences, and genome regions of *E. coli* which they hybridize. Table 3.10[94,95,98,99–105] shows the pan-fungal primers used in fungal endophthalmitis, their sequences, and the regions of *C. albicans* with which they hybridize. Figure 3.19 shows the position of the bacterial and fungal broad-range primers in the ribosomal DNA region.

Broad-range PCR

This method is used most frequently for the diagnosis of endophthalmitis because the species of microorganisms causing the infectious process is unknown, and carrying out a specific PCR for every microorganism that could produce infection would be a long, costly process. This application uses conserved sequences within phylogenetically informative genetic targets to diagnose

Nested PCR

Designed mainly to increase sensitivity, nested PCR uses two sets of amplification primers.[106] One set is used for the first round of amplification, consisting of 25–30 cycles. Products of the first reaction are then subjected to a second round of amplification with another set of primers specific for a sequence within the product of the first pairs

Table 3.9 Commonly used primers for broad-range PCR in bacterial endophthalmitis

Authors (reference)	Primers	Sequence (beginnings or ends may have been modified from the indicated references by subsequent authors)	Position on E. coli rDNA	rDNA amplified	Fragment (bp)	Original reference	Name*
Anand et al[82]	RW01	5'-AACTGGAGGAAGGTGGGGAT-3'	1168–1188	16S	370	Chen et al[84]	1194f
	DG74	5'-AGGAGGTGATCCAACCGCA-3'	1520–1539			Edwards et al[85]	1525r
Carroll et al[80]	16SF	5'-TTGGAGAGTTTGATCCTGGCTC-3'	4–25	16S	1190	Edwards et al[85]	27f
	16SR	5'-ACGTCATCCCCACCTTCCTC-3'	1175–1194			Chen et al[84]	1175r
	NF	5'-GGCGGCAKGCCTAAYACATGCAAGT-3'	42–66	16S	1000	Hykin et al[87]	66f
	NR	5'-GACGACAGCCATGCASCACCTGT -3'	1044–1067			Okhravi et al[88]	1044r
Hykin et al[87]	U1	5'-TTGGAGAGTTTGATCCTGGCTC-3'	4–25	16S	800	Edwards et al[85]	27f
	rU4	5'-GGACTACCAGGGTATCTAA-3	789–806			Wilson et al[89]	787r
	U2	5'-GCCGTGCTTAACACATGCAAGTCG-3'	41–64	16S	500	Hykin et al[87]	64f
	rU3	5'-GCGGCTGGCACGTAGTTAG-3'	506–528			Lane et al[90]	515r
Kerkhoff et al[91]	16S8FEVAR1	5'-AGAGTTTGATCMTGGTCCAG-3'	8–25	16S	570	Edwards et al[85]	27f
	16S556RBVAR2	5'-CGCTTTAGCCCCARTNASTCCG-3'	556–578			Bergmans et al[92]	556r
Knox et al[93]	8FLP	5'-AGTTTGATCCTGGCTCAG-3'	8–25	16S	800	Edwards et al[85]	27f
	806R	5'-GGACTACCAGGGTATCTAAT-3'	787–806			Wilson et al[89]	787r
	MF16	5'-TTGAACGCTGGCGGCAGGCCT-3'	16–36	16S	500	Edwards et al[85]	27f
	B515	5'-TGCGTGCGCTTTACGCCCAGT-3'	516–533			Lane et al[90]	515r
	515FPL	5'-GTGCCAGCAGCCGCGGTAA-3'	515–533	16S	870	Lane et al[82]	533f
	13B	5'-AGGCCCGGGAACGTATTCAC-3'	1371–1390			Relman et al[90]	1371r
	MF91	5'-ACTCAAATGAATTGACGGGGGC-3'	911–930	16S	480	Lane et al[82]	926f
	13B	5'-AGGCCCGGGAACGTATTCAC-3'	1371–1390			Chen et al[84]	1371r
Lohmann et al[94]	Bakt F2	5'-CAAACAGAGATTAGATACCC-3'	778–796	16S	600	Chen et al[84]	806f
	Bakt rev3	5'-CCCGGGAACGTATTCACCG-3'	1368–1386			Wilson et al[89]	1371r
Lohmann et al[95]	RW01	5'-AACTGGAGGAAGGTGGGGAT-3'	1168–1188	16S	370	Chen et al[84]	1194f
	DG74	5'-AGGAGGTGATCCAACCGCA-3'	1520–1539			Chen et al[84]	1525r
Okhravi et al[96]	16SF	5'-TTGGAGAGTTTGATCCTGGCTC-3'	4–25	16S	1190	Edwards et al[85]	27f
	16SR	5'-ACGTCATCCCCACCTTCCTC-3'	1175–1194			Chen et al[84]	1175r
Okhravi et al[88]	16SF	5'-TTGGAGAGTTTGATCCTGGCTC-3'	4–25	16S	1190	Edwards et al[85]	27f
	16SR	5'-ACGTCATCCCCACCTTCCTC-3'	1174–1194			Chen et al[84]	1175r
	NF	5'-GGCGGCAKGCCTAAYACATGCAAGT-3'	42–66	16S	1000	Hykin et al[87]	66f
	NR	5'-GACGACAGCCATGCASCACCTGT -3'	1044–1067			Okhravi et al[88]	1044r
Therese et al[97]	U1	5'-TTGGAGAGTTTGATCCTGGCTC-3'	4–25	16S	800	Edwards et al[85]	27f
	rU4	5'-GGACTACCAGGGTATCTAA-3	789–806			Wilson et al[89]	787r
	U2	5'-GGCGTGCTTAACACATGCAAGTCG-3'	41–64	16S	500	Hykin et al[87]	64f
	rU3	5'-GCGGCTGGCACGTAGTTAG-3'	506–528			Lane et al[82]	515r
						Reiman et al[90]	

*Names are based on the 3' nucleotide position and the orientation (f, forward; r, reverse) according to Lane[90]

Table 3.10 Commonly used primers for broad-range PCR in fungal endophthalmitis

Authors (reference)	Primers	Sequence	Position on Candida albicans rDNA	rDNA amplified	Fragment (bp)	Original reference	Name[a]
Anand et al[99]	U1	5'-GTGAAATTGTTGAAAGGGAA-3'	404–423 (28S)	28S	260	Sandhu et al[100]	423f
	U2	5'-GACTCCTTGGTCCGTGTT-3'	646–663 (28S)				646r
Ferrer et al[101]	ITS1	5'-TCCGTAGGTGAACCTGCGG-3'	1759–1777 (18S)	ITSs-5.8S	550	White et al[102]	1777f
	ITS4	5'-TCCTCCGCTTATTGATATGC-3'	40–59 (28S)				40r
Ferrer et al[103]	ITS1	5'-TCCGTAGGTGAACCTGCGG-3'	1759–1777 (18S)	ITSs-5.8S	550	White et al[102]	1777f
	ITS4	5'-TCCTCCGCTTATTGATATGC-3'	40–59 (28S)				40r
Jaeger et al[104]	Pffor	5'-AGGGATGTATTTATTAGATAAAAAATCAA-3'	196–224 (18S)	18S	740	Jaeger et al[104]	224f
	Pfrev2	5'-CGCAGTAGTTAGTCTTCAGTAAATC-3'	900–924 (18S)				900r
Lohmann et al[94]	B2 F	5'-ACTTTCGATGGTAGGATAG-3'	314–332 (18S)	18S	650	Makimura et al[105]	332f
	B4 R	5'-TGATCGTCTTCGATCCCCTA-3'	968–987 (18S)				987r
Lohman et al[95]	P1	5'-ATCAATAAGCGGAGGAAAAG -3'	45–64 (28S)	28S	800	Sandhu et al[100]	64f
	P2	5'-CTCTGGCTTCACCCTATTC -3'	825–843 (28S)				825r

[a]Names are based on the 3' nucleotide position and the orientation (f, forward; r, reverse) according to Lane.[98]

Table 3.11 Methods used for detection and identification of bacterial DNA in bacterial endophthalmitis

Authors (reference)	Year of publication	Target region	Product size (bp)	Type of assay	Method of detection	Level of identification	Method of identification
Hykin et al[87]	1994	16S	760	Single-step PCR	Agarose	*Propionibacterium acnes*	Nested PCR
Lohmann et al[95]	1998	16S	370	Single-step PCR	Agarose	Species level	DNA sequencing
Therese et al[97]	1998	16S	470	Nested PCR	Agarose	*Propionibacterium acnes*	Nested PCR
Knox et al[93]	1999	16S	800	Two PCR	Agarose	Species level	DNA sequencing
Anand et al[83]	2000	16S	370	Single-step PCR	Agarose	Gram reaction	Hybridization
Carroll et al[86]	2000	16S	1200	Nested PCR	Agarose	Gram reaction	Nested PCR
Lohmann et al[94]	2000	16S	600	Single-step PCR	Agarose	Species level	DNA sequencing
Okhravi et al[96]	2000	16S	1200	Single-step PCR	Agarose	Species level	DNA sequencing
Okhravi et al[88]	2000	16S	1000	Nested PCR	Agarose	Species level	RFLP DNA sequencing
Ferrer et al[103]	2001	16S	760	Single-step PCR	Agarose	*Propionibacterium acnes*	Nested PCR
Kerkhoff et al[91]	2003	16S	570	Single-step PCR	Biotinylated primer	*Neisseria meningitidis*	Microtiter assay
Ferrer et al[108]	2004	16S	954	Single-step PCR	Agarose	*Corynebacterium macginleyi*	DNA sequencing

Table 3.12 Methods used for detection and identification of fungal DNA in fungal endophthalmitis

Authors (reference)	Year of publication	Target region	Product size (bp)	Type of assay	Method of detection	Level of identification	Method of identification
Alexandrakis et al[109]	1996	Cutinase gene of *Fusarium*	196	Single-step PCR	Agarose	*Fusarium solani*	Specific PCR Southern blot hybridization
Lohmann et al[95]	1998	28S rDNA	800	Single-step PCR	Agarose	Not done	Not done
Okhravi et al[75]	1998	Cytochrome P450 L$_1$ A$_1$ gene of *Candida*	1000	Single-step PCR	Agarose	Species of *Candida*	Nested PCR RFLP
Hidalgo et al[77]	2000	Random	Variable (500–3200)	Random PCR	Agarose	*Candida albicans*	Length polymorphism of amplified products
Jaeger et al[104]	2000	18S rDNA	740	Single-step PCR	Agarose	*Candida albicans* *Aspergillus fumigatus* *Fusarium solani*	Nested PCR
Anand et al[99]	2001	28S rDNA	260	Single-step PCR	Agarose	Not done	Not done
Ferrer et al[102]	2001	ITS2	250	Nested PCR	Agarose	Species level	DNA sequencing
Ferrer et al[101]	2003	ITSs-5.8S rDNA	550	Single-step PCR	Agarose	Species level	DNA sequencing

of primers.[106,107] Nested PCR is highly sensitive because of the large number of total cycles. The major disadvantage of nested amplification is the high risk of contamination during transfer of first-round amplification products to a second tube. This technique has been used frequently in the diagnosis of bacterial endophthalmitis, not only to increase the sensitivity but also to differentiate Gram-positive from Gram-negative bacteria,[86] and to identify *P. acnes*, once the first PCR has detected bacterial DNA[87,97,103] (Tables 3.11[83,86–88,91, 93–97,103,108] and Table 3.12[75,77,95,99,101,103,104,109]).

Multiplex PCR

Multiplex PCR is an amplification reaction in which two or more sets of primers specific for different targets are put in the same tube, allowing multiple target sequences to be amplified simultaneously. For diagnostic purposes, multiplex PCR can be used for detecting internal controls and for detecting multiple pathogens in a single specimen.[110,111] This technique has been used in the diagnosis of intraocular inflammation, keratitis, and conjunctivitis for detected HSV-I, HSV-II, and VZV.[112–114]

Random PCR

A random amplified polymorphic DNA assay involves the use of a single, short, arbitrarily chosen primer to amplify genomic DNA under low stringency conditions.[115] Usually various DNA fragments with different sizes are amplified by random PCR, showing a specific pattern of bands for a determinate species or strain. It is useful in determining whether two isolates of the same species are epidemiologically related. This technique is not very useful in the diagnosis of endophthalmitis[77] because of the question of reproducibility between runs and among laboratories.

Real-time PCR

Recently, a modification of the traditional PCR, real-time PCR, has been developed; its efficacy in

the diagnosis of infectious ocular diseases has yet to be determined. In real-time PCR, the amplification and detection take place in the same reaction chamber or tube, often simultaneously.[116,117] This method vastly reduces the handling of the amplicon (and therefore the risk of carryover contamination). A thermocycler is combined with a fluorimeter, allowing the detection and quantification of PCR products the moment they are produced. These PCR products can be used as highly sensitive qualitative detection methods or as quantitative tests.

Visualization of the amplified project

After PCR, the millions of target DNA copies that accumulate are invisible to the eye. We need a way of visualizing the results of amplification assays. The most frequently used technique is by electrophoresis and ethidium bromide staining. The DNA fragments are separated according to their size in an agarose gel: the smaller DNA molecules move faster toward the anode than large DNA molecules (Tables 3.11 and 3.12). Another method used by Kerkoff et al is to label one of the primers with biotin.[91] PCR products are captured onto streptavidin (SA-microtiter wells). DNA is denatured by the addition of NaOH. Capture strands are detected by hybridization of a specific oligonucleotide probe which contains a label that can be detected by a conjugate and a colorimetric substrate reaction.

Current techniques for amplification, detection, and identification of pathogens in endophthalmitis by molecular methods are shown in Tables 3.11 and 3.12.

Identification of the pathogen

Once the DNA region has been amplified, various molecular techniques can be used to identify the pathogen, including utilization of genus or species-specific primers and oligonucleotide probes, length polymorphism of amplified DNA, restriction fragment length polymorphism (RFLP) analysis, and direct sequence analysis of amplified DNA.

Genus- or species-specific PCR

In this method, detection and identification are simultaneous. PCR is carried out with genus- or species-specific primers. Usually, a PCR with universal or broad-range primers is performed first, and when bacterial or fungal DNA is detected, a second PCR (nested PCR) is carried out with specific primers. This technique is frequently used for detection of *P. acnes* DNA in delayed endophthalmitis (see Table 3.11).[87,97,103] PCR with universal fungal primers and subsequent nested PCR using species-specific primers to differentiate *C. albicans, Aspergillus fumigatus,* and *Fusarium solani*[104] or the first PCR with genus-specific primers and nested PCR with species-specific primers for different *Candida* species,[75] have been used in the diagnosis of delayed fungal endophthalmitis (see Table 3.12).

Hybridization analysis of PCR products with genus- or species-specific oligonucleotide probes

The most common way to investigate the sequence obtained by PCR is to hybridize it to one or more oligonucleotide probes. The best known method is Southern blotting, which involves transferring DNA from an electrophoresis gel to a solid support (membrane). Once the DNA is immobilized on the membrane (nylon or nitrocellulose), it can be readily probed by hybridization, enabling fragments of DNA with a similar sequence to the labeled DNA probe to be identified. This technique allows the identification of the pathogen at genus or species level according to probes used by hybridization. PCR with broad-range primers followed by hybridization with oligonucleotide probes has been reported for the differentiation between Gram-positive and Gram-negative bacteria by Anand et al.[83] Another hybridization method of identification used in endogenous endophthalmitis explained above is by microtiter assay (see Table 3.11).

Restriction fragment length polymorphism analysis

After amplification, the sequence composition of a PCR product can be investigated by restriction enzyme-mediated digestion of amplified DNA. Digestion of PCR products by restriction endonucleases may generate multiple fragments, which can be resolved by gel electrophoresis. The endonucleases recognize a specific sequence of nucleotides (4–8 nucleotides) and when found, cleave the DNA. Variations of the compositions of the fragment alter the restriction site; the endonuclease may not recognize the site and will fail to digest the DNA, resulting in different sized restriction fragments and an alteration of the restriction fragment length polymorphism (RFLP) profile. Figure 3.20 shows a schematic representation of the ITS-5.8S rDNA fragment cut with three restriction endonucleases. RFLP analysis has been used by Okhravi et al for identification at species level of bacteria[88] and fungi[75] causing endophthalmitis (see Tables 3.11 and 3.12).

For all of these methods, clinical suspicion of the causative agent is mandatory, because of the inherent limitation caused by the selection of specific primers or probes.

Nucleic acid sequence analysis

This technique provides the most information, given that in this case the size, nucleotide composition, and order of this nucleotide are taken into account. The technique is based on the synthesis of new DNA strands synthesized from the purification PCR amplicon, beginning with one sequencing primer, and each strand having one more nucleotide. This technique is made possible by use of limited concentrations of dideoxynucleoside triphosphates (ddNTPs) into which four different fluorescent dyes have been incorporated, mixed with unlabeled deoxynucleotides (dNTPs). Synthesis terminates whenever a ddNTP is incorporated into the strand. Accumulated fragments are separated by size using electrophoresis. During electrophoresis, labeled products are visualized by fluorescence, with each of the four fluorescent dyes indicating which of the terminal ddNTPs has been incorporated. Combining the terminal ddNTP information with the fragment size allows the determination of sequence information (Figure 3.21).

Nucleic acid sequence analysis is preferable because it provides a definitive diagnosis. This technique has been used by numerous authors to

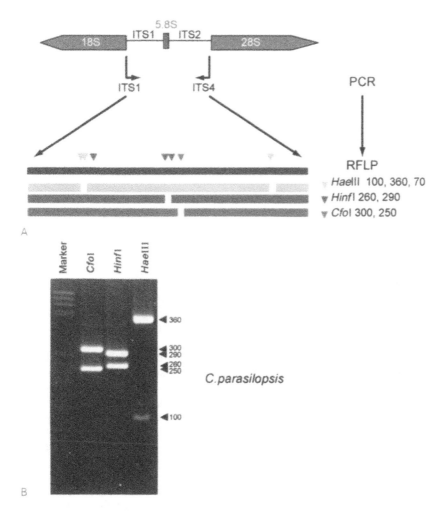

Figure 3.20

(A) Schematic representation indicating the points of cleavage of the restriction endonucleases HaeIII, HinfI, and CfoI of the ITS-5.8S rDNA region of *C. parapsilosis*. (B) Gel showing the band patterns for *C. parapsilosis* after digestion of the fragment by the endonucleases.

identify the microorganism causing the infection in both bacterial endophthalmitis[88,93–96,108] (Table 3.11) and fungal endophthalmitis (Table 3.12).[95,101,103]

New fastidious or uncultivated pathogens have been identified directly from infected human tissue or blood by this method and in the case of endophthalmitis there is evidence of bacterial involvement in eyes with suspected intraocular infections.[96]

Discussion

There are significant limitations to culture methods.[72] *In vitro* growth of an organism may be a lengthy process (possibly days to months), and may require subculture for final characterization, resulting in further delays. As a result of the fastidious nature of many organisms, specialized media or culture conditions may be necessary, thus making routine screening of specimens impractical and severely limiting the identification of disease associations. **The sensitivity and specificity that are desirable in a clinical assay are often lacking in these methods. In fact, it is now thought that only a small proportion of all bacterial species can be grown on artificial media.**[72,118] Valuable information, both diagnostic and in the study of disease pathogenesis, may be missed.

Many chronic endophthalmitis cases have an unknown cause (negative culture) and are

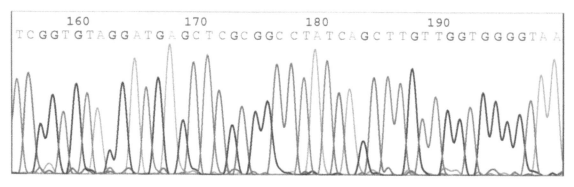

160   170   180   190
T C G G T G T A G G A T G A G C T C G C G G C C T A T C A G C T T G T T G G T G G G G T A A

Figure 3.21

Result of direct sequence analysis generated from a 16S rDNA amplification product from a vitreous sample of a patient.

diagnosed as 'sterile' endophthalmitis. Although the infection improves with antimicrobial therapy, most likely a microorganism caused this clinical picture and the culture was negative because of the specific growth requirements of the species: bacteria are sequestrated on solid surfaces[119] or located inside macrophages (Chapter 6).[120,121] PCR has detected new microorganisms in endophthalmitis, demonstrating evidence of various species of bacteria involved in the infection, whereas none or only one of the species detected by PCR grew in culture.[96] In addition, in some studies, the pathogen was identified at the species level using molecular techniques, contributing to the knowledge of the microbial spectrum causing endophthalmitis.[96,101]

Molecular methods aid identification of microorganisms involved in endophthalmitis and their pathogenetic mechanisms. Molecular biology techniques are used by a growing number of laboratories to support microbiological diagnosis and/or solve some of its limitations (Tables 3.13,[83,86–88,91,93–97,108,122–126] and Table 3.14[75,77, 95,99,101,103,104,109]). This circumstance requires special attention to avoid false results. The greatest disadvantages of molecular diagnosis are the false-positive results, the high cost, and the lack of standardization of the techniques.

False results can be divided into three groups according to the origin:

- From the sample. Any disturbance while collecting the sample may produce both false positives and false negatives. The false positives that appear in bacterial and fungal PCR may be produced by contamination during ocular surface puncture with the needle, or from contaminated air or equipment.

- From the laboratory. Contamination has been reported not only from specimens that have been processed adjacent to one another but also from sources such as contaminated instruments, clothing, room air, and even skin particles from laboratory workers. PCR assays have a reputation for producing false-positive reactions if there is specimen contamination or amplicon carryover. Negative controls must be processed at every step to exclude false positives; it is essential that samples are extracted, amplified, and visualized in separate rooms using equipment designated for each area (including pipettes) to minimize the possibility of specimen contamination. Ultraviolet irradiation has been used to help destroy nucleic acids on laboratory surfaces.[127–129]

- From reagents. Some authors have described contamination problems in commercially available laboratory reagents. It is widely known that many commercial polymerases have remains of bacterial DNA.[130,131] When nested PCR is carried out with bacterial universal primers, false-positive results can appear as a result of these DNA remains or amplicon carryover. Decontamination measures have included the use of topical agents, such as sodium hypochlorite, and of decontaminants within mixes of PCR, such as isopsorelins and uracil-n-glycosylase.[132–137]

Table 3.13 Polymerase chain reaction (PCR) for diagnosis of bacterial endophthalmitis

Reference	Year of publication	Type of endophthalmitis (no. of infected patients)	Type of bacterium (no. of patients)	Molecular assay	Place
Hykin et al[87]	1994	Postoperative • Delayed (19)	P. acnes (5) S. epidermidis (3) S. aureus (1) Streptococcus sp. (1) Citrobacter freundii (1)	Nested PCR	London, UK
Grenzebach et al[122]	1996	Postoperative (1)	Mycobacterium sp. (1)	PCR	Munster, Germany
Dockholm-Dworniczak et al[123]	1996		Mycobacteria (1)	PCR	Munster, Germany
Knox et al[124]	1998	Retinitis (38)	10 CMV, 8 VCV and 6 HSV	PCR	San Francisco, USA
Lohmann et al[85]	1998	Postoperative • Acute (10) • Delayed (6)	S. aureus (9) P. acnes (3) A. israelii (3) Streptococci (1)	DNA sequencing	Regensburg, Germany
Therese et al[97]	1998	Postoperative (36) Posttraumatic (13) Endogenous (6)	Eubacterial genome (17)* P. acnes (9)	Nested PCR	Chennai, India
Knox et al[93]	1999	Postoperative • Acute (5)	Serratia marcescens (1) S. epidermidis (2) Streptococcus defectivus (1) Leuconostoc sp. (1)	PCR DNA sequencing	San Francisco, USA
Lohmann et al[125]	1999	Endogenous	Listeria monocytogenes (1)	PCR	Regensburg, Germany
Anand et al[83]	2000	Postoperative • Acute (16) • Delayed (13)	S. epidermidis (2) S. aureus (4) Strep. viridans (2) E. faecalis (4)	PCR DNA probe hybridization to detect Gram stain of bacterium	Chennai, India
		Posttraumatic (22)	Bacillus sp. (3) Neisseria subflava (1) Klebsiella sp. (1) Ps. aeruginosa (3) P. stutzeri (1)		
		Endogenous (4)	Achromobacter sp. (2) Acinetobacter calcoaceticus (1) Alkaligenes faecalis (1) Flavobacterium sp. (1)		
Carroll et al[86]	2000	Postoperative • Acute (1) • Delayed (1)	Strep. pneumoniae (1) S. aureus (1)	Nested PCR	London, UK
		Endogenous (1)	Gram-positive (1)		

continued overleaf

Table 3.13 Polymerase chain reaction (PCR) for diagnosis of bacterial endophthalmitis – continued

Reference	Year of publication	Type of endophthalmitis (no. of patients)	Type of bacterium (no. of patients)	Molecular assay	Place
Lohmann et al[84]	2000	Postoperative • Delayed (25)	S. epidermidis (6) A. israelii (5) P. acnes (14)	PCR DNA sequencing	Regensburg, Germany
Okhravi et al[96]	2000	Indeterminate (25)	P. acnes (1) E. coli (1) B. cereus (1) Staphylococcus spp. (4) Pseudomonas spp. (4) Aeromonas spp. (1) Enterococcus (Strep.) faecalis (3) Proteobacteria (10) Unidentifiable bacteria (8)	PCR RFLP DNA sequencing	London, UK
Okhravi et al[88]	2000	• Acute (2)	E. coli (1) Staphylococcus spp. (1)	PCR RFLP DNA sequencing	London, UK
Goldstein et al[128] Kerkhoff et al[91]	2001 2003	Endogenous (1) Endogenous (1)	Bartonella henselae (1) Neisseria meningitidis (1)	Semi-nested PCR Microtiter	Chicago, USA Veldhoven, Holland
Ferrer et al[108]	2004	Postoperative	Corynebacterium macginleyi (1)	PCR DNA sequencing	Alicante, Spain

*PCR positive in 20 culture-positive patients and 17 culture-negative patients.

Table 3.14 Polymerase chain reaction (PCR) for diagnosis of fungal endophthalmitis

Reference	Year of publication	Type of endophthalmitis (no. of infected patients)	Type of fungus (no. of patients)	Molecular assay	Place
Alexandrakis et al[109]	1996	Endogenous (1)	*Fusarium* spp. (1)	PCR Southern blot hybridization	New Haven, CT, USA
Okhravi et al[75]	1998	Indeterminate (3)	*Candida albicans* (3)	Nested PCR RFLP	London, UK
Lohmann et al[96]	1998	Postoperative (1)	Fungus (1)	PCR	Regensburg, Germany
Jaeger et al[104]	2000	Endogenous (2)	*Candida albicans* (2)	Nested PCR	London, UK
Hidalgo et al[77]	2000	Endogenous (3) Posttraumatic (1)	*Candida albicans* (4)	Random PCR	Michigan, USA
Ferrer et al[103]	2001	Postoperative (2)	*Candida parapsilosis* (2)	PCR DNA sequencing	Alicante, Spain
Anand et al[99]	2001	Postoperative (13)	*Aspergillus flavus* (4) *Aspergillus fumigatus* (1) *Aspergillus niger* (1) Unidentified (2) Culture negative (5)	PCR	Chennai, India
		Endogenous (12)	*Aspergillus falciforme* (2) *Aspergillus flavus* (1) *Aspergillus fumigatus* (1) *Nigrospora* sp. (1) *Penicillium* sp. (1) *Candida albicans* (1) Culture negative (10)		
		Posttraumatic (2)	*Chrysosporium* sp. (1) Culture negative (1)		
Ferrer et al[101]	2003	Posttraumatic (1)	*Alternaria infectoria* (1)	PCR DNA sequencing	Alicante, Spain

The high cost of PCR is related to the high degree of expertise needed to develop, run, and interpret the results of tests; expensive physical space is required to set up and run the assays, and high capital and operating costs are associated with many of the reagents.

The final disadvantage of molecular diagnosis is the lack of standardization resulting from recently developed techniques that are still not optimized. Early investigations into the molecular diagnosis of ocular infections were based on DNA species-specific regions that tend to be unicopy genes and detect only one species, usually *Candida*,[75] *Fusarium*,[109] or *Aspergillus*.[138] Later studies established the ribosomal genes as the basis of phylogenetics and taxonomy and as the target for the detection and diagnosis of the infection process. Ribosomal genes have begun to be used as a target, thus increasing the sensitivity of the method (multicopy genes) and the spectrum detectable. This expanded ability is extremely important because ocular samples are limited in size; the determination of whether the origin of the infection is bacterial or fungal is imperative. For the application of species-specific primers, unless it is clear which species is the cause of infection, it is preferable to extend the target to be able to detect any species of bacteria or fungi and then identify it by molecular techniques.

Various groups are working with ribosomal genes as a target for the diagnosis of ocular infections. In bacterial endophthalmitis, all groups work with 16S rDNA (Table 3.11), although they differ in the amplified zone. There is a greater variety of ribosomal genes used to

Table 3.15 Number of patients, type of sample, culture, and PCR results in diagnosis of bacterial endophthalmitis

Reference	Year of publication	No. of samples (no. patients)	Type of sample	Culture positive PCR positive	Culture negative PCR positive	Culture positive PCR negative	Target DNA
Hykin et al[87]	1994	23 (19)	23V	9	8	–	16S rDNA
Grenzebach et al[122]	1996	1 (1)	1V	–	1	–	16S rDNA
Lohmann et al[95]	1998	32 (16)	16V, 16A	8	22	–	16S rDNA
Therese et al[97]	1998	58 (55)	30V, 28A	20	17	–	16S rDNA
Knox et al[93]	1999	5 (5)	5V	2	1	2	16S rDNA
Lohmann et al[125]	1999	1 (1)	1A	–	1	–	16S rDNA
Anand et al[83]	2000	57 (55)	40V, 17A	32	20	–	16S rDNA
Carroll et al[86]	2000	4 (3)	3V, 1A	3	1	–	16s rDNA
Lohmann et al[94]	2000	50 (25)	25V, 25A	6	38	–	16S rDNA
Okhravi et al[96]	2000	37 (25)	15V, 22A	20	17	–	16S rDNA
Okhravi et al[88]	2000	2 (2)	2V	1	1	–	16S rDNA
Ferrer et al[103]	2001	4 (3)	1V, 3A	3	1	–	16S rDNA
Goldstein et al[126]	2001	1 (1)	1V	–	1	–	Antigen gene
Frelich et al[139]	2003	1 (1)	1V	–	1	–	16S rDNA
Kerkhoff et al[91]	2003	1 (1)	1A	–	1	–	16S rDNA
Asensio Sanchez et al[140]	2003	1 (1)	1V	–	1	–	Indeterminate
Ferrer et al[108]	2004	2 (1)	2A	0	2	–	16S rDNA

Table 3.16 Number of patients, type of sample, culture and PCR results in diagnosis of fungal endophthalmitis

Reference	Year of publication	No. of samples (no. patients)	Type of sample	Culture positive PCR positive	Culture negative PCR positive	Culture positive PCR negative	Target DNA
Alexandrakis et al[109]	1996	1 (1)	Formalin-fixed ocular tissue	–	1	–	Cutinase gene
Okhravi et al[75]	1998	4 (4)	4V, 2A	2	1	–	Cytochrome P450 L₁ A₁ gene
Lohmann et al[95]	1998	2 (1)	1V, 1A	–	2	–	28S rDNA
Hidalgo et al[77]	2000	4 (4)	4V, 1A	2	2	–	Random
Jaeger et al[104]	2000	2 (2)	2V	1	1	–	18S rDNA
Ferrer et al[103]	2001	3 (2)	1V, 2A	2	–	–	ITS-5.8S rDNA
Anand et al[99]	2001	43 (30)	29V, 14A	16	16	1	28S rDNA
Ferrer et al[101]	2003	1 (1)	Corneal scraping	1	–	–	ITS-5.8S rDNA

diagnose fungal endophthalmitis (Table 3.12). Anand and Lohmann use the 28S rDNA as target DNA,[95,99] Jaeger (Okhravi group) uses the 18S rDNA,[104] and Ferrer works with the ITS/5.8S rDNA region.[101,103] In all cases, the sensitivity is higher than by culture whatever the amplified region (Table 3.15[83,86–88,91–97,103,108,122,125,126,139,140] and Table 3.16[75,77,95,99,101,103,104,109]). However, the sensitivity of detection by PCR does not depend only on the amplified ribosomal gene but also on the primers and the specific conditions for each primer. Figure 3.22 shows how sensitivity varies according to the primers used, where in both cases the amplified region is 16S rDNA of *Ps. aeruginosa* but the zone and the primers are different.

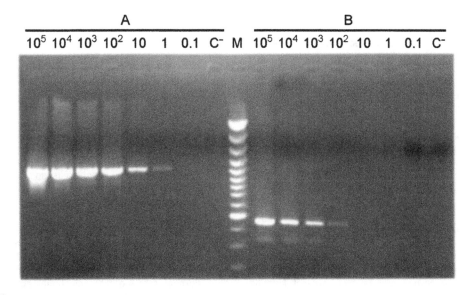

Figure 3.22

Sensitivity of the PCR with *Pseudomonas aeruginosa* cells. M represents the ladder marker GeneRuler 100 bp DNA Ladder Plus. (A) Primers used: 66f/1044r; (B) primers used: 66f/490r.

A wide range of techniques is used for the identification of the microorganism causing the infection, as shown in Tables 3.11 and 3.12. Depending on the type of infection produced, any of the techniques of molecular identification can be applied. In delayed bacterial endophthalmitis, specific primers are often used to detect DNA of *P. acnes*[87,94,97] or in the case of endogenous endophthalmitis caused by *Candida* and *Aspergillus,* we can apply techniques (nested, RFLP) that detect and directly differentiate their species.[77,104,138] In these cases, the identification can be based on techniques that limit the suspects to a series of species, given that the spectrum produced by this infection is quite restricted.

However, in other types of endophthalmitis and particularly in the case of posttraumatic endophthalmitis, the spectrum of possible causative organisms broadens; unless broad-range primers are used for their detection and the identification is performed by sequencing, it is highly unlikely that the pathogen causing the infection will be identified. Although the broadest spectrum of pathogens is found in keratitis and posttraumatic endophthalmitis, the causal agent in a high number of cases of postoperative endophthalmitis remains a mystery.[96,99]

Molecular biology can provide a rapid method to detect and identify ocular pathogens at a species level. Bacterial and fungal speciation constitutes an important aid for effective treatment, facilitating the application of species-specific therapy, avoiding problems of drug resistance, and establishing a more precise epidemiology. The lack of species identification in infections reported in the literature prevents precise knowledge as to the efficacy of antimicrobial therapy and species epidemiology. Therefore, the use of universal or broad-range primers to detect DNA of the pathogen and identification by sequencing of the DNA is recommended. Use of PCR combined with automated DNA sequencing provides great advantages compared with other forms of molecular identification.

References

1. Seal DV, Bron AJ, Hay J. *Ocular Infection – Investigation and Treatment in Practice* (Martin Dunitz: London, 1998): 1–275.
2. Pillar CM, Hazlett LD, Hobden JA. Alkaline protease-deficient mutants of *Pseudomonas aerug-*

inosa are virulent in the eye, *Curr Eye Res* (2000) **21**:730–9.

3. Chen LD, Hazlett LD. Perlecan in the basement membrane of corneal epithelium serves as a site for *P. aeruginosa* binding, *Curr Eye Res* (2000) **20**:260–7.

4. Kernacki KA, Barrett RP, McClellan SA et al. Aging and PMN response to *P. aeruginosa* infection, *Invest Ophthalmol Vis Sci* (2000) **41**:3019–25.

5. Kernackni KA, Fridman R, Hazlett LD et al. In vivo characterization of host and bacterial protease expression during *Pseudomonas aeruginosa* corneal infections in naive and immunized mice, *Curr Eye Res* (1997) **16**:289–97.

6. Chen L, Hobden JA, Masinick SA et al. Environmental factors influence *P. aeruginosa* binding to the wounded mouse cornea, *Curr Eye Res* (1998) **17**:231–7.

7. Masinick SA, Montgomery CP, Montgomery PC et al. Secretory IgA inhibits *Pseudomonas aeruginosa* binding to cornea and protects against keratitis, *Invest Ophthalmol Vis Sci* (1997) **38**:910–18.

8. Gupta SK, Masinick SA, Hobden JA et al. Bacterial proteases and adherence of *Pseudomonas aeruginosa* to mouse cornea, *Exp Eye Res* (1996) **62**:641–50.

9. Wu X, Gupta SK, Hazlett LD. Characterization of *P. aeruginosa* pili binding human corneal epithelial proteins, *Curr Eye Res* (1995) **14**:969–77.

10. Eggar SF, Huber-Spitzy V, Scholda C et al. Bacterial contamination during extracapsular cataract surgery. Prospective study on 200 consecutive patients, *Ophthalmologica* (1994) **208**:77–81.

11. Beigi B, Westlake W, Chang B et al. The effect of intracameral, per-operative antibiotics on microbial contamination of anterior chamber aspirates during phacoemulsification, *Eye* (1998) **12**:390–4.

12. Mistlberger A, Ruckhofer J, Raithel E et al. Anterior chamber contamination during cataract surgery with intraocular lens implantation, *J Cataract Refract Surg* (1997) **23**:1064–9.

13. Leong JK, Shah R, McCluskey PJ et al. Bacterial contamination of the anterior chamber during phacoemulsification cataract surgery, *J Cataract Refract Surg* (2002) **28**:826–33.

14. Kresloff MS, Castellarin AA, Zarbin MA. Endophthalmitis, *Surv Ophthalmol* (1998) **43**: 193–224.

15. Colleaux KM, Hamilton WK. Effect of prophylactic antibiotics and incision type on the incidence of endophthalmitis after cataract surgery, *Can J Ophthalmol* (2000) **35**:373–8.

16. Ciulla TA, Starr MB, Masket S. Bacterial endophthalmitis prophylaxis for cataract surgery. An evidence-based update, *Ophthalmology* (2002) **109**:13–24.

17. Montan PG, Wejde G, Koranyi G et al. Prophylactic intracameral cefuroxime. Efficacy in preventing endophthalmitis after cataract surgery, *J Cataract Refract Surg* (2002) **28**:977–81.

18. Han DP, Wisniewski SR, Wilson LA et al. Spectrum and susceptibilities of the microbiologic isolates in the Endophthalmitis Vitrectomy Study, *Am J Ophthalmol* (1996) **112**:1–17 [erratum appears in *Am J Ophthalmol* (1996) **122**:920].

19. Parkkari M, Paivarinta H, Salminen L. The treatment of endophthalmitis after cataract surgery: review of 26 cases, *J Ocul Pharmacol Ther* (1995) **11**:349–59.

20. Murray BE. The life and times of the *Enterococcus*, *Clin Microbiol Rev* (1990) **3**:46–65.

21. Moellering RC Jr. Emergence of *Enterococcus* as a significant pathogen, *Clin Infect Dis* (1992) **14**:1173–6.

22. Schaberg DR, Culver DH, Gaynes RP. Major trends in the microbial etiology of nosocomial infection, *Am J Med* (1991) **91**(Suppl 3B):72S–75S.

23. Yorston D, Foster A. Cutaneous anthrax leading to corneal scarring from cicatricial ectropion, *Br J Ophthalmol* (1989) **73**:809–11.

24. Soysal HG, Kiratli H, Recep OF. Anthrax as the cause of preseptal cellulitis and cicatricial ectropion, *Acta Ophthalmol Scand* (2001) **79**:208–9.

25. Romsaitong DP, Grasso CM. *Clostridium perfringens* endophthalmitis following cataract surgery, *Arch Ophthalmol* (1999) **117**:970–1.

26. Iyer MN, Kranias G, Daun ME. Post-traumatic endophthalmitis involving *Clostridium tetani* and *Bacillus* spp, *Am J Ophthalmol* (2001) **132**:116–17.

27. Nangia V, Hutchinson C. Metastatic endophthalmitis caused by *Clostridium perfringens*, *Br J Ophthalmol* (1992) **76**:252–3.

28. Insler MS, Karcioglu ZA, Naugle T Jr. *Clostridium septicum* panophthalmitis with systemic complications, *Br J Ophthalmol* (1985) **69**:774–7.

29. Eliott D, O'Brien TP, Green WR et al. Elevated intraocular pressure, pigment dispersion and dark hypopyon in endogenous endophthalmitis from *Listeria monocytogenes*, *Surv Ophthalmol* (1992) **37**:117–24.

30. Mames RN, Friedman SM, Stinson WG et al. Positive vitreous cultures from eyes without signs of infectious endophthalmitis, *Ophthalmic Surg Lasers* (1997) **28**:365–9.

31. Dickens A, Greven CM. Posttraumatic endophthalmitis caused by *Lactobacillus*, *Arch Ophthalmol* (1993) **111**:1169.

32. Hull DS, Patipa M, Cox F. Metastatic endophthalmitis: a complication of meningococcal meningitis, *Ann Ophthalmol* (1982) **14**:29–30.

33. Saperstein DA, Bennett MD, Steinberg JP et al. Exogenous *Neisseria meningitidis* endophthalmitis, *Am J Ophthalmol* (1997) **123**:135–6.

34. Barnard T, Das A, Hickey S. Bilateral endophthalmitis as an initial presentation of meningococ-

cal meningitis, *Arch Ophthalmol* (1997) **115**: 1472–3.

35. Abousaesha F, Dogar GF, Young BJ et al. Endophthalmitis as a presentation of meningococcal septicaemia, *Ir J Med Sci* (1993) **162**:495–6.

36. Margo CE, Mames RN, Guy JR. Endogenous *Klebsiella* endophthalmitis. Report of two cases and review of the literature, *Ophthalmology* (1994) **101**:1298–301.

37. Joondeph HC, Nothnagel AF. *Serratia rubidae* endophthalmitis following penetrating ocular injury, *Ann Ophthalmol* (1983) **15**:1138–40.

38. Lam DS, Kwok AK, Chew S. Post-keratoplasty endophthalmitis caused by *Proteus mirabilis*, *Eye* (1998) **12** (Pt I):139–40.

39. Cunningham ET Jr, Whitcher JP, Kim RY. *Morganella morganii* postoperative endophthalmitis, *Br J Ophthalmol* (1997) **81**:170–1.

40. Recchia FM, Baumal CR, Sivalingam A et al. Endophthalmitis after pediatric strabismus surgery, *Arch Ophthalmol* (2000) **118**:939–44.

41. Pach JM. Traumatic *Haemophilus influenzae* endophthalmitis, *Am J Ophthalmol* (1988) **106**: 497–8.

42. Al Faran MF. *Brucella melitensis* endogenous endophthalmitis, *Ophthalmologica* (1990) **201**: 19–22.

43. Penland RL, Boniuk M, Wilhelmus KR. Vibrio ocular infections on the U.S. Gulf Coast, *Cornea* (2000) **19**:26–9.

44. Mindel JS, Rosenberg EW. Is *Helicobacter pylori* of interest to ophthalmologists? *Ophthalmology* (1997) **104**:1729–30.

45. Kountouras J, Mylopoulos N, Boura P et al. Relationship between *Helicobacter pylori* infection and glaucoma, *Ophthalmology* (2001) **108**:599–604.

46. Gopal L, Ramaswamy AA, Madhavan HN et al. Postoperative endophthalmitis caused by sequestered *Acinetobacter calcoaceticus*, *Am J Ophthalmol* (2000) **129**:388–90.

47. Prashanth K, Ranga MP, Rao VA et al. Corneal perforation due to *Acinetobacter junii*: a case report, *Diagn Microbiol Infect Dis* (2000) **37**:215–17.

48. Crawford PM Jr, Conway MD, Peyman GA. Trauma-induced *Acinetobacter lwoffi* endophthalmitis with multi-organism recurrence: strategies with intravitreal treatment, *Eye* (1997) **11** (Pt 6):863–4.

49. Melki TS, Sramek SJ. Trauma-induced *Acinetobacter lwoffi* endophthalmitis, *Am J Ophthalmol* (1992) **113**:598–9.

50. Mark DB, Gaynon MW. Trauma-induced endophthalmitis caused by *Acinetobacter anitratus*, *Br J Ophthalmol* (1983) **67**:124–6.

51. Roussel TJ, Olson ER, Rice T et al. Chronic postoperative endophthalmitis associated with *Actinomyces* species, *Arch Ophthalmol* (1991) **109**:60–2.

52. Kouyoumdjian GA, Larkin TP, Blackburn PJ et al. Optic disk edema as a presentation of *Propionibacterium acnes* endophthalmitis, *Am J Ophthalmol* (2001) **132**:259–61.

53. Hamza HS, Loewenstein A, Haller JA. Fungal retinitis and endophthalmitis. *Ophthalmol Clin North Am* (1999) **12**:89–108.

54. Patel AS, Hemady RK, Rodrigues M et al. Endogenous *Fusarium* endophthalmitis in a patient with acute lymphocytic leukemia, *Am J Ophthalmol* (1994) **117**:363–8.

55. Goldblum D, Frueh BE, Zimmerli S et al. Treatment of post-keratitis *Fusarium* endophthalmitis with amphotericin B lipid complex, *Cornea* (2000) **19**:853–6.

56. Weissgold DJ, Maguire AM, Brucker AJ. Management of postoperative *Acremonium* endophthalmitis, *Ophthalmology* (1996) **103**:749–56.

57. Pettit TH, Olson RJ, Foos RY et al. Fungal endophthalmitis following intraocular lens implantation. A surgical epidemic, *Arch Ophthalmol* (1980) **98**: 1025–39.

58. Kozarsky AM, Stulting RD, Waring GO III et al. Penetrating keratoplasty for exogenous *Paecilomyces* keratitis followed by postoperative endophthalmitis, *Am J Ophthalmol* (1984) **98**: 552–7.

59. Scott IU, Flynn HW Jr, Miller D et al. Exogenous endophthalmitis caused by amphotericin B-resistant *Paecilomyces lilacinus*: treatment options and visual outcomes, *Arch Ophthalmol* (2001) **119**: 916–19.

60. Orgel IK, Cohen KL. Postoperative zygomycetes endophthalmitis, *Ophthalmic Surg* (1989) **20**: 584–7.

61. Dugel PU, Rao NA, Forster DJ et al. *Pneumocystis carinii* choroiditis after long-term aerosolized pentamidine therapy, *Am J Ophthalmol* (1990) **110**:113–17.

62. Foster RE, Lowder CY, Meisler DM et al. Presumed *Pneumocystis carinii* choroiditis. Unifocal presentation, regression with intravenous pentamidine, and choroiditis recurrence, *Ophthalmology* (1991) **98**:1360–5.

63. Weinberg RS. Uveitis. Update on therapy, *Ophthalmol Clin North Am* (1991) **12**: 71–81.

64. Brooks RG. Prospective study of *Candida* endophthalmitis in hospitalized patients with candidemia, *Arch Int Med* (1989) **149**: 2226–8.

65. Scherer WJ, Lee K. Implications of early systemic therapy on the incidence of endogenous fungal endophthalmitis, *Ophthalmology* (1997) **104**: 1593–8.

66. Donahue SP, Greven CM, Zuravleff JJ et al. Intraocular candidiasis in patients with candidemia. Clinical implications derived from a prospective

multicenter study, *Ophthalmology* (1994) **101**: 1302–9.

67. Donahue SP, Hein E, Sinatra RB. Ocular involvement in children with candidemia, *Am J Ophthalmol* (2003) **135**: 886–7.

68. Thomas PA. Current perspectives on ophthalmic mycoses, *Clin Microb Rev* (2003) **16**:730–97.

69. Mullis KB, Faloona FA. Specific synthesis of DNA in vitro via a polymerase-catalyzed chain reaction, *Methods Enzymol* (1987) **155**:335–50.

70. Saiki RK, Gelfand DH, Stoffel S et al. Primer-directed enzymatic amplification of DNA with a thermostable DNA polymerase, *Science* (1988) **239**:487–91.

71. Saiki RK, Scharf S, Faloona F et al. Enzymatic amplification of beta-globin genomic sequences and restriction site analysis for diagnosis of sickle cell anemia, *Science* (1985) **230**:1350–4.

72. Fredricks DN, Relman DA. Application of polymerase chain reaction to the diagnosis of infectious diseases, *Clin Infect Dis* (1999) **29**: 475–86.

73. White TJ, Madej R, Persing DH. The polymerase chain reaction: clinical applications, *Adv Clin Chem* (1992) **29**:161–96.

74. Kan VL. Polymerase chain reaction for the diagnosis of candidemia, *J Infect Dis* (1993) **168**:779–83.

75. Okhravi N, Adamson P, Mant R et al. Polymerase chain reaction and restriction fragment length polymorphism mediated detection and speciation of *Candida* spp causing intraocular infection, *Invest Ophthalmol Vis Sci* (1998) **39**:859–66.

76. Nosek J, Tomaska L, Rycovska A et al. Mitochondrial telomeres as molecular markers for identification of the opportunistic yeast pathogen *Candida parapsilosis*, *J Clin Microbiol* (2002) **40**:1283–9.

77. Hidalgo JA, Alangaden GJ, Eliott D et al. Fungal endophthalmitis diagnosis by detection of *Candida albicans* DNA in intraocular fluid by use of a species-specific polymerase chain reaction assay, *J Infect Dis* (2000) **181**:1198–201.

78. Klappenbach JA, Saxman PR, Cole JR et al. rrndb: the ribosomal RNA operon copy number database, *Nucleic Acids Res* (2001) **29**:181–4.

79. Maleszka R, Clark-Walker GD. Yeasts have a four-fold variation in ribosomal DNA copy number, *Yeast* (1993) **9**:53–8.

80. Kolbert CP, Persing DH. Ribosomal DNA sequencing as a tool for identification of bacterial pathogens, *Curr Opin Microbiol* (1999) **2**:299–305.

81. Woese CR. Bacterial evolution, *Microbiol Rev* (1987) **51**:221–71.

82. Lane DJ, Pace B, Olsen GJ et al. Rapid determination of 16S ribosomal RNA sequences for phylogenetic analyses, *Proc Natl Acad Sci USA* (1985) **82**:6955–9.

83. Anand AR, Madhavan HN, Therese KL. Use of polymerase chain reaction (PCR) and DNA probe hybridization to determine the Gram reaction of the infecting bacterium in the intraocular fluids of patients with endophthalmitis, *J Infect* (2000) **41**:221–6.

84. Chen K, Neimark H, Rumore P et al. Broad range DNA probes for detecting and amplifying eubacterial nucleic acids, *FEMS Microbiol Lett* (1989) **48**:19–24.

85. Edwards U, Rogall T, Blocker H et al. Isolation and direct complete nucleotide determination of entire genes. Characterization of a gene coding for 16S ribosomal RNA, *Nucleic Acids Res* (1989) **17**:7843–53.

86. Carroll NM, Jaeger EE, Choudhury S et al. Detection of and discrimination between gram-positive and gram-negative bacteria in intraocular samples by using nested PCR, *J Clin Microbiol* (2000) **38**:1753–7.

87. Hykin PG, Tobal K, McIntyre G et al. The diagnosis of delayed post-operative endophthalmitis by polymerase chain reaction of bacterial DNA in vitreous samples, *J Med Microbiol* (1994) **40**:408–15.

88. Okhravi N, Adamson P, Matheson MM et al. PCR-RFLP-mediated detection and speciation of bacterial species causing endophthalmitis, *Invest Ophthalmol Vis Sci* (2000) **41**:1438–47.

89. Wilson KH, Blitchington RB, Greene RC. Amplification of bacterial 16S ribosomal DNA with polymerase chain reaction, *J Clin Microbiol* (1990) **28**:1942–6. [Erratum appears in *J Clin Microbiol* (1991) **29**:666]

90. Relman DA, Falkow S. Identification of uncultured microorganisms: expanding the spectrum of characterized microbial pathogens, *Infect Agents Dis* (1992) **1**:245–53.

91. Kerkhoff FT, van der Zee A, Bergmans AM et al. Polymerase chain reaction detection of *Neisseria meningitidis* in the intraocular fluid of a patient with endogenous endophthalmitis but without associated meningitis, *Ophthalmology* (2003) **110**:2134–6.

92. Bergmans AM, Groothedde JW, Schellekens JF et al. Etiology of cat scratch disease: comparison of polymerase chain reaction detection of *Bartonella* (formerly *Rochalimaea*) and *Afipia felis* DNA with serology and skin tests, *J Infect Dis* (1995) **171**:916–23.

93. Knox CM, Chandler D, Short GA et al. Polymerase chain reaction-based assays of vitreous samples for the diagnosis of viral retinitis. Use in diagnostic dilemmas, *Ophthalmology* (1998) **105**:37–44.

94. Lohmann CP, Linde HJ, Reischl U. Improved detection of microorganisms by polymerase chain reaction in delayed endophthalmitis after cataract surgery, *Ophthalmology* (2000) **107**:1047–51.

95. Lohmann CP, Heeb M, Linde HJ et al. Diagnosis of infectious endophthalmitis after cataract surgery by polymerase chain reaction, *J Cataract Refract Surg* (1998) **24**:821–6.

96. Okhravi N, Adamson P, Carroll N et al. PCR-based evidence of bacterial involvement in eyes with suspected intraocular infection, *Invest Ophthalmol Vis Sci* (2000) **41**:3474–9.

97. Therese KL, Anand AR, Madhavan HN. Polymerase chain reaction in the diagnosis of bacterial endophthalmitis, *Br J Ophthalmol* (1998) **82**:1078–82.

98. Lane DJ. 16S/23S rRNA sequencing. In: Stackebrandt E, Goodfellow M, eds. *Nucleic Acid Techniques in Bacterial Systematics* (John Wiley & Sons: Chichester, UK, 1991) 115–75.

99. Anand A, Madhavan H, Neelam V et al. Use of polymerase chain reaction in the diagnosis of fungal endophthalmitis, *Ophthalmology* (2001) **108**:326–30.

100. Sandhu GS, Kline BC, Stockman L et al. Molecular probes for diagnosis of fungal infections, *J Clin Microbiol* (1995) **33**:2913–19. [Erratum appears in *J Clin Microbiol* (1996) **34**:1350]

101. Ferrer C, Montero J, Alio JL et al. Rapid molecular diagnosis of posttraumatic keratitis and endophthalmitis caused by *Alternaria infectoria*, *J Clin Microbiol* (2003) **41**:3358–60.

102. White TJ, Bruns T, Lee S et al. PCR protocols. A guide to methods and applications. In: Innins MA, Gelfand DH, Sninsky JJ, White TJ, eds. *Amplification and Direct Sequencing of Fungal Ribosomal RNA Genes for Phylogenetics* (Academic Press: San Diego, 1990) 315–22.

103. Ferrer C, Colom F, Frases S et al. Detection and identification of fungal pathogens by PCR and by ITS2 and 5.8S ribosomal DNA typing in ocular infections, *J Clin Microbiol* (2001) **39**:2873–9.

104. Jaeger EE, Carroll NM, Choudhury S et al. Rapid detection and identification of *Candida*, *Aspergillus*, and *Fusarium* species in ocular samples using nested PCR, *J Clin Microbiol* (2000) **38**:2902–8.

105. Makimura K, Murayama SY, Yamaguchi H. Detection of a wide range of medically important fungi by the polymerase chain reaction, *J Med Microbiol* (1994) **40**:358–64.

106. Haqqi TM, Sarkar G, David CS et al. Specific amplification with PCR of a refractory segment of genomic DNA, *Nucleic Acids Res* (1988) **16**:11844.

107. Schmidt B, Muellegger RR, Stockenhuber C et al. Detection of *Borrelia burgdorferi*-specific DNA in urine specimens from patients with erythema migrans before and after antibiotic therapy, *J Clin Microbiol* (1996) **34**:1359–63.

108. Ferrer C, Ruiz-Moreno JM, Rodriguez AE et al. Postoperative *Corynebacterium macginleyi* endophthalmitis, *J Cataract Refract Surg* (in press).

109. Alexandrakis G, Sears M, Gloor P. Postmortem diagnosis of *Fusarium* panophthalmitis by the polymerase chain reaction, *Am J Ophthalmol* (1996) **121**:221–3.

110. Bej AK, Mahbubani MH, Miller R et al. Multiplex PCR amplification and immobilized capture probes for detection of bacterial pathogens and indicators in water, *Mol Cell Probes* (1990) **4**:353–65.

111. Geha DJ, Uhl JR, Gustaferro CA et al. Multiplex PCR for identification of methicillin-resistant staphylococci in the clinical laboratory, *J Clin Microbiol* (1994) **32**:1768–72.

112. Chichili GR, Athmanathan S, Farhatullah S et al. Multiplex polymerase chain reaction for the detection of herpes simplex virus, varicella-zoster virus and cytomegalovirus in ocular specimens, *Curr Eye Res* (2003) **27**:85–90.

113. Elnifro EM, Cooper RJ, Klapper PE et al. Multiplex polymerase chain reaction for diagnosis of viral and chlamydial keratoconjunctivitis, *Invest Ophthalmol Vis Sci* (2000) **41**:1818–22.

114. Jackson R, Morris DJ, Cooper RJ et al. Multiplex polymerase chain reaction for adenovirus and herpes simplex virus in eye swabs, *J Virol Methods* (1996) **56**:41–8.

115. Welsh J, McClelland M. Fingerprinting genomes using PCR with arbitrary primers, *Nucleic Acids Res* (1990) **18**:7213–18.

116. Whitcombe D, Newton CR, Little S. Advances in approaches to DNA-based diagnostics, *Curr Opin Biotechnol* (1998) **9**:602–8.

117. Whitcombe D, Brownie J, Gillard HL et al. A homogeneous fluorescence assay for PCR amplicons: its application to real-time, single-tube genotyping, *Clin Chem* (1998) **44**:918–23.

118. Amann RI, Ludwig W, Schleifer KH. Phylogenetic identification and in situ detection of individual microbial cells without cultivation, *Microbiol Rev* (1995) **59**:143–69.

119. Pinna A, Sechi LA, Zanetti S et al. Adherence of ocular isolates of *Staphylococcus epidermidis* to ACRYSOF intraocular lenses. A scanning electron microscopy and molecular biology study, *Ophthalmology* (2000) **107**:2162–6.

120. Abreu JA, Cordoves L, Mesa CG et al. Chronic pseudophakic endophthalmitis versus saccular endophthalmitis, *J Cataract Refract Surg* (1997) **23**:1122–5.

121. Margo CE, Pavan PR, Groden LR. Chronic vitritis with macrophagic inclusions. A sequela of treated endophthalmitis due to a coryneform bacterium, *Ophthalmology* (1988) **95**:156–61.

122. Grenzebach UH, Busse H, Totsch M et al. Endophthalmitis induced by atypical mycobacterial infection, *Ger J Ophthalmol* (1996) **5**:202–6.

123. Dockholm-Dworniczak B, Grenzebach UH, Totsch M et al. [Detection of atypical mycobacterial

endophthalmitis by PCR], *Pathologe* (1996) **17**:115 [in German].

124. Knox CM, Cevallos V, Margolis TP et al. Identification of bacterial pathogens in patients with endophthalmitis by 16S ribosomal DNA typing, *Am J Ophthalmol* (1999) **128**:511–12.

125. Lohmann CP, Gabel VP, Heep M et al. *Listeria monocytogenes*-induced endogenous endophthalmitis in an otherwise healthy individual: rapid PCR-diagnosis as the basis for effective treatment, *Eur J Ophthalmol* (1999) **9**:53–7.

126. Goldstein DA, Mouritsen L, Friedlander S et al. Acute endogenous endophthalmitis due to *Bartonella henselae*, *Clin Infect Dis* (2001) **33**:718–21.

127. Fairfax MR, Metcalf MA, Cone RW. Slow inactivation of dry PCR templates by UV light, *PCR Methods Appl* (1991) **1**:142–3.

128. Cone RW, Fairfax MR. Protocol for ultraviolet irradiation of surfaces to reduce PCR contamination, *PCR Methods Appl* (1993) **3**:S15–S17.

129. Ou CY, Moore JL, Schochetman G. Use of UV irradiation to reduce false positivity in polymerase chain reaction, *Biotechniques* (1991) **10**:442, 444, 446.

130. Hughes MS, Beck LA, Skuce RA. Identification and elimination of DNA sequences in Taq DNA polymerase, *J Clin Microbiol* (1994) **32**:2007–8.

131. Rand KH, Houck H. Taq polymerase contains bacterial DNA of unknown origin, *Mol Cell Probes* (1990) **4**:445–50.

132. Cimino GD, Metchette KC, Tessman JW et al. Post-PCR sterilization: a method to control carryover contamination for the polymerase chain reaction, *Nucleic Acids Res* (1991) **19**:99–107.

133. Isaacs ST, Tessman JW, Metchette KC et al. Post-PCR sterilization: development and application to an HIV-1 diagnostic assay, *Nucleic Acids Res* (1991) **19**:109–16.

134. Espy MJ, Smith TF, Persing DH. Dependence of polymerase chain reaction product inactivation protocols on amplicon length and sequence composition, *J Clin Microbiol* (1993) **31**:2361–5.

135. Rys PN, Persing DH. Preventing false positives: quantitative evaluation of three protocols for inactivation of polymerase chain reaction amplification products, *J Clin Microbiol* (1993) **31**:2356–60.

136. Meier A, Persing DH, Finken M et al. Elimination of contaminating DNA within polymerase chain reaction reagents: implications for a general approach to detection of uncultured pathogens, *J Clin Microbiol* (1993) **31**:646–52.

137. Sharma S, Das D, Anand R et al. Reliability of nested polymerase chain reaction in the diagnosis of bacterial endophthalmitis, *Am J Ophthalmol* (2002) **133**:142–4.

138. Anand AR, Madhavan HN, Sudha NV et al. Polymerase chain reaction in the diagnosis of *Aspergillus* endophthalmitis, *Indian J Med Res* (2001) **114**:133–40.

139. Frelich VS, Murray DL, Goei S et al. *Neisseria meningitidis* endophthalmitis: use of polymerase chain reaction to support an etiologic diagnosis, *Pediatr Infect Dis J* (2003) **22**:288–90.

140. Asensio Sanchez VM, Perez Flandez FJ, Gil Fernandez E. [Endogenous *Serratia marcescens* endophthalmitis diagnosis with PCR], *Arch Soc Esp Oftalmol* (2003) **78**:281–3 [in Spanish].

4

Epidemiology

In the investigation of risk factors for infectious diseases, a basic understanding of epidemiological methods is required in order to avoid misinterpretation when comparing the results of one study with another. For example, crude rates should not be used to compare populations of different structure without definition. Similarly, it is not appropriate to draw population-related conclusions from studies of limited size and power. Criticism can also be made of those people producing population-based judgments from the results of a limited study sample; this is always dangerous. Definitions are summarized below.

Definitions

- *Epidemiology* is the study of disease in relation to populations. All findings must relate to a defined population. Epidemiology relates the pattern of disease to the population in which it occurs and requires study of both diseased and healthy persons. For epidemiology, incidence and prevalence rates form the basis for comparison between defined population groups.
- A *population* for epidemiology is a defined group of people including both *diseased* and *healthy* subjects, about whose health some statement is to be made.
- *Group orientation.* Clinical appearances determine decisions about individual patients. Epidemiological observations determine decisions about groups and are the basis for preventive medicine.
- *Incidence* is the proportion (1 in 1000) or percentage (%) with *new* disease, in a defined group occurring within a given time period. It is annualized unless otherwise expressed, but may be stated over any time period.

- *Prevalence* is the proportion or percentage with disease (including both *old* and *new*) of a defined group occurring at or over a specific time (may take place over a day, week, or month, etc.).
- *Error.* In epidemiology, statistical inference is valid only if the sample is truly representative of the population, and thus random, accepting that each individual has defined criteria. In addition, the control groups must have no inherent bias. One way of achieving this is to choose a sample at random from the whole population; however, this process is difficult without a sampling frame which is a list of the whole population. Hence, a selection has to be made and this is where error frequently arises.
- Implications of variability in epidemiology include random error and biased error:
  - In *random* error, individuals are apt to be incorrectly assessed or misclassified; this error is serious in clinical practice but is not so serious in epidemiology which is concerned with group decisions.
  - In *biased* error, the wrong groups are selected (usually the controls), which then distort comparisons – *an epidemiological disaster which cannot be corrected by statistics!* Using hospital-based rather than community-based controls for patients admitted to the hospital from the community often causes bias and should be avoided.
- In epidemiology, computed information is usually used. These data can have errors from:
  - *Imprecision* – information correctly entered into the computer but the data are wrong.
  - *Unreliability* – correct data entered into the computer incorrectly.

Disease outcome has to be assessed accurately. Clinical experience alone cannot predict prognosis and outcome. Important causes of bias which frequently occur are bias in the selection of cases, bias in the choice of medical therapy or surgical technique, and bias resulting from incomplete follow-up with unconfirmed assumptions about final outcomes.

Within a drug trial, sources of error that must be avoided include misallocation of interventions (wrong drug given to the wrong person) and poor compliance with drug administration (failure to give the drug as expected). These two sources of error should be prevented by careful study design and protocol enforcement with repeated quality assurance visits by the trial co-ordinator. Poor compliance means that the expected effect will not be realized.

Retrospective and prospective studies

Epidemiological methods for retrospective or prospective surveys are described below.

Descriptive study

A descriptive study lists a number of cases of infection, such as postcataract surgery (extracapsular cataract extraction [ECCE] or phacoemulsification) endophthalmitis, in a particular place over a time period and is often retrospective. The observations may suggest a variety of different causes for increased or decreased infection such as a reduced infection rate of postcataract surgery endophthalmitis with introduction of a foldable sterile intraocular lens (IOL) inserted through a sterile injector.[1] The authors identified the power limitations of their study but considered that their findings warranted further analysis in a large multicenter trial.

Others have suggested various risk factors for endophthalmitis following cataract surgery based on retrospective descriptive studies. Chitkara and Smerdon examined a large series of ECCE to determine risk factors for posterior capsule rupture with vitreous loss; risk factors included pseudoexfoliation, diabetes mellitus, and a traumatic etiology.[2] Norregaard et al in Denmark identified 19,426 patients who had first eye

cataract surgery between 1985 and 1987 of whom 61 (0.31%) had presumed clinical endophthalmitis following ECCE. Advanced age and male sex were associated risk factors.[3]

A descriptive study can be a useful start to investigate a particular problem, such as endophthalmitis following cataract surgery, but does not record the incidence or prevalence in the population at large. The assessment of risk factors is open to bias by the population attending the particular hospital and the surgical techniques used, i.e. the sample is not representative of the population at large. This type of study does provide a useful basis, however, on which to plan a case-control or cohort study; it is also cheap to perform. If the population from which the cases have been collected is known, it may be possible to calculate an approximate incidence figure from a large retrospective study such as that performed by Javitt et al in the USA (1991 Medicare Study).[4] The authors used cases of postoperative infection reported to the US Medicare funding organization as the numerator, and the total number of cataract surgeries that had been paid for as the denominator. The overall incidence of endophthalmitis following ECCE was 0.12%.

In another retrospective study in 1998, Aaberg et al reviewed the incidence of acute culture-proven postoperative (ECCE and phacoemulsification) endophthalmitis (occurring within 6 weeks of surgery) in their hospital over the previous 10 years from 1984 to 1994 when a rate was found of 0.082% (34 of 41,654 operations); 5 culture-negative patients who were not included comprised 12.8% of the total number of patients with presumed clinical endophthalmitis. The incidence was higher after secondary IOL implantation.[5] In Holland, a descriptive study based on a questionnaire survey in 2000 (refer to 'Use of Questionnaire Reporting Surveys' below), estimated the incidence of endophthalmitis after cataract surgery to be 0.11%; however, there was only a 51% response to the survey.[6] The authors attempted to estimate bias by under-reporting and calculated an expected nationwide incidence of 0.15%.

Other descriptive studies have suggested that the 'clear cornea' incision used in phacoemulsification cataract surgery might be associated with increased postoperative endophthalmitis, with incidence rates of 0.13% (5 cases out of 3886) and 0.66% (6 cases out of 912) for clear cornea incisions and 0.05% (5 cases out of 10,000) and 0.25% (1 case out of 397) for scleral tunnel incisions, respectively; however, these results were not statistically significant.[7,8] In addition, these studies were retrospective and not random-ized and so were open to bias in the choice of the incision by the surgeon. The two studies have also produced very different incidence rates. Such studies lack statistical power to draw population-based conclusions but can be improved by comparison between and within each other using a meta-analysis technique.[9]

Taban has recently performed such a meta-analysis.[9] He decided to compare postoperative rates of endophthalmitis following cataract surgery with those following penetrating kerato-plasty (PK, corneal graft) as a control group, assuming that changes in infection rates associ-ated with PK would reflect the changing practices and drugs used for antibiotic prophylaxis. Taban obtained 5000 papers on cataract surgery and 1900 reports on PK and selected 215 papers on cataract surgery, including 3 million patients, and 66 studies on PK including over 90,000 opera-tions, that fulfilled the study selection criteria; these studies were considered to be most repre-sentative of all the reports found. The overall endophthalmitis rate was three times higher for PK (0.38%) than for cataract surgery (0.13%).

Taban compared the endophthalmitis rate for cataract surgery before and after 1992, when Howard Fine introduced the clear cornea incision, and pre- and post-2000, by which time many cataract surgeons, perhaps half of them, were practicing with it. His analysis showed a correla-tion between increased use of the clear cornea incision and increased risk of endophthalmitis. This correlation was evident both qualitatively, using a weighted linear regression analysis and determination of the slope coefficient of plots of infection rates over time, as well as quantitatively, based on a relative risk comparison of pooled estimates of endophthalmitis rates between study periods and of different cataract incision techniques. There was a gradual trend downward of postcataract surgery endophthalmitis rates between 1961 and 1991 which was reversed between 1992 and 2003. In contrast, the opposite pattern was seen in the slope coefficients for the graphs of endophthalmitis following PK over time.

For the period 2000–2003, the rate of endoph-thalmitis after cataract surgery and use of the clear cornea incision reached 0.27%, representing a 2.5-fold increase over earlier years that was statisti-cally significant. However, there was no significant difference in the rates of endophthalmitis after cataract surgery with the limbal and scleral tunnel approaches for the same period.

Taban commented that his findings should be confirmed in a large-scale, prospective trial with defined inclusion criteria, which is being pursued currently by the ESCRS (see 'Longitudinal study' below). He accepted that there was bias resulting from the review of studies submitted or accepted for publication that can potentially affect the results of a meta-analysis which is inevitably retrospective. It can at best produce a hypothesis for further testing. This hypothesis includes the suggestion of poorer stability of the clear cornea wound than that of the scleral tunnel.

While these approaches within a health care system or specific hospital provide a guideline figure for historical incidence rates, they are unreliable for recording late-presenting cases of endophthalmitis and others that may be missed such as 'hypopyon uveitis' in which the diagno-sis is postoperative inflammation, which may itself be due to capsule bag (or saccular) infection with *Propionibacterium acnes* (Chapter 6). In addition, care must be taken in presenting results of descriptive studies as they are derived from the population sampled which may not be represen-tative of the population as a whole.

Case-control study

A case-control study compares those with and without the disease who are suitably matched. The study should include only incident cases of disease, i.e. *new* cases of infection that develop during the study and not chronic cases of long duration before the study started. Case-control studies are usually prospective but may be retro-spective as well. Diagnostic criteria must be well defined and, for cases of infection, should be Gram- or other stain-positive and/or culture-positive or involve microbial antigen recognition (antibody-based or DNA by a polymerase chain reaction [PCR technique, Chapter 3]). Patients who have developed a disease such as postoper-ative endophthalmitis are compared with controls who have not developed the disease when risk factors can be identified reliably.[10,11] A case-control study permits estimation of odds ratio statistics but not the population attributable risk.[12]

Allowance must be made for potential confounding factors. The most important point to note is that the controls *must* match the patients, so that for example if the patients enter the hospital from a UK-wide community, then the controls must be selected likewise. If those selected as controls are all from the hospital or its local area, there will be potentially serious bias. Controls are best matched to each patient for age, sex, and location of residence; however, some studies, such as those of contact lens wearers, require controls to be matched as well for educational status, income, and type of housing.[13]

Use of a case-control study to compare different groups of people developing endophthalmitis after cataract surgery is effective for investigating different risk factors within a defined group, and is not too costly. However, it does *not* identify the frequency of the infection in the population, i.e. neither the number of new cases (incidence) nor the proportion present at any time (prevalence) is measured.

If risk factors of postoperative endophthalmitis are predicted from a case-control study, such as those listed by Menikoff et al[10] and Montan et al,[11] including rupture of the posterior capsule to give communication with the vitreous cavity, use of IOLs with haptics made of polypropylene, immunosuppressive treatment, wound abnormality, and the use of IOLs without a heparinized surface, then the findings need corroboration in a population-based study. A population-based study is needed because of confounding factors that include possible bias both in the controls selected and in the population of patients being investigated. In some studies, this may relate to geographical location (high or low altitude), climate (humid or dry and hot, warm or cold), and the insect population. It is dangerous to extrapolate the findings of a case-control study in one place to the population at large: the results only apply to the precise population studied and other inferences can be unreliable. For example, fungus infections are much more common in a hot, wet climate but not in a hot urban, high-density, built-up environment such as Kowloon and Shatin, Hong Kong.[14]

A case-control study is best conducted prospectively with random selection of patients and controls for the procedures to be used. For example, Nagaki et al[15] compared rates of postoperative endophthalmitis following phacoemulsification surgery between those who were operated on through a 'clear cornea' incision with those who were operated on through a scleral tunnel in a prospectively planned study in their hospital. They found that there was a postoperative endophthalmitis rate of 0.29% (11 presumed [9 culture-proven] out of 3831 eyes) for the clear temporal cornea incision group (A) and 0.05% (4 presumed [4 culture-proven] out of 7764 eyes) for those who had surgery via a superior scleral tunnel approach (groups B and C). The relative risk of postoperative endophthalmitis proven by culture in the scleral tunnel group was 4.6 times lower than the clear cornea group (p = 0.037). Their findings infer that the clear cornea incision is a risk factor for postoperative infection. They also compared an acrylic IOL (Alcon, MA60BM) with a silicone IOL (Allergan, SI-40NB) and found no difference with the use of these two materials in influencing the postoperative endophthalmitis rate. However, as the authors only had approximately 4000 patients in each of three groups, the statistical power of their study was limited so that the results, although of great interest, require confirmation in a larger multicenter trial.

The application of a case-control study is also given in the section below on 'Statistical methods to analyze clusters of cases of endophthalmitis following cataract surgery.'

Longitudinal study

A longitudinal study examines associations between exposure to suspected causes of disease and morbidity (the actual disease). The simplest type of longitudinal study is the cohort study, when those subjects exposed to one or a number of risk factors and those not exposed are followed up prospectively in a defined community-based population study over a period of time. This method measures the incidence of disease in each group in the community and can therefore measure the relative risk of the different exposures, together with the population attributable risk.[16] Cohort studies are time-consuming, costly, and therefore reserved for testing precisely formulated hypotheses that have been previously explored by descriptive and/or case-control studies, which are used for initial exploratory investigations.

A cohort study concentrates on risk factors related to the development of disease. The length of the study depends on the number of new cases of disease and on the duration of the induction period between risk and the occurrence of the disease; large numbers are needed to gain sufficient statistical power to detect the smallest effect of interest. Retrospective cohort studies may be possible if the necessary data have already been collected from the population.

The European Society of Cataract and Refractive Surgeons (ESCRS) study is prospective, randomized, multicenter and partially placebo-controled, with a classic Fisher 2×2 factorial design[16] similar to that used for the Endophthalmitis Vitrectomy Study (EVS).[17,18] This study compares the use of perioperative 0.9% saline drops with topical 0.5% levofloxacin drops and use of intracameral cefuroxime (1 mg in 0.1 ml) versus no injection, and the combination of each. The ESCRS study started in October 2003 and will last 2 years. The study, which is taking place in 16 operating centers in 8 European countries, will involve about 30,000 patients having phacoemulsification cataract surgery randomized into blocks of 12, with each of four treatment regimes replicating three times within each block. Data collection is electronic and includes full surgical details to assess the effect of incision and IOL type on the postoperative endophthalmitis rate as well as many other details. Finally, this study will provide a reliable figure for endophthalmitis rates following phacoemulsification surgery for the first time.

Cross-sectional study

A cross-sectional study measures the prevalence of any disease, condition, functional impairment, or health outcome in a population at a point in time or over a short period. The prevalence is the proportion afflicted by that defined clinical state at any one point in time. Prevalence is estimated using sample surveys which can introduce bias, as discussed below.[19]

Sampling involves selection of a representative fraction of the population. For example, it can be used to assess the prevalence (that is, the proportion) of ischemic heart disease in different workers in a factory in order to alter their risk of myocardial infarction by reducing the stress of those with the highest prevalence figure. The cross-sectional study considers *existing* disease, as contrasted with the *development* of disease in a cohort study. Care is required in detecting known existing cases because they may not be representative of all cases of the disease, i.e. in the example above, detection of myocardial insufficiency is dependent on the test method used and does not necessarily predict those who will develop acute disease (in this example, myocardial infarction). Furthermore, cases of chronic disease of long duration are over-represented in a cross-sectional study.[19]

A cross-sectional study may be used to initiate a cohort study by defining the population at risk such as the type of contact lens worn or ocular trauma suffered prior to the development of microbial keratitis; it does not replace the cohort study, which measures the incidence and risk factors of *new* cases of the disease under study.

Use of questionnaire reporting surveys

Current standards of practice for cataract surgery in the aging population involve the full range of choice from nonuse of antibiotics to their application pre-, intra-, and postoperatively, delivered either intra- or extraocularly. There is considerable debate over the possible effectiveness of antibiotic prophylaxis. As yet, there has been no result of a large prospective randomized multicenter study in either Europe or the USA, so that all results to date of antibiotic prophylaxis have been limited in statistical power or else open to bias in selection of patient, surgical technique, environment, or drug.[20,21]

There have been questionnaire reporting surveys of antibiotic use for prophylaxis of endophthalmitis following cataract surgery in Germany,[22] the USA,[23] and Australia[24] in the last 5 years but only approximately 66% of surgeons polled by post returned their questionnaire, with the exception of the Australians, for whom the figure was 89%. Two of these three surveys did suggest that subconjunctival antibiotics as commonly given immediately after cataract surgery did not significantly reduce the incidence of endophthalmitis, further corroborated by the evidence-based review of Ciulla et al.[21] This finding of 'no' evidence to support the use of subconjunctival antibiotics in preventing endophthalmitis is disputed by the findings of Colleaux et al[7] in their retrospective review which found 1 case out of 8856 surgeries (0.011% incidence rate) using subconjunctival antibiotics and 9 out of 5030 surgeries (0.179% incidence rate) in those not using subconjunctival antibiotics. This was statistically significant (p < 0.009) but open to bias as regards the type of incision used and type of patient included, as it was not a prospective randomized study. A similar experience, however, is described below.[25]

These questionnaire surveys also suggested that the use of intraocular antibiotics during surgery, given as a supplement in the irrigation fluid, often with vancomycin (20 mg/l) and/or gentamicin (8 mg/l), produced the lowest (unproven) incidence rates of postoperative endophthalmitis. The Australian survey found an incidence rate of postoperative endophthalmitis of 0.11% with no relationship with antibiotic prophylaxis; however, more experienced surgeons had fewer cases of postoperative endophthalmitis.

The danger with a low response rate to a survey, where the sample surveyed has been carefully chosen to be representative of the population under study, is that it may introduce *non response* bias.[19] An absurd but extreme example of this would be to conduct a survey investigating death rates during a year and to ask the question, 'Are you still alive?' All those responding would say 'Yes,' but it would not be safe to infer from this questionnaire survey that the death rate was zero.

A less extreme example would be to ask, 'Have you ever used illicit drugs?' It is very likely that those people who have made use of the drugs will be less willing to respond affirmatively and more likely to lie than those people who have not used them. Nonresponse bias will reinforce the bias already present because of the tendency to lie.

Questionnaire surveys distributed by post do not usually provide a response rate above 66%. Without some check of the likely effect of nonresponse bias, the results of such surveys will remain 'questionable' in many cases. One way to validate such a survey is to choose a manageably small but representative sample of all those surveyed who failed to respond initially and to obtain responses from them. From the results of this exercise, an estimate of the nonresponse bias in the full survey can be made and used to correct the crude results. In addition, this estimate of the nonresponse bias will itself be subject to random sampling error as well as nonresponse bias, which will lead to further loss of precision in the final corrected estimates from the full survey. Wormald has commented that the minimum response rate should be 80% and that all non responders needed to be pursued.[19] He also stated that the survey organizer should be aware of the characteristics of those who persistently fail to respond and of the bias that this introduces to the survey.

Any result from a questionnaire reporting survey with only a 66% response rate that has not been corrected as discussed above, which gives a 'significant' result at the 95% level (p < 0.05), should be regarded as 'highly suspect.' This situation arises because of the chance that the non responders would, if included, give results which would mean that this significance level would not be achieved. A 99% significance level (p < 0.01) should be considered the minimum level to be acceptable from an uncorrected questionnaire reporting survey with only a 66% response rate. Even then, the study should have included a poll of nonresponders. If the nonresponse bias remains unknown, then the results of a questionnaire reporting survey with only a 66% response rate can be considered 'interesting' but not statistically or epidemiologically valid.

Is 'no' evidence of a beneficial effect as good as evidence?

Low rates of postoperative endophthalmitis of 0.06% have been produced in Sweden in over 50,000 patients using cefuroxime 1 mg in 0.1 ml as an intracameral injection into the anterior chamber at the end of cataract surgery.[26] This study for the introduction of intracameral cefuroxime was a retrospective analysis which was not randomized or placebo-controlled. As there has been no reliable prospective randomized placebo-controlled study, these figures for prophylaxis by an intraocular antibiotic and those from other studies, including subconjunctival use of gentamicin and cefazolin,[7] have been considered 'unreliable' in a recent review of evidence-based medicine on this subject.[21] The study by Colleaux et al was the first to find a difference between no use and subconjunctival use of antibiotics for cataract surgery, with postoperative endophthalmitis rates of 0.179% and 0.011%, respectively, but the size of the study was too limited to justify these figures without doubt.[7]

Based on the lack of evidence for the beneficial effect of prophylactic antibiotics as described above and from 'apparent' results of the questionnaire reporting surveys, as well as the experience of patients developing postoperative endophthalmitis who had received subconjunctival injections of antibiotics, one surgeon recently withdrew the routine use of prophylactic subconjunctival cefuroxime 125 mg given at the end of surgery;[25] in addition, no preoperative or postoperative antibiotics were used but povidone iodine prophylaxis was given at the time of surgery to disinfect the ocular surface. The result was 7 cases of postoperative cataract surgery endophthalmitis out of 427 patients compared with 0 out of 1073 patients operated on by colleagues in the same unit who continued giving subconjunctival injections of cefuroxime immediately after surgery.

The surgeon stopped operating, reviewed surgical technique, and then restarted with reintroduction of subconjunctival cefuroxime, after which there were no further cases of postoperative endophthalmitis after another 1350 operations.[25] This interesting situation demonstrates that while a questionnaire reporting survey with a response rate of 66% or a literature review of evidence-based medicine may fail to provide evidence of the effectiveness of prophylactic antibiotics, this does not mean that such antibiotic prophylaxis is in fact of no benefit. The likely problem here was the lack of reliability of the questionnaire reporting survey as an epidemiological tool, as described above. In addition, the variable effect of surgical technique for a clear cornea incision or scleral tunnel approach was not properly considered in the evidence reviewed,[21] because of a lack of relevant studies on which the evidence-based review depends; this lack is the weak link in the latter type of study.

The clear cornea incision used for phacoemulsification has since been suggested to be possibly more likely to be associated with postoperative endophthalmitis.[8,9] This type of incision may thus benefit from prophylactic antibiotics more than the scleral tunnel approach. This example emphasizes the need to constantly evaluate epidemiological and study-based data for inherent errors either in the study design or the methods being used, or their application in practice which will produce misleading results for others to practice. Clinicians should always question studies that fail to show any benefit of a particular technique; it may be the study and not the technique that is at fault.

Assessment of statistical associations

When a significant result is obtained, the following questions should always be considered.

- Was the result due to bias? Have the wrong controls been selected? Have hospital controls been used for community patients? Is there bias in patient selection or in patient referral to the hospital? Is there bias in the selection of the controls? In a questionnaire study, is there nonresponse bias?
- Could the result be due to chance? The confidence intervals should always be calculated and the degree of statistical significance considered. Statistics define the degree of chance but do not abolish it altogether.
- Are there any unsuspected confounding factors at play? These factors may involve unsuspected secondary microbial contamination such as bacterial contamination of sterile instruments, perhaps because they are not being washed properly. Where and why patients become infected must always be considered. Is the organism or the host at fault?
- Does the significance level calculated represent a real effect for a risk factor or a confounding one that may be associated with the infection but is not the primary cause of it? Have the correct statistical methods been used? Should the data have been stratified before analysis? Is there a better statistical model by which to analyze the results of the study? Are the results suitable for analysis by

multivariate or logistical regression analysis? Would Bayesian methods be more applicable than frequentist ones?

Statistical methods to analyze clusters of cases of endophthalmitis following cataract surgery

An increasing number of cases of postoperative endophthalmitis after cataract surgery present an urgent situation for a surgeon. There is an immediate need to establish whether the numbers of cases are caused by chance or by the development of an outbreak due to a particular cause, such as a sterilization failure. Samples of aqueous humor or vitreous should be collected for both microbiology and molecular biology examinations and the organism should be identified if at all possible (Chapter 3). Typically, different types of coagulase-negative staphylococci (CNS), a *Staphylococcus aureus* and a streptococcus may be isolated from such patients (Chapters 3 and 6).

Statistical analysis is needed to evaluate the number of cases of endophthalmitis considering the number of operations performed. There is a long-standing argument for a frequentist[27] versus a Bayesian[25,28–32] approach. In either case, comparison is made with the expected postoperative endophthalmitis rate experienced by others which may itself vary by technique and country. The classical approach starts from a null hypothesis that the infection process follows a given model (say the binomial distribution or a Poisson approximation to it) with a given assumed rate. From this the probability of a result as extreme as that observed is calculated (the p-value) and if this is smaller than some threshold significance level the null hypothesis is rejected and it is taken that the rate is different from the expected norm.

To make this determination more simple, Tables 4.1–4.5 have been constructed for postoperative endophthalmitis rates of 0.05, 0.1, 0.2, 0.3, and 0.5%, for between 50 and 5000 operations, and for 1 to 6 cases of postoperative endophthalmitis.[27] The number of cases of postoperative endophthalmitis for the number of operated patients can then be found in the appropriate table and the probability gained (p value) for the occurrence being the result of chance. A figure of

Table 4.1 Probabilities of observing X cases (or more) during N operations, where cases are expected to occur with a Poisson frequency at a rate of 5 per 10,000 operations (1:2000 or 0.05%)

No. of operations	Cases observed (X or more)					
	$X \geq 1$	$X \geq 2$	$X \geq 3$	$X \geq 4$	$X \geq 5$	$X \geq 6$
50	0.0247	0.0003	0.0000	0.0000	0.0000	0.0000
100	0.0488	0.0012	0.0000	0.0000	0.0000	0.0000
150	0.0723	0.0027	0.0001	0.0000	0.0000	0.0000
200	0.0952	0.0047	0.0002	0.0000	0.0000	0.0000
250	0.1175	0.0072	0.0003	0.0000	0.0000	0.0000
300	0.1393	0.0102	0.0005	0.0000	0.0000	0.0000
350	0.1605	0.0136	0.0008	0.0000	0.0000	0.0000
400	0.1813	0.0175	0.0011	0.0001	0.0000	0.0000
450	0.2015	0.0218	0.0016	0.0001	0.0000	0.0000
500	0.2212	0.0265	0.0022	0.0001	0.0000	0.0000
550	0.2404	0.0315	0.0028	0.0002	0.0000	0.0000
600	0.2592	0.0369	0.0036	0.0003	0.0000	0.0000
700	0.2953	0.0487	0.0055	0.0005	0.0000	0.0000
800	0.3297	0.0616	0.0079	0.0008	0.0001	0.0000
900	0.3624	0.0754	0.0109	0.0012	0.0001	0.0000
1000	0.3935	0.0902	0.0144	0.0018	0.0002	0.0000
2000	0.6321	0.2642	0.0803	0.0190	0.0037	0.0006
3000	0.7769	0.4422	0.1912	0.0656	0.0186	0.0045
4000	0.8647	0.5940	0.3233	0.1429	0.0527	0.0166
5000	0.9179	0.7127	0.4562	0.2424	0.1088	0.0420

Table 4.2 Probabilities of observing X cases (or more) during N operations, where cases are expected to occur with a Poisson frequency at a rate of 10 per 10,000 operations (1:1000 or 0.1%)

No. of operations	Cases observed (X or more)					
	X≥1	X≥2	X≥3	X≥4	X≥5	X≥6
50	0.0488	0.0012	0.0000	0.0000	0.0000	0.0000
100	0.0952	0.0047	0.0002	0.0000	0.0000	0.0000
150	0.1393	0.0102	0.0005	0.0000	0.0000	0.0000
200	0.1813	0.0175	0.0011	0.0001	0.0000	0.0000
250	0.2212	0.0265	0.0022	0.0001	0.0000	0.0000
300	0.2592	0.0369	0.0036	0.0003	0.0000	0.0000
350	0.2953	0.0487	0.0055	0.0005	0.0000	0.0000
400	0.3297	0.0616	0.0079	0.0008	0.0001	0.0000
450	0.3624	0.0754	0.0109	0.0012	0.0001	0.0000
500	0.3935	0.0902	0.0144	0.0018	0.0002	0.0000
550	0.4231	0.1057	0.0185	0.0025	0.0003	0.0000
600	0.4512	0.1219	0.0231	0.0034	0.0004	0.0000
700	0.5034	0.1558	0.0341	0.0058	0.0008	0.0001
800	0.5507	0.1912	0.0474	0.0091	0.0014	0.0002
900	0.5934	0.2275	0.0629	0.0135	0.0023	0.0003
1000	0.6321	0.2642	0.0803	0.0190	0.0037	0.0006
2000	0.8647	0.5940	0.3233	0.1429	0.0527	0.0166
3000	0.9502	0.8009	0.5768	0.3528	0.1847	0.0839
4000	0.9817	0.9084	0.7619	0.5665	0.3712	0.2149
5000	0.9933	0.9596	0.8753	0.7350	0.5595	0.3840

Table 4.3 Probabilities of observing X cases (or more) during N operations, where cases are expected to occur with a Poisson frequency at a rate of 20 per 10,000 operations (1:500 or 0.2%)

No. of operations	Cases observed (X or more)					
	X≥1	X≥2	X≥3	X≥4	X≥5	X≥6
50	0.0952	0.0047	0.0002	0.0000	0.0000	0.0000
100	0.1813	0.0175	0.0011	0.0001	0.0000	0.0000
150	0.2592	0.0369	0.0036	0.0003	0.0000	0.0000
200	0.3297	0.0616	0.0079	0.0008	0.0001	0.0000
250	0.3935	0.0902	0.0144	0.0018	0.0002	0.0000
300	0.4512	0.1219	0.0231	0.0034	0.0004	0.0000
350	0.5034	0.1558	0.0341	0.0058	0.0008	0.0001
400	0.5507	0.1912	0.0474	0.0091	0.0014	0.0002
450	0.5934	0.2275	0.0629	0.0135	0.0023	0.0003
500	0.6321	0.2642	0.0803	0.0190	0.0037	0.0006
550	0.6671	0.3010	0.0996	0.0257	0.0054	0.0010
600	0.6988	0.3374	0.1205	0.0338	0.0077	0.0015
700	0.7534	0.4082	0.1665	0.0537	0.0143	0.0032
800	0.7981	0.4751	0.2166	0.0788	0.0237	0.0060
900	0.8347	0.5372	0.2694	0.1087	0.0364	0.0104
1000	0.8647	0.5940	0.3233	0.1429	0.0527	0.0166
2000	0.9817	0.9084	0.7619	0.5665	0.3712	0.2149
3000	0.9975	0.9826	0.9380	0.8488	0.7149	0.5543
4000	0.9997	0.9970	0.9862	0.9576	0.9004	0.8088
5000	1.0000	0.9995	0.9972	0.9897	0.9707	0.9329

Table 4.4 Probabilities of observing X cases (or more) during N operations, where cases are expected to occur with a Poisson frequency at a rate of 30 per 10,000 operations (1:333 or 0.3%)

No. of operations	Cases observed (X or more)					
	X≥1	X≥2	X≥3	X≥4	X≥5	X≥6
50	0.1393	0.0102	0.0005	0.0000	0.0000	0.0000
100	0.2592	0.0369	0.0036	0.0003	0.0000	0.0000
150	0.3624	0.0754	0.0109	0.0012	0.0001	0.0000
200	0.4512	0.1219	0.0231	0.0034	0.0004	0.0000
250	0.5276	0.1734	0.0405	0.0073	0.0011	0.0001
300	0.5934	0.2275	0.0629	0.0135	0.0023	0.0003
350	0.6501	0.2826	0.0897	0.0222	0.0045	0.0008
400	0.6988	0.3374	0.1205	0.0338	0.0077	0.0015
450	0.7408	0.3908	0.1546	0.0482	0.0124	0.0027
500	0.7769	0.4422	0.1912	0.0656	0.0186	0.0045
550	0.8080	0.4911	0.2296	0.0859	0.0265	0.0070
600	0.8347	0.5372	0.2694	0.1087	0.0364	0.0104
700	0.8775	0.6204	0.3504	0.1614	0.0621	0.0204
800	0.9093	0.6916	0.4303	0.2213	0.0959	0.0357
900	0.9328	0.7513	0.5064	0.2859	0.1371	0.0567
1000	0.9502	0.8009	0.5768	0.3528	0.1847	0.0839
2000	0.9975	0.9826	0.9380	0.8488	0.7149	0.5543
3000	0.9999	0.9988	0.9938	0.9788	0.9450	0.8843
4000	1.0000	0.9999	0.9995	0.9977	0.9924	0.9797
5000	1.0000	1.0000	1.0000	0.9998	0.9991	0.9972

Table 4.5 Probabilities of observing X cases (or more) during N operations, where cases are expected to occur with a Poisson frequency at a rate of 50 per 10,000 operations (1:200 or 0.5%)

No. of operations	Cases observed (X or more)					
	X≥1	X≥2	X≥3	X≥4	X≥5	X≥6
50	0.2212	0.0265	0.0022	0.0001	0.0000	0.0000
100	0.3935	0.0902	0.0144	0.0018	0.0002	0.0000
150	0.5276	0.1734	0.0405	0.0073	0.0011	0.0001
200	0.6321	0.2642	0.0803	0.0190	0.0037	0.0006
250	0.7135	0.3554	0.1315	0.0383	0.0091	0.0018
300	0.7769	0.4422	0.1912	0.0656	0.0186	0.0045
350	0.8262	0.5221	0.2560	0.1008	0.0329	0.0091
400	0.8647	0.5940	0.3233	0.1429	0.0527	0.0166
450	0.8946	0.6575	0.3907	0.1906	0.0780	0.0274
500	0.9179	0.7127	0.4562	0.2424	0.1088	0.0420
550	0.9361	0.7603	0.5185	0.2970	0.1446	0.0608
600	0.9502	0.8009	0.5768	0.3528	0.1847	0.0839
700	0.9698	0.8641	0.6792	0.4634	0.2746	0.1424
800	0.9817	0.9084	0.7619	0.5665	0.3712	0.2149
900	0.9889	0.9389	0.8264	0.6577	0.4679	0.2971
1000	0.9933	0.9596	0.8753	0.7350	0.5595	0.3840
2000	1.0000	0.9995	0.9972	0.9897	0.9707	0.9329
3000	1.0000	1.0000	1.0000	0.9998	0.9991	0.9972
4000	1.0000	1.0000	1.0000	1.0000	1.0000	0.9999
5000	1.0000	1.0000	1.0000	1.0000	1.0000	1.0000

0.05 (5% chance) is just significant, 0.02 (2% chance) more so, and 0.01 (1% chance) or less is highly significant and suggests a problem with an autoclave or other sterility failure with bacterial contamination of instruments as one possibility.

A new approach to investigate the problem of ongoing or increasing numbers of postoperative endophthalmitis cases uses the concept of 'traffic lights' as targets.[27] The 'traffic light system' is based on the statistical theory above which states that if an event is occurring randomly at a specified rate, then the probability of observing a given number of cases is defined by the Poisson distribution. The practical application involves referring to one of the five tables (Tables 4.1–4.5), according to the expected postoperative infection rate, and discontinuing surgery when a threshold has been reached for the probability being due to chance of less than 2%. Investigation of the infection control procedures and sterilization of instruments should take place, consideration should be given to the use of prophylactic antibiotics (Chapters 5, 6 and 11), and then surgery is recommenced. If further cases occur, then the 'traffic light system' is applied again and surgery continues until the likelihood of its occurrence being the result of chance is less than 2%, again by referring to Tables 4.1–4.5. In this way the decision to stop or start performing surgery can be based on probability levels that exclude cases that might be the result of random chance.

An additional approach used to investigate the above study[27] was to perform a case-control study by comparing the 11 cases of postoperative endophthalmitis with 49 controls, randomly selected from the possible 1212 patients who had similar operations in the unit but did not develop postoperative endophthalmitis. A series of univariate analyses was carried out using Fisher's exact test followed by stepwise logistic regression using both forward and backward conditional methods to examine the independent effect of each variable on endophthalmitis. These analyses showed that there was a higher risk of endophthalmitis associated with being female, having a vitrectomy or a previous history of respiratory disease. A similar predominance of female patients was found by Montan et al in the Swedish prophylaxis study using intracameral cefuroxime.[26]

An alternative approach is to use Bayesian methodology[25,28–32] that involves establishing a 'prior,' a 'likelihood,' and a 'posterior distribution.' For a 'prior' to be taken seriously, its evidential basis must be given explicitly.[28] In addition to defining their prior, investigators should quote briefly (with some technical detail) the algebra involved, and what analytical form was used for the prior distribution. They should choose, for example, from a Weibull distribution or a Gamma distribution or other possibilities. Bayesian methods are appropriate for use here; however, they involve a completely different methodological approach. Nevertheless, these methods, if properly applied, have a logical consistency about them which, with proper grounds on which to base a prior, may be superior to the traditional frequentist approach, but full details must be explicitly given.

The recent outbreak study in Scotland used the traditional frequentist approach[27] while that in England used the alternative Bayesian approach.[25] The authors of the latter study criticized the use of the Poisson approximation to the binomial distribution used in the former study but freely admitted that use of this approximation is satisfactory. They found that use of the Bayesian method for the exact distribution led to the same conclusion as using the Poisson approximation. The use of the Poisson approximation has allowed the calculation of values given in Tables 4.1–4.5, allowing readers to quickly establish if their cases are likely due to an outbreak when surgery should stop for assessment.[27] The Bayesian/frequentist debate is a long-standing one and is not easy to resolve.

References

1. Mayer E, Cadman D, Ewings P et al. A 10 year retrospective study of cataract surgery and endophthalmitis in a single eye unit: injectable lenses lower the incidence of endophthalmitis, *Br J Ophthalmol* (2003) **87**:867–9.

2. Chitkara DK, Smerdon DL. Risk factors, complications, and results in extracapsular cataract extraction, *J Cataract Refract Surg* (1997) **23**:570–4.

3. Norregaard JC, Thoning H, Bernth-Petersen P et al. Risk of endophthalmitis after cataract extraction: results from the International Cataract Surgery Outcomes study, *Br J Ophthalmol* (1997) **81**:102–6.

4. Javitt JC, Vitale S, Canner JK et al. National outcomes of cataract extraction. Endophthalmitis

following inpatient surgery, *Arch Ophthalmol* (1991) **109**:1085–9.

5. Aaberg TM Jr, Flynn HW Jr, Schiffman J et al. Nosocomial acute-onset postoperative endophthalmitis survey. A 10-year review of incidence and outcomes, *Ophthalmology* (1998) **105**:1004–10.

6. Versteegh MFL, van Rij G. Incidence of endophthalmitis after cataract surgery in the Netherlands: several surgical techniques compared, *Doc Ophthalmol* (2000) **100**:1–6.

7. Colleaux KM, Hamilton WK. Effect of prophylactic antibiotics and incision type on the incidence of endophthalmitis after cataract surgery, *Can J Ophthalmol* (2000) **35**:373–8.

8. Thurber LT, Chalfin S, Kavanagh JT. Incidence of postoperative endophthalmitis in clear corneal and scleral tunnel incisions for phacoemulsification cataract surgery. Presented at the Association for Research in Vision and Ophthalmology, Fort Lauderdale, FL, 2003. Abstract 189.

9. Taban M. Clear cornea incisions implicated in endophthalmitis: a meta-analysis. Presented at the American Academy of Ophthalmology, Anaheim, CA, 2003, and reported in Escrs Eurotimes Jan 2004.

10. Menikoff JA, Speaker MG, Marmor M et al. A case-control study of risk factors for postoperative endophthalmitis, *Ophthalmology* (1991) **98**: 1761–8.

11. Montan PG, Koranyi G, Setterquist HE et al. Endophthalmitis after cataract surgery: risk factors relating to technique and events of the operation and patient history: a retrospective case-control study, *Ophthalmology* (1998) **105**:2171–7.

12. Friedman GD. *Primer of Epidemiology*, 4th edn (McGraw-Hill: New York, 1994.)

13. Lam DS, Houang E, Fan DS et al. Incidence and risk factors for microbial keratitis in Hong Kong: comparison with Europe and North America, *Eye* (2002) **16**: 608–18.

14. Houang E, Lam D, Fan D et al. Microbial keratitis in Hong Kong – relationship to climate, environment and contact-lens disinfection, *Trans R Soc Trop Med Hyg* (2001) **95**:361–7.

15. Nagaki Y, Hayasaka S, Kadoi C et al. Bacterial endophthalmitis after small-incision cataract surgery. Effect of incision placement and intraocular lens type, *J Cataract Refract Surg* (2003) **29**:20–6.

16. Fisher RA. *The Design of Experiments*, 1st edn (Oliver & Boyd: London, 1935).

17. Endophthalmitis Vitrectomy Study Group. Results of the Endophthalmitis Vitrectomy Study. A randomized trial of immediate vitrectomy and of intravenous antibiotics for the treatment of postoperative bacterial endophthalmitis, *Arch Ophthalmol* (1995) **113**:1479–96.

18. Han DP, Wisniewski SR, Wilson LA et al. Spectrum and susceptibilities of microbiologic isolates in the Endophthalmitis Vitrectomy Study, *Am J Ophthalmol* (1996) **122**:1–17 [erratum appears in *Am J Ophthalmol* (1996) **122**:920].

19. Wormald R. Assessing the prevalence of eye disease in the community, *Eye* (1995) **9**:674–6.

20. Liesegang TJ. Prophylactic antibiotics in cataract operations, *Mayo Clin Proc* (1997) **72**:149–59.

21. Ciulla TA, Starr MB, Masket S. Bacterial endophthalmitis prophylaxis for cataract surgery. An evidence-based update, *Ophthalmology* (2002) **109**:13–24.

22. Schmitz S, Dick HB, Krummenauer F et al. Endophthalmitis in cataract surgery. Results of a German survey, *Ophthalmology* (1999) **106**: 1869–7.

23. Masket S. Questionnaire survey of cataract surgery practice in the USA. Presented to the Annual Meeting of the ASCRS, 1998.

24. Morlet N, Gatus B, Coroneo M. Patterns of perioperative prophylaxis for cataract surgery: a survey of Australian ophthalmologists, *Aust NZ J Ophthalmol* (1998) **26**:5–12.

25. Mandal K, Hildreth A, Farrow M et al. An investigation into post-operative endophthalmitis and lessons learned, *J Cataract Refract Surg* (2004) **30**:1960–5.

26. Montan PG, Wejde G, Koranyi G et al. Prophylactic intracameral cefuroxime. Efficacy in preventing endophthalmitis following cataract surgery, *J Cataract Refract Surg* (2002) **28**:977–81.

27. Allardice GM, Wright EM, Peterson M et al. A statistical approach to an outbreak of endophthalmitis following cataract surgery at a hospital in the West of Scotland, *J Hosp Infect* (2001) **49**:23–9.

28. Spiegelhalter DJ, Myles JP, Jones DR et al. Bayesian methods in health technology assessment: a review, *Health Technol Assess* (2000) **4**: 1–130.

29. Spiegelhalter DJ, Myles JP, Jones DR et al. Methods in health service research. An introduction to Bayesian methods in health technology assessment, *BMJ* (1999) **319**: 508–12.

30. Bland JM, Altman DG. Bayesians and frequentists, *BMJ* (1998) **317**:1151–60.

31. Matthews RAJ. Why should clinicians care about Bayesian methods? *J Statist Plan Infer* (2001) **94**:43–58; discussion 59–71.

32. Lee PM. *Bayesian Statistics: An Introduction*, 2nd edn (Arnold: London, 1997).

Further reading

Berger JO, Boukai B, Wang W. Unified frequentist and Bayesian testing of precise hypotheses, *Statist Sci* (1997) **12**:133–60.

Coggon D, Rose G, Barker DJP. *Epidemiology for the Uninitiated,* 5th edn (BMJ Publishing Group: London, 2003).

Johnson GA, Minassian D, Weale R et al. *Epidemiology of Eye Disease*, 2nd edn (Arnold: London, 2003).

Jones B, Teather D, Wang J et al. A comparison of various estimators of a treatment difference for a multi-centre clinical trial, *Stat Med* (1998) **17**:1767–77, 1799–800.

Lewsey JD, Leyland AH, Murray GD et al. Using routine data to complement and enhance the results of randomised controlled trials, *Health Technol Assess* (2000) **4**:1–55.

Lilford RJ, Braunholtz D. The statistical basis of public policy: a paradigm shift is overdue, *BMJ* (1996) **313**:603–7.

Matthews DE, Farewell VT. *Using and Understanding Medical Statistics*, 3rd edn (Karger: Basel, 1996).

O'Hagan A. *Kendall's Advanced Theory of Statistics, Vol. 2B: Bayesian Inference* (Arnold: London, 1994).

Puri BK. *Statistics in Practice. An Illustrated Guide to SPSS* (Arnold: London, 1996).

Rowntree D. *Statistics Without Tears* (Penguin Books: London, 1991).

Selke T, Bayarri MJ, Berger JO. Calibration of p-values for testing precise null hypotheses, *American Statistician* (2001) **55**:62–71.

Whitehead J. A unified theory for sequential clinical trials, *Stat Med* (1999) **18**:2271–86.

5

Pharmacokinetics

The science of pharmacokinetics mathematically describes drug behavior in living tissue, providing a basis for understanding how best to achieve a desired pharmacological response. Drug penetration into the eye is influenced by many factors, including characteristics of the antibiotic administered (e.g. lipophilicity versus hydrophilicity), route of drug administration, frequency of dosing, degree of ocular inflammation, and surgical status of the eye.

For a pharmacological review of individual antibiotics, the reader is referred to Chapter 11 'Pharmacology'.

Lipophilicity/hydrophilicity

Antibiotics, like other drugs, are chemical compounds that can be characterized as to their solubility in water. A coefficient named the lipid/water solubility coefficient (or ether/water solubility coefficient) describes to what extent the compound is freely soluble in either kind of solvent.

The greater the lipophilicity of the compound, the greater the penetration will be through the lipid-containing membranes of cell walls. However, to administer a drug with a very high lipid/water solubility ratio requires dissolution in a solvent that is not aqueous; these solvents themselves are usually toxic to cell membranes and would also be noxious when administered via the bloodstream. Therefore, dissolution of highly lipophilic compounds in specific solvents is feasible in the laboratory, but not feasible for intravenous administration in clinical medicine.

Familiar examples of relatively lipophilic antibiotics are chloramphenicol, levofloxacin, and clarithromycin, but highly lipophilic antibiotics are fewer in number than the relatively hydrophilic antibiotics used extensively in clinical medicine. The penicillins, cephalosporins, and aminoglycosides are relatively water-soluble and these comprise the majority of antibiotics commonly used. The new group of quinolone antibiotics (ciprofloxacin, ofloxacin, levofloxacin, gatifloxacin, and moxifloxacin) is relatively more lipophilic than the cephalosporins, but data specific to each antibiotic should guide the clinical use and expectations surrounding any new drug.

Fortunately, antibiotics and other drugs usually exhibit some degree of both water and lipid solubility characteristics, and this again is expressed by their lipid/water solubility coefficient. In fact, some degree of both lipid and water solubility is most desirable for drugs administered by any route. This solubility ratio determines how well the drug will penetrate cell membranes and be retained within compartments, how easily it can be dissolved in nontoxic solvents for human use, how safely it can be administered, and what the pharmacokinetic characteristics will be in regard to a specific targeted tissue.

Diffusion

Simple diffusion is the most common method of drug transfer from one space or tissue of the body to another or from one compartment to another. It involves the movement of solute particles from an area of higher concentration to one of lower concentration by transfer through tissues and interfaces. Once diffusion has occurred, drug concentrations within adjacent compartments become stabilized according to the drug's partition coefficient (Figure 5.1).

Diffusion is affected by factors such as the concentration of drug presented at a tissue interface (concentration gradient), molecular weight of

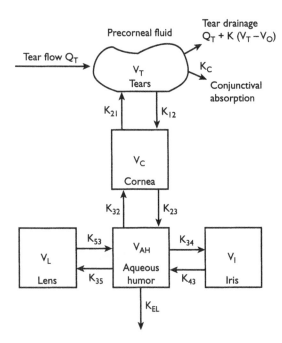

Figure 5.1

Partition coefficients (K) for drug transfer from topical drops to aqueous humor. Adapted from: Patton TF. Ocular drug disposition characteristics. In: *Ophthalmic Drug Delivery Systems* (American Pharmaceutical Association: Washington, DC, 1980) 28–55.

the drug, membrane permeability (inflamed or noninflamed), tissue binding, active transport mechanisms, surgical status of the eye, and others including formulation of the drug itself. A complete discussion of pharmacokinetics as it pertains to drug delivery and behavior in the eye is available elsewhere.[1]

Epithelial barrier

The epithelia of the bulbar conjunctiva and cornea are relatively impermeable to even water-soluble agents of small molecular size applied topically. Proprietary ophthalmic preparations such as gentamicin sulfate are available as drops (0.3%) or ointments at high concentrations (e.g. 0.3–1.0%) relative to their effective antimicrobial concentration and are thus active in the treatment of surface ocular infection (e.g. conjunctivitis).

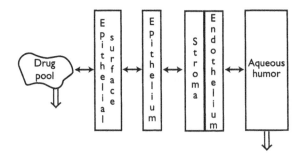

Figure 5.2

Barriers to drug penetration. Adapted from: Patton TF. Ocular drug disposition characteristics. In: *Ophthalmic Drug Delivery Systems* (American Pharmaceutical Association: Washington, DC, 1980) 28–55.

Antibiotics with a relatively high lipid/water solubility coefficient (such as chloramphenicol, the poorly dissociated sulfonamides, levofloxacin, and moxifloxacin) can penetrate the conjunctiva and cornea much better to enter deeper tissues at more effective concentrations. For a topically applied antibiotic to penetrate to the aqueous humor, it has to pass through the various layers of the cornea as illustrated in Figure 5.2.

If the surface epithelium is breached, as with corneal ulceration, water-soluble drugs can diffuse into the anterior segment of the eye in high concentrations; diffusion is enhanced by the use of fortified eye drops whose concentrations exceed those of commercial preparations. **However, this route is ineffective in providing useful concentrations in the posterior segment of the eye (e.g. vitreous) because there is a diffusion barrier across the lens-zonules compartment and across the anterior vitreous.**

The barrier offered by the epithelium of the ocular surface can be circumvented therapeutically by delivering a bolus of drug under the conjunctiva (subconjunctival injection, Table 5.1[2–24]) or more deeply into the orbit (sub-Tenon's injection). These periocular routes will deliver effective antimicrobial concentrations into the anterior segment of the eye (cornea and anterior chamber) and to some extent into the posterior segment (the vitreous) but should *not* be relied upon to deliver a sufficiently high concentration of antibiotic to treat bacterial endophthalmitis satisfactorily.

Table 5.1 Aqueous humor levels of antibiotics achieved by the subconjunctival and topical routes

Antibiotic	Subconjunctival injection/aqueous humor level achieved	Topical administration/aqueous humor level achieved
Gentamicin[2,3]	10–40 mg, gave 4 µg/ml in aqueous for 4 h. Suggested dose is 40 mg	3 mg/ml (0.3%), TL in cornea and AC for 1 h
Amikacin[4]	25 mg, gave 19 µg/ml in aqueous for 4 h	Level far below TL of *Pseudomonas* infections (10 µg/ml)
Penicillin G[5]	300–600 mg (1 × 10⁶ units), gave persistent TL in AC for 12–24 h	NP
Methicillin[6]	20–40 mg, gave TL for 4 h. Can give 100 mg	10% solution, no TL achieved
Oxacillin[7]	100 mg, gave 70 µg/ml in aqueous for 4 h	NP
Dicloxacillin[8]	50 mg, gave levels almost 100 × MIC for *S. aureus* at 4 h. Can give 100 mg	NP
Ampicillin[9–14]	2.5–250 mg, gave TL up to 4–6 h. Suggested dose is 100 mg	0.5% solution, aqueous levels better than systemic administration, compares favorably to subconjunctival administration
Cephaloridine[15]	50 mg, gave extremely high TL for 4 h. Can give 100 mg	NP
Cefuroxime[16]	125 mg, gave 20 µg/ml	NP
Ceftazidime[17]	100 mg	NP
Erythromycin[18]	10–20 mg, gave excellent TL but caused persistent chemosis	2.5% solution – TL 4 h without significant local reaction
Lincomycin[19,20]	75 mg, gave excellent TL for 12 h	NP
Clindamycin[21]	34 mg	NP
Vancomycin[22]	25 mg, gave TL > 4 h with mild chemosis (can be irritating)	50 mg/ml (5% solution), AC levels similar to subconjunctival injection results
Chloramphenicol[23]	1.2 mg gave good TL for at least 30 min	2.5–50 mg/ml (0.25–5%) gave various TL depending on conditions and investigator
Ciprofloxacin[24]	1 mg, gave level of 0.9 µg/ml after 1 h; level of 0.009 µg/ml after 10 h	NP

AC, anterior chamber; NP, not performed; TL, therapeutic level.

Penetration of the different quinolone antibiotics into the anterior chamber

Penetration of the different quinolone antibiotics (ciprofloxacin, ofloxacin, levofloxacin, moxifloxacin, and gatifloxacin) into the anterior chamber from the topical drop route or by oral therapy is given in Table 5.2.[25–37] The rates vary widely between the different compounds, with levofloxacin and moxifloxacin achieving the highest levels in the aqueous humor because of their relative lipophilicity. These two drugs are considered in detail later in this chapter (page 93).

Table 5.2 Aqueous humor levels of quinolones following oral and topical doses

Quinolone drug	Oral dose preoperatively	Topical dose preoperatively	AC levels (µg/ml)	Number of replicates
GAT[25]	400 mg GAT 16 and 4 h before sampling		1.34 (1.36 vitreous) (5.14 serum)	n = 24
LVFX[26]		5 drops LVFX 0.5% over 2 h (30-min intervals)	0.68 LVFX	n = 32
LVFX[26]	200 mg LVFX 2 h		0.42 LVFX	n = 35
LVFX[26]	3 × 200 mg LVFX 18, 6 and 2 h		1.3 LVFX	n = 34
LVFX[26]	3 × 200 mg LVFX 18, 6 and 2 h	5 drops LVFX 0.5% over 2 h (30-min intervals)	1.86 LVFX	n = 35
LVFX[27] OFX		4 drops 0.5% LVFX over 1 h (15-min intervals) 4 drops 0.3% OFX over 1 h (15-min intervals)	1.14 LVFX 0.62 OFX	n = 69
LVFX[28] CIP		4 drops 0.5% LVFX over 1 h (15-min intervals) 4 drops 0.3% CIP over 1 h (15-min intervals)	0.92 LVFX 0.12 CIP	n = 59
CIP[29] LVFX MOX	2 × 500 mg CIP 24 and 12 h, 1 × 500 mg LVFX 6 h, 1 × 400 mg MOX 6 h		0.5 CIP 1.5 LVFX 2.33 MOX	n = 42
MOX[30] OFX		1 drop 30 min prior to collection in rabbits with 0.3% MOX or 0.3% OFX	1.8 MOX 0.8 OFX	n = 10
LVFX[31]	1 × 400 mg LVFX on day of surgery		0.78 LVFX	n = 35
LVFX[32] LOM		6 drops 0.5% LVFX or 0.3% LOM over 1.5 h (15-min intervals)	0.6 LVFX 0.23 LOM	n = 59
LVFX[33] CIP		8 drops 0.5% LVFX or 0.3% CIP over 2 days (6-h intervals) 5 drops 0.5% LVFX or 0.3% CIP over 1 h (12-min intervals) and the combination	0.28 LVFX 0.07 CIP 1.14 LVFX 0.19 CIP 1.62 LVFX 0.24 CIP	n = 93
LVFX[34]	2 × 500 mg LVFX 12 h		1.9 LVFX	n = 17
LVFX[35]		3 drops of LVFX 0.3% (15-min intervals)	1.49 LVFX	
LVFX[36] LVFX[37]	200 mg 4–5 h	3 drops of LVFX 0.5% at 15-min intervals × 6 before surgery	0.68 LVFX Stromal levels (µg/ml) 4.63 LVFX 2.74 LOM 1.33 NOR	n = 14

CIP, ciprofloxacin; GAT, gatifloxacin; LVFX, levofloxacin; LOM, lomefloxacin; MOX, moxifloxacin; NOR, norfloxacin; OFX, ofloxacin.

Blood–ocular barriers

Barriers influencing the entry of drugs into the eye

There are two main barrier systems in the eye.[38,39] The first regulates exchange between blood and aqueous humor in which inward movement predominates: the blood–aqueous barrier (Figure 5.3). Aqueous humor is secreted into the posterior chamber by the ciliary processes and flows through the pupil into the anterior chamber to leave via the trabecular meshwork. Important diffusional solute exchange takes place between

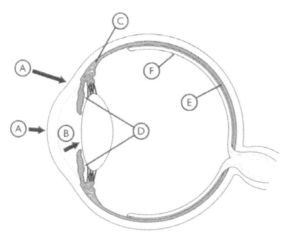

Figure 5.3

Barriers to penetration of antibiotics into the eye: A, epithelial; B, aqueous–vitreous; C and D, blood–aqueous; E, external blood–retinal (pigment epithelium); F, internal blood–retinal (capillary endothelium). Derived from Cunha-Vaz JG. The blood-ocular barriers, *Surv Ophthalmol* (1979) **23**: 79–296 and Cunha-Vaz JG. The blood-ocular barriers: past, present, and future, *Doc Ophthalmol* (1997) **93**:149–57.

the aqueous and not only the surrounding tissues but also the vitreous.

The blood–aqueous barrier is formed by two layers of cells, the endothelium of the iris blood vessels and the nonpigmented inner layer of the ciliary epithelium. These cell layers impair transport of blood proteins to maintain an osmotic and chemical equilibrium. However, the ciliary vascular endothelium is permeable to blood-borne solutes that give a concentration of 1% of proteins found in the plasma. The ciliary body has a pivotal role in regulating all inner ocular fluids via its large surface covered by the ciliary processes. There is active secretory transport of sodium, chloride, and bicarbonate providing the osmotic force for the production of the aqueous as well as maintaining ascorbic acid at a higher level than in plasma. The ciliary body is also responsible for a free continuous flow of ions, amino acids, and vitamins from the aqueous into the vitreous.

- Epithelial barrier. The corneal epithelium restricts the entry of water-soluble drugs into the cornea and aqueous humor. The barrier is breached by an epithelial defect and, if the epithelium is intact, is bypassed by a subconjunctival injection.

- Bulk flow of aqueous humor from the eye, and the presence of an intact lens and zonules retard the diffusion of drugs from the anterior chamber into the vitreous humor.
- The blood–aqueous barrier limits the entry of drugs from the blood into the aqueous.
- The epithelia of the iris and ciliary body pump anionic drugs out of the aqueous.
- The blood–retinal barrier limits the entry of drugs into the vitreous from the systemic circulation.
  - Externally is the pigment epithelial barrier.
  - Internally the blood–retinal barrier is the retinal capillary endothelial barrier. There is an outward pumping of anions across the retina by the retinal pigment epithelium (RPE).

The internal barrier in the posterior segment affects outward movement from the retina into the blood: the blood–retinal barrier (see Figure 5.3), which is responsible for the homeostasis and microenvironment of the retina.[40,41] This barrier also serves to remove waste products of metabolic activity from within the eye. There are no diffusional barriers between the extracellular fluid of the retina and the adjacent vitreous or with the posterior chamber or the anterior segment. The endothelial cells of the retina have functional and morphological differences compared with those of other organs. They have narrow tight junctional structures composed of a complex called the zonulae occludentes. The RPE cells impair cellular transport of hydrophilic compounds. The RPE is in the outer blood–retinal barrier and is also sealed with extensive zonulae occludentes. High activities of barrier-selective enzymes contribute to a protective function but essential nutrients are transported into the vitreous by carrier-selective mechanisms.

Equally important are the active transport mechanisms to remove ions from the vitreous. The microenvironment of the retina, which resembles the extracellular fluid of the brain, is regulated by active transport processes located within the barrier cells. These three main sites of transport exiting the eye are the endothelial cells of the retinal vessels, the RPE, and the ciliary epithelium. Within the retinal barrier, potassium is actively transported to the blood with a net magnesium flux in the opposite direction. Organic anions such as prostaglandins and

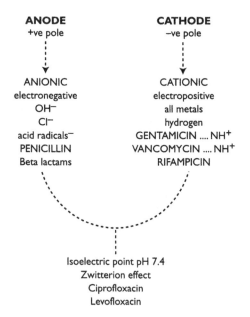

Figure 5.4

Ionicity of antibiotics.

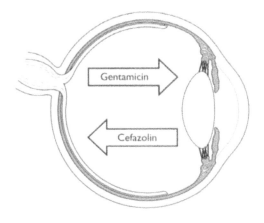

Figure 5.5

Active (cefazolin) and passive (gentamicin) transport of antibiotics out of the eye.

related compounds that are produced but not metabolized within the eye, anionic drugs such as penicillins and cephalosporins, and zwitterions such as ciprofloxacin are removed from the extracellular fluid of the retina by active transport across the blood–retinal barrier cells similarly to the renal tubular clearance mechanism.

This active transport system is inhibited by probenecid which can be used to maintain higher levels of anionic drugs in the eye but this may interfere with outward transport of prostaglandins (Chapters 1 and 2). Use of oral probenecid (500 mg every 12 hours) retards outward transport of penicillins, cephalosporins, and ciprofloxacin across the retinal capillary endothelial cells, thus extending the half-life of these drugs within the vitreous. This finding was demonstrated in normal monkey eyes when the half-life of cefazolin was extended from 7 to 30 hours.[42] Probenecid also raises the plasma level by blocking secretion of these drugs by the proximal renal tubule.

Cationic compounds and drugs such as the aminoglycosides (gentamicin and tobramycin), vancomycin, erythromycin, and rifampicin are not actively transported out of the eye by the blood–retinal barrier and have to leave the posterior compartment by diffusing forward into the anterior chamber and aqueous humor. Ciprofloxacin and the other quinolones are removed by both the active and passive transport systems (Figure 5.4).

The blood–ocular barriers (see Figure 5.3) do not exist for other orbital structures. Thus infections within the orbit or ocular adnexae (the eyelids, lacrimal gland, and nasolacrimal system) are readily treatable with systemic antibiotics.

The result of the blood–retinal barrier described above is an active transport system for the anionic drugs (penicillin and cephalosporins) out of the eye, giving a half-life of approximately 8 hours when given intravitreally, as opposed to the passive diffusion forward of the cationic drugs (gentamicin and other aminoglycosides, vancomycin, rifampicin, and erythromycin), giving a half-life of 24 hours. These results mean that a combination injection given intravitreally of a cephalsporin versus ceftazidime and an aminoglycoside or vancomycin have different half-lives that must be considered in the management of the clinical infection (Figure 5.5). However, in the inflamed eye, an actively absorbed drug has a longer half-life than in a noninflamed eye, for reasons discussed below. A passively transported drug with forward diffusion has enhanced removal in an inflamed eye; therefore, a combination injection is acceptable in practice for the treatment of the acutely infected and inflamed eye.

Table 5.3 Intravitreal doses of antibiotics*

Antibiotic	Intravitreal injection (μg)	Duration (h)	Effective intravenous dose (mg)
Amikacin	200	24–48	15 mg/kg/24 h
Ampicillin	500	24	1 g/4 h
Amphotericin	5 or 10	24–48	0.1–1.0 mg/kg/24 h
Carbenicillin	2000	16–24	3 g/4 h
Cefazolin	2000	16	1 g/4 h
Ceftazidine	2000	16–24	1.5 g/6 h
Cefuroxime	2000	16–24	1.5 g/6 h
Chloramphenicol	2000	20	0.75 g/6 h
Clindamycin	1000	16–24	0.75 g/8 h
Ciprofloxacin	200†	–	0.2 g/12 h
Erythromycin	500	24	0.5 g/6 h
Gentamicin	200	48	5 mg/kg/24 h
Methicillin	2000	40	1 g/4 h
Miconazole	10	20	0.6–3.6 g/24 h
Oxacillin	500	24	2 g/4 h
Vancomycin	1000	72	1 g/12 h

*Maximum intravitreal injection volume for each antibiotic is usually 0.1 ml. USE THE INTRATHECAL PREPARATION WHEN AVAILABLE.
†Very limited use only; not used by the authors.

Effects of inflammation

These barriers affect the ocular distribution of drugs, including the potential of systemically administered drugs to enter the vitreous as well as the retention of drugs after direct delivery by intravitreal injection. In the uninflamed eye, the highest aqueous concentration using the systemic route will be achieved by lipid-soluble drugs such as chloramphenicol or the quinolones (ciprofloxacin, ofloxacin, levofloxacin, gatifloxacin, and moxifloxacin). Negligible concentrations will be achieved using water-soluble drugs, particularly those in anionic form (such as the penicillins and cephalosporins) that are actively transported out of the eye.

In the inflamed eye, the concentrations achieved in the ocular compartments are increased, owing to partial breakdown of the blood–aqueous barrier, so that effective antimicrobial concentrations may be reached in the aqueous. However, concentrations reached in the vitreous with parenteral therapy are always much lower than those achieved in the aqueous, even in the inflamed eye with endophthalmitis. Vitreous concentrations after high-dose systemic therapy in such situations will be subtherapeutic (see Figure 6.8(A–C) in Chapter 6) and lower than those achievable by subconjunctival injection. The highest levels are gained by direct injection into the vitreous which is always favored in the treatment of serious endophthalmitis (Table 5.3 and Chapter 8, 'Management and treatment'). However, administration of the *same* antibiotic by the intravenous route as that given by intravitreal injection will prolong effective levels in the vitreous and should be practiced in the treatment of acute bacterial endophthalmitis.

Infectious endophthalmitis creates sufficient intraocular inflammation to compromise the function of the retinal pump mechanism that helps to eliminate antibiotics such as cefazolin, thereby prolonging their half-life in the vitreous of the normal eye from 6.5 to 10.4 hours. At the same time, surgical alteration of the eye such as lensectomy and/or vitrectomy altogether change the inner anatomy of the eye that affects overall elimination characteristics. The relative effects of inflammation, aphakia, and vitrectomy on the half-life of cefazolin are best studied in experimental animal models that simulate these conditions (Tables 5.4[43] and 5.5,[44,45] Figures 5.6–5.9). It

Table 5.4 Rabbit model of half-life for cefazolin under different conditions[43]

Conditions	Half-life (h)
Uninflamed phakic eye	6.5
Inflamed phakic eye	10.4
Uninflamed aphakic eye	8.3
Inflamed aphakic eye	9
Uninflamed aphakic, vitrectomized eye	6
Inflamed aphakic vitrectomized eye	6.7

Table 5.5 Rabbit models of half-life for gentamicin under different conditions

Conditions	Half-life (h)
Uninflamed phakic eye[44]	20/24
Inflamed phakic eye	10
Uninflamed phakic eye[45]	32
Inflamed phakic eye	19
Uninflamed aphakic eye[45]	12
Inflamed aphakic eye	14

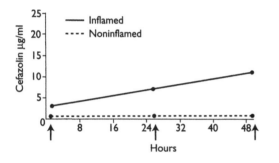

Figure 5.6

Antibiotic levels in vitreous of inflamed and noninflamed phakic eyes of rabbits given **intravenous** cefazolin.

can be seen that the half-life prolongation given by inflammation in the phakic eye does not occur after the combination of aphakia and vitrectomy (see Table 5.4).

Low levels of cefazolin were found within the vitreous cavity of uninflamed albino rabbit eyes after intravenous administration; however, with inflammation, much higher levels were achieved (see Figures 5.6 and 5.8), regardless of the surgical status of the eye. It should be noted that after repeated systemic doses with the inflamed eye (see Figure 5.8), intravitreal antibiotic levels rise, approaching therapeutic levels, and these intravitreal antibiotics may be considered useful as an adjunct to the declining drug levels seen within the vitreous cavity after an intravitreal injection. The use of repeated systemic doses and an increase in dose (where safe and tolerable to the patient) are factors often overlooked in clinical treatment strategies for infectious endophthalmitis.

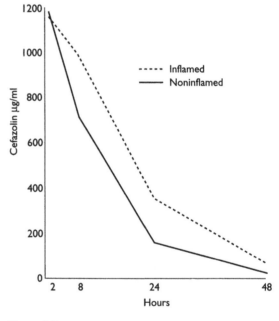

Figure 5.7

Antibiotic levels in vitreous of inflamed and noninflamed phakic eyes of rabbits given **intravitreal** cefazolin.

In contrast, gentamicin, which is not removed by the retinal pump mechanism, does not show any prolongation of half-life in the vitreous of the inflamed or infected eye but instead has a reduction of 50% from 20 to 10 hours (see Table 5.5). A similar reduction is given with aphakia but this is not further increased with inflammation or infection. This finding was also repeated with vancomycin, when aphakia and vitrectomy were

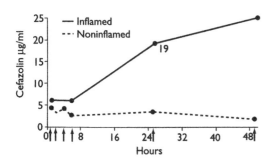

Figure 5.8

Antibiotic levels in vitreous of inflamed and noninflamed aphakic vitrectomized eyes of rabbits given **intravenous** cefazolin.

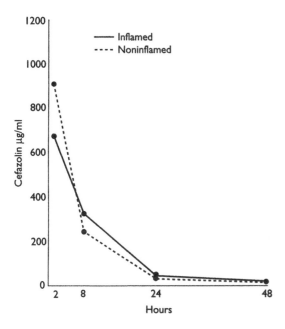

Figure 5.9

Antibiotic levels in vitreous of inflamed and noninflamed aphakic vitrectomized eyes of rabbits given **intravitreal** cefazolin.

found to reduce vitreous vancomycin levels, compared with phakic nonvitrectomized eyes, so that only 25 μg/ml remained out of a dose of 2 mg given 48 hours earlier.[46] This finding of the shortest half-life occurring with aphakia and vitrectomy was also shown by Case et al with clearance studies of 3H-fluorouracil.[47]

A clinical parallel to the treatment of infectious endophthalmitis is seen in the treatment of meningitis, where higher cerebrospinal fluid drug levels are also achieved through an inflamed meninges and after repeated systemic doses. Here, also, penetration of the drug through the meninges is proportional to its degree of lipophilicity.

Repeated systemic dosing

When serum levels of an antibiotic can be increased or sustained by repeated intravenous administration of high but safe doses, vitreous drug penetration is further increased. Repeated, or higher, systemically administered doses raise the 'concentration gradient,' that is, the concentration of antibiotic present in the serum that interfaces with the tissues of the blood–eye barrier. Together with inflammation, intravitreal penetration of an antibiotic can be increased.

The exact increments in drug penetration, or precise intraocular antibiotic levels, are not quantified because the degree of ocular inflammation caused by infection is difficult, if not impossible, to standardize in experimental animal models of endophthalmitis. Therefore, drug levels commonly reported in the literature often reflect assays after only a single systemic antibiotic dose has been administered, a situation that is not analogous to the clinical setting. While useful, these reports do not adequately describe the penetration of antibiotics after multiple doses have been given.

Intravitreal injection of antibiotics, vitrectomy, and toxicity

Many factors are described above that severely limit the levels of antibiotic achievable in the vitreous cavity after intravenous administration; this is also the case for topical, subconjunctival, and intramuscular dosing with both gentamicin and amikacin in the normal and aphakic eye, which do not produce levels that are sufficiently high for effective bactericidal therapy in the vitreous although they may do so in the aqueous.[48,49]

Direct intravitreal antibiotic injection is now the 'standard of practice' for treatment of infectious endophthalmitis. Direct intravitreal injection of an antibiotic in the highest nontoxic dose (see Table 5.3) delivers high, instantaneous antibiotic levels where they are needed: at the focus of infection inside the vitreous space (see Figures 5.7 and 5.9).[50] 'Debulking' of the vitreous with surgery (partial or full vitrectomy) will also remove part of the infectious load and allow the antibiotic to diffuse easily within the cavity. The goal of intravitreal antibiotic injection is to sterilize the vitreous cavity as early as possible to reduce the destructive effect of the bacteria on the retina.

Antibiotic levels delivered intravitreally are bactericidal, at least for a period of time. These high antibiotic levels are needed for eradication of bacteria in this closed, avascular space. The purpose of injecting the highest dose that can be safely injected is to ensure that antibiotic levels destructive to bacteria are delivered in a single injection, and that they are maintained above a subtherapeutic level for as long as possible, while the intravitreal level of antibiotic is declining. Bacteria kill rates are a function not only of drug concentration but of contact time with the bacterium as well as the numbers involved. An early diagnosis with a low number of actively replicating bacterial cells will provide a better response than a late diagnosis with large numbers of static bacterial cells, quite apart from inflammation and damage that may exist within the retina. Treatment at a late stage involves a different environment with pH change, hypoxia, nutrient shortage, and nonreplicating bacteria, reducing the effectiveness of the antibiotic.

The concentration of antibiotic in the vitreous cavity after an intravitreal injection is generally calculated by dividing the dose injected by the volume of the vitreous in humans (4.5 ml). However, the presence of infection and/or inflammation, aphakia, and vitrectomy all affect the immediate and early antibiotic levels distributed throughout the vitreous space after intravitreal injection.

After instantaneous antibiotic levels are established by intravitreal injection, the drug half-life then determines the rate of decline or reduction of drug levels within the vitreous space (see Figures 5.7 and 5.9). Drug elimination is affected by factors including the degree of inflammation, the elimination route for the antibiotic in question

(anterior or posterior), tissue binding of drug, and the surgical status of the eye such as aphakia or vitrectomy (see Tables 5.4 and 5.5).

Inflammation prolongs the half-life of cefazolin after intravitreal injection in the nonsurgical eye. In this instance, as described above, damage to the retinal pump mechanism actually serves to prolong the retention of those drugs within the vitreous cavity that are eliminated via the posterior route. However, drugs eliminated via the anterior route are not subject to this effect, and inflammation will decrease their half-life or retention after an intravitreal injection, as will removal of the cataractous lens.

In aphakic, vitrectomized eyes, the rate of antibiotic decline in the vitreous space can still be faster (see Figure 5.9). The vitreous gel that sequesters the injected bolus of drug and promotes gradual diffusion throughout the vitreous cavity has been removed. Figures 5.7 and 5.9 demonstrate the more rapid decline in antibiotic level in phakic vitrectomized eyes. In phakic eyes, the relative retention of cefazolin is seen in inflamed eyes.

Interpretation of these models suggests that the use of a cephalosporin and an aminoglycoside (gentamicin) or vancomycin in combination by the intravitreal route to treat endophthalmitis in the aphakic, vitrectomized eye will yield approximately similar half-lives of 10 hours. This level can be supplemented by the intravenous route because there is better penetration in the inflamed eye (see Figures 5.6 and 5.8). By 48 hours, however, most of the antibiotic will have been removed, so if there is a limited clinical response, repeat intravitreal injection should be therapeutic and safe at this time.

The increasing use of vitrectomy demands that the toxicity of the injected dose and the method of intravitreal injection be reconsidered. When injected into the vitreous gel, gradual diffusion of antibiotic occurs. However, where vitrectomy has been performed, the injection should be given slowly so that these relatively high concentrations of antibiotic, or their vehicles, are not 'squirted' with force onto the retina itself. This precaution is especially important with gentamicin. The gentamicin dose of 0.4 mg in 0.1 ml has been reduced to 0.2 mg because of suspected macular infarction due to toxicity[51] as has the dose of amikacin (0.2 mg), although it is not equipotent and amikacin is less effective per milligram as a bactericidal drug than gentamicin. Gentamicin and other antibiotics should be reduced in concentration by a further 50% (for gentamicin to 0.1 mg) if given intravitreally when a full vitrectomy is performed.

Most cases of gentamicin toxicity occurred after a 0.4-mg dose in eyes that had undergone a vitrectomy. The retinal toxicity of gentamicin may have been exacerbated due to the methods used to prepare the intraocular injection in some places. By irregular means of creating the intraocular injection (drawing up concentrated commercial products within one tuberculin syringe in 'series' – in poor order) in the syringe, and not going through the more cumbersome serial dilutions first in separate vials that also dilute out the preservative in the vehicle, clinicians have deviated in the past from standard clinical procedures and recommendations.

However, a more recent survey of retinal specialists has suggested that amikacin or low-dose gentamicin can still cause macular toxicity.[52] To investigate this issue further, critical details were investigated from 13 patients who received intravitreous injections of 0.2–0.4 mg of amikacin sulfate or 0.1–0.2 mg of gentamicin sulfate for prophylaxis or treatment of endophthalmitis and who suffered toxicity.[52] These cases suggest that amikacin and low-dose gentamicin can cause macular infarction. The causative dose cannot be ascertained in any of the cases but the dilutions were prepared by hospital pharmacists using typewritten protocols, a practice that helps to prevent errors. Several cases differed from previously reported cases of aminoglycoside toxicity in that the involvement of the macula was quite discrete. Most of the patients suffered severe visual loss, but two patients, in whom most of the nonperfusion was adjacent to the macula and in whom some of the perifoveal capillaries were spared, recovered 20/50 visual acuity. These cases emphasize the potential hazards of the intravitreous use of aminoglycosides. A toxic reaction can occur even when injection of low doses is intended and precautions are taken to avoid dilution errors. A localized increase in concentration in dependent areas of the retina may play a role in aminoglycoside toxicity. If some of the perifoveal capillaries are spared, retention of some central vision is possible. Consideration should be given to substituting ceftazidime for aminoglycosides (gentamicin) for the treatment and prophylaxis of endophthalmitis.

Liposomal preparation of drugs

Drugs such as amphotericin B can be incorporated into liposomes to enhance drug transport into the retina (and brain) by the intravenous route; however, the disadvantage of this technique is the rapid uptake of the liposomes by the liver, lungs, and spleen. It is debatable whether to treat fungal endophthalmitis with intravitreal amphotericin B and systemic use of liposomal amphotericin B (AmBizone) instead of deoxycholate amphotericin (Fungizone) (see fungus treatment in Chapters 7 and 9 and pharmacology in Chapter 11). A recent study, using a rabbit model of inflammatory uveitis, has found that liposomal amphotericin B penetrated better to the cornea (mean concentration of amphotericin 2.4 ± 1.5 µg/g) compared with deoxycholate amphotericin B (the standard IV preparation) which yielded only 0.5 ± 0.2 µg/g.[53] No amphotericin could be detected in the corneas of noninflamed eyes with either preparation. Amphotericin can be repeated intravitreally every 72 hours according to the clinical response as well as being injected into the anterior chamber (intracameral route) at 10 µg in 0.1 ml.

Intracellular and extracellular levels of antibiotics

Once an antibiotic or another drug reaches a particular tissue within the eye, its concentration will be partitioned between the cellular and extracellular space. There is a big difference in cellular penetration between the various antibiotics that surprisingly is not related to their ionic charge (see Figure 5.4). Their values are listed in Table 5.6.[54–61] PMN cells are used in laboratory experiments and are representative of levels expected within macrophages.

The antibiotics can be classified according to whether their PMN/extracellular tissue ratio is less than or greater than 1. Those antibiotics with a ratio of less than 1 have a lower concentration within the cell than within the extracellular tissue. In contrast, those antibiotics with a ratio of greater than 1 become concentrated within the cell. The penicillins, cephalosporins, and all the aminoglycosides have a ratio of less than 1. The ratio is highest for azithromycin (226),

Table 5.6 Experimental concentrations of drugs (μg/ml) within polymorphonuclear (PMN) cells and extracellular tissue[a]

	Amp-icillin	Cephalo-thin	Cloxa-cillin	Fusidic acid	Peni-cillin	Genta-micin	Chloram-phenicol	Rifamp-icin	Cipro-floxacin[a]/Lome-floxacin[a]	Levo-floxacin[a,b]/Ofloxa-cin[a]	Gemi-floxacin[b]/Moxi-floxacin[b]	Erythro-mycin	Clinda-mycin	Azithro-mycin/Clarithro-mycin
PMN cells	8	<1	32.5	16	5	15	22	47	10.0	30	55	254	434	2260
Extracellular tissue	100	10	100	40	10	18	10	20	2.7	5	5	18	10	10
Ratio PMN/extracellular	0.08	<0.1	0.33	0.4	0.5	0.8	2.2	2.4	3.7	6	8/10.9	14	43	226/200

clarythromycin (220) and clindamycin at 43, erythromycin at 14, and the various quinolones at between 10.9 and 3.7. Chloramphenicol, which has been much used in the past because of its lipophilicity cell membrane penetration, only has a ratio of 2.2.

Chronic low-grade infection, often presenting as a 'hypopyon uveitis' that develops 6 weeks or more after extracapsular cataract extraction or phacoemulsification cataract surgery and lasts for months, can be due to 'saccular', plaque, or capsular bag endophthalmitis (Chapter 6). The bacteria causing this type of infection are usually *Propionibacterium acnes*, diphtheroids or coagulase-negative staphylococci. They are found within macrophages lining the capsule fragment.[62–66] In order to eradicate these intracellular bacteria, illustrated in Chapter 6, antibiotics are required that penetrate well into macrophages, such as the erythromycin derivatives azithromycin and clarithromycin (Chapter 11). Clarithromycin was first used for this purpose in an individual case of 'saccular' (plaque) endophthalmitis, confirmed by polymerase chain reaction (PCR), that responded well to treatment and resulted in a quiet eye without the need for any surgical removal of the intraocular lens.[67] Since then, clarithromycin has been used similarly by others[68] and in a randomized trial of therapy for chronic subacute endophthalmitis,[69] in which patients responded much better to this therapy than those who did not receive clarithromycin.

Clarithromycin is given orally as 500 mg every 12 hours and is well absorbed. It penetrates well into both the anterior and posterior segments[70] and is then concentrated into macrophages at up to 200-fold (see Table 5.6). In order to examine the penetration of clarithromycin in ocular tissues, 21 patients who underwent elective cataract surgery received a single, oral 500-mg dose of clarithromycin preoperatively.[70] The concentrations of clarithromycin in the aqueous fluid 4, 8, 10, 12, and 22 hours after administration were (mean ± standard deviation [SD]): 0.13 ± 0.05, 0.137 ± 0.11, 0.074 ± 0.03, 0.06 ± 0.02, and 0.074 ± 0.04 µg/ml, respectively.[70] This is compatible with the 2-hour turnover of the aqueous humor (volume 0.2 ml) in the anterior chamber, giving an approximate 2-hour half-life with 6 hours of bactericidal activity.

Another 21 patients who underwent elective vitreoretinal surgery received 500 mg every 12 hours orally for 3 days preoperatively.[70] The concentrations in vitreous 3, 6, 8, 11, and 24 hours after administration were (mean ± SD): 0.11 ± 0.02, 0.257 ± 0.13, 0.27 ± 0.21, 0.307 ± 0.26, and 0.108 ± 0.07 µg/ml, respectively. The mean concentration of clarithromycin in the iris was 6.2 µg/g, demonstrating the drug's concentration into cells.[70]

Effect of different doses of quinolones on aqueous humor levels

There is currently great interest in the use of the quinolones, particularly levofloxacin and moxifloxacin, given by the topical route for prophylaxis of endophthalmitis following phacoemulsification cataract surgery. Levofloxacin is a second-generation quinolone that is both lipophilic and hydrophilic (water-soluble), allowing it to penetrate the corneal epithelial barrier into the stroma and anterior chamber (Chapter 11). Different regimens have been investigated prior to cataract surgery with use of frequent drop therapy, oral therapy, or the combination which has penetrated well both into the stroma and into the anterior chamber (see Table 5.2). Samples of aqueous humor were collected at the time of cataract surgery for assay of quinolones by high-performance liquid chromatography.

These studies have consistently shown that levofloxacin is better absorbed into the anterior chamber by the topical or oral route than ofloxacin by a two-fold factor and by a 4–8-fold factor greater than ciprofloxacin. Levofloxacin is the levoracemer of ofloxacin and is the active component.

A frequent drop regime of levofloxacin 0.5%, four times every 15 minutes in the hour prior to cataract surgery, has given levels of 1.1 µg/ml in the aqueous humor (Table 5.2) which can be boosted by additional oral therapy to 1.8 µg/ml. Graves et al have found the minimum inhibitory concentration $(MIC)_{90}$ of most bacteria causing corneal infection, and hence a source of postoperative infection, to be less than 1.0 µg/ml.[71] More recent work has found lower MIC levels for levofloxacin from 1.0 µg/ml (*S. pneumoniae*) to 0.03 µg/ml (*Haemophilus* sp.).[72] Effective levels are maintained in the tears and conjunctiva for up to 6 hours or more (Figure 5.10).[73]

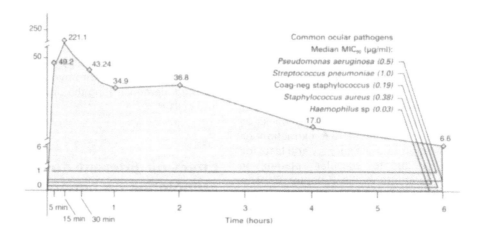

Figure 5.10

Graph of levofloxacin concentration in tears with time over 6 hours (Raizman et al.[73]) in relation to MICs of common ocular pathogens (Kowalski et al.[72])

In addition, levofloxacin has a rapid action that can be expected to reduce the bacterial count on the conjunctiva prior to surgery, when applied two or four times every 15 minutes, by up to 2 $\log_{10}$ or 100-fold. It also penetrates the epithelium to the corneal stroma and into the anterior chamber, resulting in a depot effect for the conjunctiva (see Figure 5.10).

Moxifloxacin has given good penetration, equal to levofloxacin. Moxifloxacin is a new quinolone that has some effect against methicillin-resistant *Staphylococcus aureus* (MRSA), which is not susceptible to levofloxacin, and has better activity against streptococci (MIC 0.15 µg/ml). Moxifloxacin prevented experimental *S. aureus* endophthalmitis in the rabbit when given by the topical route as 0.5% drops, four times every 15 minutes, prior to inoculation of the anterior chamber with bacterial cells.[74] In addition, recent evidence has shown that moxifloxacin 0.5% has better penetration into the anterior chamber than gatifloxacin 0.3% (the alternative 'fourth' generation quinolone) following topical therapy (1d qid for 24 hours then 1d one hour before surgery) with aqueous humor levels of 1.93 ± 0.87 and 0.26 ± 0.09 µg/ml respectively.[75] Other recent evidence has found aqueous humor levels for topically-applied moxifloxacin 0.5% and gatifloxacin 0.3% (1d qds for 3 days then every 15 mins for one hour before surgery) of 1.31 and 0.63 µg/ml respectively,[76] with 1.44 ± 0.8 or 1.19 ± 0.32 µg/ml for moxifloxacin used alone.[77]

It is our belief, however, that moxifloxacin should be reserved for treatment of keratitis or endophthalmitis because of the existence of bacteria resistant to other antibiotics, and that levofloxacin, which penetrates well into the eye, should be used for surgical prophylaxis. There is good scientific reason to argue for such separate use of these two quinolones.

A multicenter, prospective, randomized, placebo-controlled study in 30,000 patients having phacoemulsification cataract surgery in 18 units is currently taking place (January 2004 to December 2005) in Europe under the auspices of the European Society of Cataract and Refractive Surgeons (ESCRS). This study is comparing use of topical levofloxacin 0.5% intensively before and after surgery (one drop every 30 minutes twice before surgery and one drop every 5 minutes three times immediately after surgery) with intracameral injection of 1 mg cefuroxime (in 0.1 ml saline) at the end of surgery[78,79] with the combination and with neither, using a Fisher 2 × 2 factorial design. All patients receive postoperative levofloxacin 0.5% drops every 6 hours for 6 days starting the day after surgery. This allows 18 hours without antibiotics either during or after surgery in the control group, in order to establish whether the intraoperative use of antibiotics can reduce the incidence of postoperative endophthalmitis following phacoemulsification cataract surgery. All patients receive antiseptic preparation of the

Table 5.7 The expected antibiotic sensitivities (MICs) of pathogenic bacteria for causing endophthalmitis

	Peni-cillin	Amp/Amoxi-cillin	Flu/cloxa-cillin	Cefur-oxime	Cefta-zidime	Fusidic acid	Cipro/Leva/Gati/Moxi-floxacin*	Oxy-tetra-cycline	Chlor-amph-enicol	Vanco-mycin	Genta-micin/Amikacin	Metroni-dazole
S. aureus†‡	R	R	S (0.1)	S (4)	(S) (6)	S (0.1)	S (1)	(S) (4)	S (4)	S (2)	S (0.25)	R
CNS†‡	R	R	S (0.1)	S (4)	(S) (6)	S (0.1)	S (1)	(S) (4)	S (4)	S (2)	S (0.25)	R
Streptococci‡	S (0.03)	S (0.03)	S (0.1)	S (0.1)	S (0.25)	(S) (1–16)	(S) (4)*	(S) (2)	S (4)	S (0.2)	R	R
P. acnes and corynebacteria‡	S	S	S	S	S	S	S	S	S	S (1)	R	R
Bacillus sp.†	R	R	R	R	R	R	S (0.25)	(S)	(S)	S	S	R
N. meningitidis	S	S	S	S	S	S (0.05)	S (<0.1)	S (1)	S (2)	R	(S) (4)	R
H. influenzae	(S) (1.0)	S (0.25)	R	S (0.1)	S (0.1)	R	S (<0.1)	S (1)	S (0.5)	R	S (0.5)	R
Coliforms	R	(S) (2–R)	R	S (4)	S (0.1)	R	S (0.25)	(S) (8)	(S) (6)	R	S (0.5)	R
Ps. aeruginosa	R	R	R	R	S (4)	R	S (1)	R	R	R	S (2)	R
Anaerobic streptococci	S	S	(S)	S			R	S	S	S (0.5)	R	S
Clostridium sp.†‡	S (0.3)	S (0.3)	S (1)	(0.5)	S (1)		R	(S) (0.3/R)	S (4)	S (0.5)	R	S
Bacteroides sp.	(S) (0.1/R)	R	R	R			R	(S) (2/R)	(S) (8)	R	R	S

*Only moxifloxacin is effective against MRSA (*in vitro* rather than *in vivo*) and *Enterococcus faecalis* with enhanced activity for other streptococci.
†Sensitive to clindamycin.
‡Sensitive to erythromycin and azithromycin.

Table 5.8 The expected antibiotic sensitivities (MICs) of pathogenic fungi for causing endophthalmitis

	Polyene antibiotics amphotericin/ natamycin	Imidazole antibiotics miconazole/fluconazole/ voriconazole and others	5–Fluorocytosine
Candida albicans and yeasts	S	S	S
Aspergillus sp.	S	S	R
Fusarium sp. and filamentous fungi	(S)	(S)	R
Scedosporium apiospermum	R	S	R

cornea and conjunctival sac with 5% povidone iodine in saline for 3 minutes prior to surgery. In addition, this study will gain a reliable incidence figure for endophthalmitis following phacoemulsification cataract surgery in Europe as well as various risk factor evaluations (Chapter 6).

Minimum inhibitory concentrations and minimum bactericidal concentrations of antibiotics for pathogenic bacteria

Antibiotics have an inhibitory (bacteriostatic) and killing (bactericidal) effect on the bacterial cell. Bacteriostatic antibiotics such as chloramphenicol, tetracycline, low-dose erythromycin, and sulfonamides bind to ribosomes to inhibit messenger RNA translation and therefore protein production. The bacterial cell cannot divide but remains viable, the killing effect depending on PMN cells and macrophages. Other antibiotics such as penicillins and cephalosporins that attach to penicillin-binding proteins prevent cell wall formation, resulting in cell death. The aminoglycosides (gentamicin, tobramycin, and amikacin) bind to ribosomes irreversibly with a bactericidal effect not requiring PMNs. Laboratory testing involves assessing the minimum inhibitory concentration (MIC) and minimum bactericidal concentrations (MBC) and usually refers to the MIC_{90} and the MBC_{90} when the values quoted reflect those likely to be found for 90% of the isolates. Tables 5.7 and 5.8 quote the MIC_{90} values expected for bacteria and fungi pathogenic for the eye. These values are meant as a quick guide for the clinician but a microbiology laboratory should always be consulted for an individual case because of hospital, local, and regional differences in bacterial resistance. For bactericidal antibiotics, the MIC value is similar to the MBC in most cases, except for Lancefield group G beta-hemolytic streptococci when the MBC can be much higher than the MIC for penicillins, and clindamycin should be used adjunctively. For bacteriostatic antibiotics, there is no bactericidal effect, and killing of the static cell depends on the immune response instead. It is important to achieve the MBC level within the vitreous cavity, rather than the MIC, for gaining control of the infection.

Challenge for the future

A challenge in the medical management of infectious endophthalmitis, aside from early surgical intervention, remains the ability to administer, as soon as possible, the most effective antibiotic against the microorganism (a drug of choice), in a maximum nontoxic dose by direct intravitreal injection that may be supplemented with orally administered doses, preferably of the same antibiotic. An understanding of how a drug is likely to behave, in light of all the factors described above, will contribute to the evolution of safe and effective antibiotic regimens for the treatment of infectious endophthalmitis. In addition, the regimen will also include intravitreal corticosteroids (Chapter 8), or newer antiinflammatory drugs (Chapter 2), to suppress inflammation within the posterior segment.

Table 5.9 Frequency of volume of globe and vitreous in relation to the axial length and lens power. (Adapted from Fechner and Teichmann, 1998[81])

Frequency										
Axial length (mm)	16	18	20	22	24	26	28	30	32	34
External volume of eye (ml)	2.1	3.0	4.2	5.6	7.2	9.2	11.4	14.1	17.2	20.6
Volume of vitreous (ml)	1.7	2.4	3.4	4.5	5.8	7.4	9.1	11.3	13.8	16.5
Dioptic power			+10.8	+5.4	0	−5.4	−10.8	−16.2	−20	

(~95% across axial length 16 to 34; ~90% across axial length 18 to 32)

Globe size and intravitreal injections

Teichmann[80] and Fechner and Teichmann[81] have considered the variation in the volume of vitreous, from 1.7 to 16.5 ml, for globe sizes of axial lengths from 16 mm to 34 mm, respectively. These are given as whole globe volumes (on average 80% is vitreous) in Table 5.9 together with the expected frequency and degree of myopia or hypermetropia.

For the 90% of eyes that have an axial length between 21 mm and 26.0 mm, the expected volume of the whole globe varies from 4.2 to 9.2 ml, respectively, of which the vitreous constitutes 75% to 85%, giving an average value for the vitreous from 4.0 ml to 7.5 ml. For the average eye with an axial length of 23.5 mm, the globe volume would be 6.5 ml (vitreous volume of 5.2 ml). The effect of injecting an antibiotic would be to dilute the expected concentration in the myopic, long eye (26 mm, −7 diopters [D]) by approximately 38% and to increase the concentration in the hypermetropic, short eye (20.5 mm, +6.6 D) by approximately 38%. This range of error should be considered by the clinician but it is probably acceptable in practice, because the antibiotic toxicity studies were done in rabbit eyes with a volume of 1.4 ml, which is lower than the vitreous volume of a human hyperopic eye. Provided the correct intravitreal dose of antibiotic has been administered with proper technique, no toxicity should be expected.

References

1. Gardner S. Ocular pharmacokinetics. In: Lamberts DW, Potter DE, eds. *Clinical Ophthalmic Pharmacology* (Little Brown: Boston/Toronto, 1987) 1–55.
2. Golden B, Coppel SP. Ocular tissue absorption of gentamicin, *Arch Ophthalmol* (1970) **84**:792–6.
3. Litwack KD, Petit T, Johnson BL Jr. Penetration of gentamicin: administered intramuscularly and subconjunctivally into aqueous humor, *Arch Ophthalmol* (1969) **82**:687–93.
4. Locatcher-Khorazo D, Gutierrez EH. Postoperative infections of the eye. In Locatcher-Khorazo D, Seegal BC, eds, *Microbiology of the Eye* (CV Mosby: St Louis, 1972) 77.
5. Sorsby A, Ungar J. Distribution of penicillin in the eye after injection of 1,000,000 units by the subconjunctival retrobulbar and intramuscular routes, *Br J Ophthalmol* (1948) **32**:864.
6. Green WR, Leopold IH. Intraocular penetration of methicillin, *Am J Ophthalmol* (1965) **60**:800–4.
7. Records RE, Ellis PP. The intraocular penetration of ampicillin, methicillin, and oxacillin, *Am J Ophthalmol* (1967) **64**:135–43.
8. Records RE. Intraocular penetration of dicloxacillin in experimental animals, *Invest Ophthalmol* (1968) **7**:663–7.
9. Faris BM, Uwaydah MM. Intraocular penetration of semisynthetic penicillins: methicillin, cloxacillin, ampicillin and carbenicillin studies in experimental animals, with a review of the literature, *Arch Ophthalmol* (1974) **92**:501–5.
10. Kurose Y, Leopold IH. Intraocular penetration of ampicillin. I. Animal experiment, *Arch Ophthalmol* (1965) **73**:361–5.
11. Goldman EE, McLain JH, Smith JL. Penicillins and aqueous humor. *Am J Ophthalmol* (1968) **65**: 717–21.
12. Migita H. Experimental and clinical studies on synthetic penicillin in ocular infections, *Acta Soc Ophthalmol Jpn* (1963) **67**:1880.
13. Milano C. Richerche sperimentali sul passaggio dell'acido 6 (D-alfa-aminofenilacetamido) penicillanico in camera anteriore, *Boll Oculist* (1964) **43**: 907–15.

14. McPherson SD Jr, Presley GD, Crawford JR. Aqueous humor assays of subconjunctival antibiotics, *Am J Ophthalmol* (1968) **66**:430–5.

15. Records RE. Intraocular penetration of cephaloridine: observations in experimental animal and human eyes, *Arch Ophthalmol* (1969) **81**:331–5.

16. Jenkins CDG, Tuft SJ, Sheraidah G et al. Comparative intraocular penetration of topical and injected cefuroxime, *Br J Ophthalmol* (1996) **80**:685–8.

17. Personal communication.

18. Naib K, Hallett JW, Leopold IH. Observations on the ocular effects of erythromycin, *Am J Ophthalmol* (1955) **39**:395–9.

19. Becker EF. The intraocular penetration of lincomycin, *Am J Ophthalmol* (1969) **67**:963–5.

20. Boyle GL, Lichtig ML, Leopold IH. Lincomycin levels in human ocular fluids and serum following subconjunctival injection, *Am J Ophthalmol* (1971) **71**:1303–6.

21. Brinton GS, Topping TM, Hyndiuk RA, Aaberg TM, Reeser FH, Abrams GW. Posttraumatic endophthalmitis, *Arch Ophthalmol* (1984) **102**:547–50.

22. Personal communication.

23. Leopold IH, Nichols AC, Vogel AW. Penetration of chloramphenicol USP (chloromycetin) into the eye, *Arch Ophthalmol* (1950) **44**:22.

24. Behrens-Baumann W, Martell J. Ciprofloxacin concentration in the rabbit aqueous humor and vitreous following intravenous and subconjunctival administration. *Infection* (1988) **16**:54–7.

25. Hariprasad SM, Mieler WF, Holz ER. Vitreous and aqueous penetration of orally administered gatifloxacin in humans, *Arch Ophthalmol* (2003) **121**:345–50.

26. Kobayakawa S, Tochikubo T, Tsuji A. Penetration of levofloxacin into human aqueous humor, *Ophthalmic Res* (2003) **35**:97–101.

27. Koch HR, Kulus SC, Ropo A et al. Corneal penetration of fluoroquinolones: aqueous humour concentrations after topical application of levofloxacin 0.5% and ofloxacin 0.3% eye drops. Presented at the XXIXth International Congress of Ophthalmology, Sydney, 2002.

28. Colin J, Simonpoli S, Geldsetzer K et al. Corneal penetration of levofloxacin into the human aqueous humour: a comparison with ciprofloxacin, *Acta Ophthalmol Scand* (2003) **81**:611–13.

29. Garcia-Saenz MC, Arias-Puente A, Fresnadillo-Martinez MJ et al. Human aqueous humor levels of oral ciprofloxacin, levofloxacin and moxifloxacin, *J Cataract Refract Surg* (2001) **27**: 1969–74.

30. Robertson SM, Sanders M, Jasheway D et al. Penetration and distribution of moxifloxacin and ofloxacin into ocular tissues and plasma following topical ocular administration to pigmented rabbits. Presented at the 2003 meeting of the Association for Research in Vision and Ophthalmology (ARVO), Fort Lauderdale, FL, USA (abstract 1454).

31. Dong B, Muhtaseb M, Mearza AA et al. Aqueous level of ofloxacin following oral administration using capillary zone electrophoresis. Presented at the 2003 meeting of the Association for Research in Vision and Ophthalmology (ARVO), Fort Lauderdale, FL, USA (abstract 1458).

32. Yamada K, Mochizuki H, Yamada M et al. Aqueous humor levels of topically applied levofloxacin, norfloxacin, and lomefloxacin in the same human eyes, *J Cataract Refract Surg* (2003) **29**:1771–5.

33. Bucci FA. An in vivo comparison of the ocular absorption of levofloxacin versus ciprofloxacin prior to phacoemulsification. Presented at the 2002 meeting of the Association for Research in Vision and Ophthalmology (ARVO), Fort Lauderdale, FL, USA (abstract 1579).

34. Fiscella RG, Nguyen TKP, Cwik MJ et al. Aqueous and vitreous penetration of levofloxacin after oral administration, *Ophthalmology* (1999) **106**: 2286–90.

35. Sasaki K, Mitsui Y, Fukuda M et al. Intraocular penetration mode of five fluoroquinolone ophthalmic solutions evaluated by the newly proposed parameter of AQCmax, *Atarashii Ganka (J Eye)* (1995) **12**:787–90.

36. Inoue S, Misaki M, Matsumura K. Intraocular penetration of DR-3355, *Atarashii Ganka (J Eye)* (1992) **9**:487–90.

37. Ishikawa K, Yamada M, Mochizuki H et al. Corneal stromal penetration of topically applied levofloxacin, norfloxacin, and lomefloxacin in the same human eyes. Presented at the 2002 meeting of the Association for Research in Vision and Ophthalmology (ARVO), Fort Lauderdale, FL, USA (abstract 1578).

38. Cunha-Vaz JG. The blood-ocular barriers, *Surv Ophthalmol* (1979) **23**:279–96.

39. Cunha-Vaz JG. The blood-ocular barriers: past, present, and future, *Doc Ophthalmol* (1997) **93**:149–57.

40. Peyman GA, Spitznas M, Straatsma BR. Peroxidase diffusion in the normal and photocoagulated retina, *Invest Ophthalmol* (1971) **10**:181–9.

41. Peyman GA, Spitznas M, Straatsma BR. Chorioretinal diffusion of peroxidase before and after photocoagulation, *Invest Ophthalmol* (1971) **10**:489–95.

42. Barza M, Kane A, Baum J. Pharmacokinetics of intravitreal carbenicillin, cefazolin and gentamicin in rhesus monkeys, *Invest Ophthalmol Vis Sci* (1983) **24**:1602–6.

43. Ficker L, Meredith TA, Gardner S et al. Cefazolin levels after intravitreal injection: effects of inflammation and surgery, *Invest Ophthalmol Vis Sci* (1990) **31**:302–5.

44. Kane A, Barza M, Baum J. Intravitreal injection of

gentamicin in rabbits: effect of inflammation and pigmentation on half-life and ocular distribution, *Invest Ophthalmol Vis Sci* (1981) **20**:593–7.

45. Cobo LM, Forster RK. The clearance of intravitreal gentamicin, *Am J Ophthalmol* (1981) **92**:59–62.

46. Pflugfelder SC, Hernandez E, Fliesler SJ et al. Intravitreal vancomycin: retinal toxicity, clearance and interaction with gentamicin, *Arch Ophthalmol* (1987) **105**:831–7.

47. Case JL, Peyman GA, Barrada A et al. Clearance of intravitreal 3H-fluorouracil, *Ophthalmic Surg* (1985) **16**:378–81.

48. Peyman GA, May DR, Homer PI et al. Penetration of gentamicin into the aphakic eye, *Ann Ophthalmol* (1977) **9**:871–80.

49. Kasbeer RT, Peyman GA, May DR et al. Penetration of amikacin into the aphakic eye, *Albrecht von Graefes Arch Klin Exp Ophthalmol* (1975) **196**:85–94.

50. Peyman GA, May DR, Ericson ES et al. Intraocular injection of gentamicin: toxic effects and clearance, *Arch Ophthalmol* (1974) **97**:42–8.

51. Campochiaro PA, Conway BP. Aminoglycoside toxicity: a survey of retinal specialists. Implications for ocular use, *Arch Ophthalmol* (1991) **109**:946–50.

52. Campochiaro PA, Lim JI. Aminoglycoside toxicity in the treatment of endophthalmitis. The Aminoglycoside Toxicity Study Group, *Arch Ophthalmol* (1994) **112**:48–53.

53. Goldblum D, Rohrer K, Frueh BE et al. Corneal concentrations following systemic administration of amphotericin B and its lipid preparations in a rabbit model, *Ophthalmic Res* (2004) **36**:172–6.

54. Smith RP, Baltch AL, Franke MA et al. Levofloxacin penetrates human monocytes and enhances intracellular killing of *Staphylococcus aureus* and *Pseudomonas aeruginosa*, *J Antimicrob Chemother* (2000) **45**:483–8.

55. Vazifeh D, Bryskier A, Labro M-T. Mechanism underlying levofloxacin uptake by human polymorphonuclear neutrophils, *Antimicrob Agents Chemother* (1999) **43**:246–52.

56. Mandell GL, Coleman E. Uptake, transport, and delivery of antimicrobial agents by human polymorphonuclear neutrophils, *Antimicrob Agents Chemother* (2001) **45**:1794–8.

57. Pascual A, Garcia I, Ballesta S et al. Uptake and intracellular activity of moxifloxacin in human neutrophils and tissue-cultured epithelial cells, *Antimicrob Agents Chemother* (1999) **43**:12–15.

58. Garcia I, Pascual A, Ballesta S et al. Uptake and intracellular activity of ofloxacin isomers in human phagocytic and non-phagocytic cells, *Int J Antimicrob Agents* (2000) **15**:201–5.

59. Perea EJ, Garcia I, Pascual A. Comparative penetration of lomefloxacin and other quinolones into human phagocytes, *Am J Med* (1992) **92**:48S–51S.

60. Garcia I, Pascual A, Ballesta S et al. Intracellular penetration and activity of gemifloxacin in human polymorphonuclear leukocytes, *Antimicrob Agents Chemother* (2000) **44**: 3193–8.

61. Seal DV, Bron AJ, Hay J. *Ocular Infection – Investigation and Treatment in Practice* (Martin Dunitz: London, 1998).

62. Abreu J, Cordovés L, Mesa CG et al. Chronic pseudophakic endophthalmitis versus saccular endophthalmitis, *J Cataract Refract Surg* (1997) **23**:1122–5.

63. Abreu JA, Cordoves L. Endoftalmitis sacular, *Arch Soc Esp Oftalmol* (2001) **76**:5–6.

64. Abreu JA, Cordovés L. Chronic or saccular endophthalmitis: diagnosis and management, *J Cataract Refract Surg* (2001) **27**:650–1.

65. Warheker PT, Gupta SR, Mansfield DC et al. Postoperative saccular endophthalmitis caused by macrophage-associated staphylococci, *Eye* (1998) **12**:1019–21.

66. Kresloff MS, Castellarin AA, Zarbin MA. Endophthalmitis, *Surv Ophthalmol* (1998) **43**: 193–224.

67. Warheker PT, Gupta SR, Mansfield DC et al. Successful treatment of saccular endophthalmitis with clarithromycin, *Eye* (1998) **12**:1017–19.

68. Karia N, Aylward GW. Letter on use of clarithromycin, *Ophthalmology* (2001) **108**:634.

69. Okhravi N, Guest S, Matheson MM et al. Assessment of the effect of oral clarithromycin on visual outcome following presumed bacterial endophthalmitis, *Curr Eye Res* (2000) **21**:691–702.

70. Al-Sibai MB, Al-Kaff AS, Raines D et al. Ocular penetration of oral clarithromycin in humans, *J Ocul Pharmacol Ther* (1998) **14**:575–83.

71. Graves A, Henry M, O'Brien TP et al. In vitro susceptibilities of bacterial ocular isolates to fluoroquinolones, *Cornea* (2001) **20**:301–5. [Erratum appears in *Cornea* (2001) **20**:546.]

72. Kowalski RP, Dhaliwal DK, Karenchak LM et al. Gatifloxacin and moxifloxacin: an in vitro susceptibility comparison to levofloxacin, ciprofloxacin and ofloxacin using bacterial keratitis isolates, *Am J Ophthalmol* (2003) **136**:500-5.

73. Raizman MB, Rubin JM, Graves AL et al. Tear concentrations of levofloxacin following topical administration of a single dose of 0.5% levofloxacin ophthalmic solution in healthy volunteers, *Clin Ther* (2002) **24**:1439–50.

74. Kowalski RP, Romanowski EG, Mah FS et al. The prevention of bacterial endophthalmitis by topical moxifloxacin in a rabbit prophylaxis model. Presented at the 2003 meeting of the Association for Research in Vision and Ophthalmology (ARVO), Fort Lauderdale, FL, USA (abstract 1467).

75. McCulley JP, Surratt G, Shine WE. Fourth generation fluoroquinolone penetration into aqueous

humor in humans - post-op concentrations. Presented at the 2004 meeting of the Association for Research in Vision and Ophthalmology (ARVO), Fort Lauderdale, Fl, USA (abstract 4927).

76. Solomon R, Donnenfeld ED, Perry HD et al. Penetration of topically applied Gatifloxacin 0.3%, Moxifloxacin 0.5% and Ciprofloxacin 0.3% into the aqueous humor. Presented at the 2004 meeting of the Association for Research in Vision and Ophthalmology (ARVO), Fort Lauderdale, Fl, USA (abstract 4925).

77. Katz H, Lane S, Masket S et al. Human aqueous humor concentrations of Moxifloxacin following two multiple-dose topical ocular dosing regimes of Vigamox™. Presented at the 2004 meeting of the Association for Research in Vision and Ophthalmology (ARVO), Fort Lauderdale, Fl, USA (abstract 4926).

78. Montan PG, Wejde G, Koranyi G et al. Prophylactic intracameral cefuroxime. Efficacy in preventing endophthalmitis after cataract surgery, *J Cataract Refract Surg* (2002) **28**:977–81.

79. Montan PG, Wejde G, Setterquist H et al. Prophylactic intracameral cefuroxime. Evaluation of safety and kinetics in cataract surgery, *J Cataract Refract Surg* (2002) **28**:982–7.

80. Teichmann KD. Intravitreal injections: Does globe size matter?, *J Cataract Refract Surg* (2002) **28**: 1886–9.

81. Fechner PU, Teichmann KD. *Ocular Therapeutics – Pharmacology and Clinical Application*. (Slack Inc.: Thorofare, NJ, USA, 1998): 11,451–70.

6

Exogenous endophthalmitis

Infectious endophthalmitis is a severe intraocular inflammatory response to an infectious agent (bacteria, virus, fungus, or parasite) following ocular surgery, trauma, or systemic infection. As a result of the inflammation, periocular congestion with lid swelling, pain, hypopyon, abscess, and blurring or loss of vision occur. If the infectious source is external such as surgery or trauma, it is termed exogenous endophthalmitis; endogenous endophthalmitis occurs from systemic dissemination, especially in an immunocompromised patient (Chapter 9, Endogenous endophthalmitis). If the inflammation involves the sclera and extraocular orbital structures, it is termed 'panophthalmitis.'

Postoperative endophthalmitis

Postoperative endophthalmitis occurs most commonly as a complication of cataract extraction, but can also follow penetrating keratoplasty and squint surgery. Both acute and chronic forms of endophthalmitis are observed. Acute postoperative endophthalmitis usually occurs within 6 weeks of surgery, caused by Gram-positive bacteria (*Staphylococcus aureus, S. epidermidis*), and virulent streptococcal species including beta-hemolytic strains (*Streptococcus pyogenes*), *Strep. pneumoniae* and *S. mitis*. Chronic postoperative endophthalmitis usually occurs after 6 weeks and is associated with less virulent organisms such as corynebacteria, *Propionibacterium acnes*, coagulase-negative staphylococci (CNS), and fungi. Most of these organisms are commensals found in the normal ocular flora (lid margin, conjunctiva, and lacrimal sac).

The incidence rate of postoperative endophthalmitis has improved considerably over the last 50 years. Ophthalmologists today have the advantage of improved antibiotic prophylaxis and sterile aseptic techniques and equipment. Other factors in the reduced incidence rate include better understanding of risk factors (Box 6.1) and sterilization techniques, perioperative antibiotics and improved methods of drug delivery (subconjunctival/intracameral routes) discussed in Chapter 4.

The most important advance in preventing postoperative endophthalmitis has been the advent of a sterile surgical field. Given that most of the organisms that cause postoperative endophthalmitis are commensals that normally populate the external ocular surface, improved sterilization of the surgical field has decreased the rate of infection. To this end, several studies have demonstrated that povidone-iodine (5%) solution applied topically prior to surgery effectively reduces the count of bacterial flora by 10–100-fold and thereby reduces the chances for, and the incidence of, postoperative endophthalmitis. However, the statistics for the benefit of this antiseptic technique are only significant at the 0.05 level.[1]

Box 6.1 Risk factors for the development of postoperative endophthalmitis

- Preoperative: diabetes (especially uncontrolled diabetics), chronic steroid use, chronic bacterial blepharitis, active conjunctivitis, lacrimal drainage system infection or obstruction, contaminated eye drops.
- Operative: wound abnormalities, vitreous loss, prolonged surgery, contaminated irrigation solutions or equipment, polypropylene haptics.
- Postoperative: wound leak or dehiscence, inadequately buried sutures, vitreous incarceration in the surgical wound, the presence of a filtering bleb, contaminated eye drops.

Povidone-iodine

The role of polyvinylpyrollidone iodine (povidone-iodine) in the prophylaxis of postoperative endophthalmitis has been studied since 1984 by Apt et al[2] and Speaker and Menikoff,[1] as reviewed by Ciulla et al.[3] A formulation of 5% povidone-iodine in balanced saline solution (BSS) has been available on the American market for many years and has now been introduced into most countries in Europe. If the solution has to be made up in hospital pharmacies or operating rooms from stock solutions, special care is required because it can easily deteriorate in activity and become contaminated with resistant pseudomonads. Only fresh sterile solutions should be used for prophylaxis. Speaker and Menikoff[1] reported a large retrospective study of 40,000 patients in 1991 in New York which gave a reduction in postoperative endophthalmitis at the 0.05% level when it was used as prophylaxis in cataract surgery.

Povidone-iodine (5% in BSS) has been identified as the only type of prophylaxis proven in scientific studies to reduce postoperative endophthalmitis.[3] This beneficial effect results from a reduction by 10–100-fold of the bacterial load on the conjunctival and corneal surface as well as a reduction in the number of bacterial species that can be isolated. Povidone-iodine does not produce a sterile conjunctiva or cornea; it simply reduces the bacterial count by 1 or 2 $\log_{10}$ counts. Apt et al also showed that povidone-iodine 5% solution applied at the end of the surgery was more effective than a drop of a broad-spectrum antibiotic solution (polymyxin B sulfate-neomycin sulfate-gramicidin) at preventing an increase, which persisted for 24 hours, in the number of bacterial colony-forming units on the conjunctiva.[4] However, Mendivil Soto and Mendivil in 2001 found that 5% povidone-iodine reduced positive cultures in the aqueous humor at the end of surgery, but this reduction did not reach statistical significance.[5] On balance, povidone-iodine should be used for surgical prophylaxis but it is not as effective as claimed by some workers.

Povidone-iodine 5% in BSS is nontoxic to the conjunctiva and cornea if applied topically for 3 minutes prior to surgery when it is then diluted by the saline used to keep the surface of the eye moist. In contrast, Alp et al have shown that 5% povidone-iodine causes severe toxicity when one drop is placed in the anterior chamber.[6] Care is thus needed when using povidone-iodine to prevent inadvertent leakage into the anterior chamber. It should also be noted that povidone-iodine is 10 times more toxic for neutrophils than for bacteria. Povidone-iodine is effective against most Gram-positive bacteria, Gram-negative bacteria, acid-fast bacteria (mycobacteria), fungi including yeasts and hyaline filamentous species, nocardia, viruses (including cytomegalovirus (CMV), herpes, enteroviruses and others), and protozoa.[7] Povidone-iodine must be reserved for topical use only because it is toxic to tissue.

Preparation of the eye with povidone-iodine is best conducted in the anesthetic room but can also be performed on the operating table. The eyelids, eyebrow, nose, cheek, and forehead should be wiped carefully with povidone-iodine 5% or 10% solution in concentric rings outward from the eye (Figure 6.1A). Then, one drop of povidone-iodine 5% in BSS, ideally from a single-use sterile container or a sterile syringe, is placed onto the cornea and into the conjunctival sac (Figure 6.1B). The period of antisepsis should be timed with a stopwatch to allow a minimum of 3 minutes activity (Figure 6.1C), after which the ocular surface can be rinsed carefully with saline. Eyelashes are not trimmed preoperatively but should be carefully removed from the surgical field with sterile adhesive foil and drapes (Figure 6.1D). Further povidone-iodine may be applied but is not considered mandatory.

Clinical signs of endophthalmitis

Endophthalmitis is a potentially blinding disease with irreversible tissue damage occurring within 24–48 hours. Early diagnosis and prompt treatment are therefore essential (Figure 6.2). Symptoms of acute endophthalmitis include:

- pain
- blurring or loss of vision
- lid and conjunctival swelling
- discharge.

Signs of acute endophthalmitis include:

- reduced visual acuity, down to perception of light
- conjunctival and corneal edema (Figure 6.3A, B)

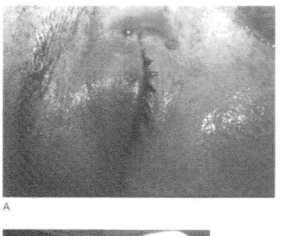

A

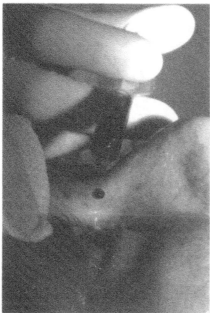

B

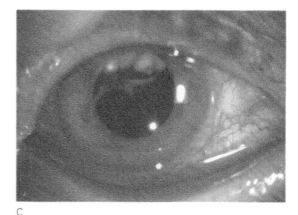

C

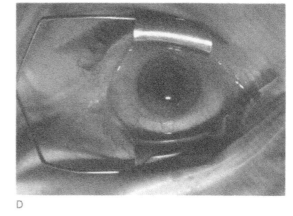

D

Figure 6.1

(A) Povidone-iodine is applied to eyelids, eyebrow, nose, cheek, and forehead preoperatively. (B) Povidone–iodine is applied to the cornea and conjunctival sac. (C) Povidone-iodine is left for 3 minutes to disinfect the ocular surface before applying drapes. (D) Eyelashes are removed from the operating site with a sterile drape and retractor to produce an 'almost sterile' surgical field.

Figure 6.2

Corneal edema, haze, and anterior chamber reaction with hypopyon at day 5 after uneventful phacoemulsification surgery – not culture-proven.

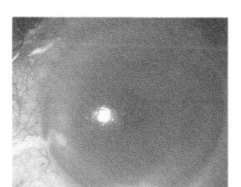

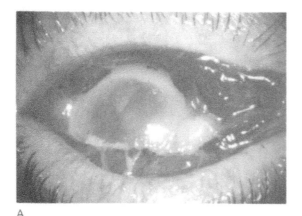

A

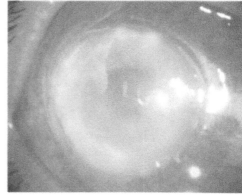

B

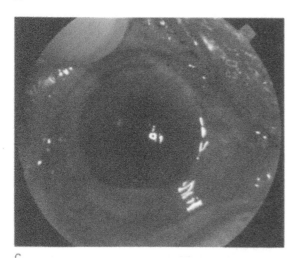

C

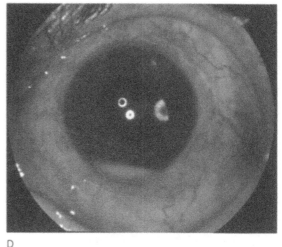

D

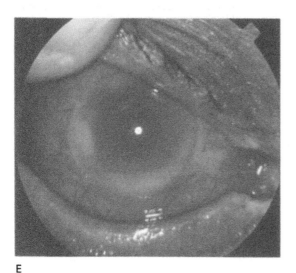

E

Figure 6.3

(A) Excessive conjunctival chemosis, corneal edema, infiltration, and exudation with ring abscess, anterior chamber reaction, and pupillary membrane formation – acute postoperative endophthalmitis due to *Pseudomonas aeruginosa* at day 4. (B) Excessive conjunctival hyperemia and corneal edema at day 6 after cataract surgery – acute postoperative endophthalmitis caused by *Staphylococcus aureus*. (C) Severe corneal edema with wound infection and anterior chamber reaction with hypopyon. The patient was referred 4 days after surgery and an intravitreal injection – not culture-proven. (D) Endophthalmitis resulting from coagulase-negative staphylococcus infection presenting with a swollen lid, chemotic conjunctiva, corneal haze, anterior chamber reaction, and hypopyon 3 weeks after combination cataract surgery. (E) After uneventful phacoemulsification surgery, infected infiltrated areas can be seen in the stab incision and phaco incision points. There is conjunctival hyperemia, corneal edema, anterior chamber reaction, and hypopyon 2 days after surgery. *Proteus* sp. was cultured from the vitreous and the patient was treated with intravitreal antibiotics.

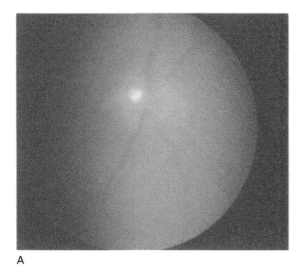

A

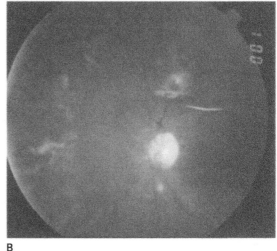

B

Figure 6.4

(A) Vitritis with retinal and papillary edema in endophthalmitis. (B) Fundus photograph after endophthalmitis with retinal detachment. Reflections of silicone oil and laser-made areas can be seen. Peripapillary edema and vascular occlusions can still be observed. Retinal surgery was performed with a circling band, pars plana vitrectomy, perfluorocarbon injection, and endolaser application on the peripheral retina with a buckling procedure and silicone oil injection.

- a cloudy cornea sometimes with an infiltrate or ring abscess (Figure 6.3C, D, E)
- a cloudy anterior chamber with cells, hypopyon, or fibrin clot
- afferent pupillary defect
- vitreous clouding (vitritis) from inflammation precluding a view of the retinal vessels; often no view of the posterior segment is possible (Figure 6.4A)
- retinitis and/or retinal periphlebitis, retinal edema, and papillary edema (Figure 6.4B)
- absent red reflex.

It is worth stressing that loss of the red reflex when the vitreous is viewed through the pupil may be a poor guide to the state of the vitreous, which may be most opaque anteriorly where the inflammatory process has begun. If the pupil is observed while the sclera is transilluminated, the red reflex may become apparent and can then form a better guide to control of the disease.

Ocular echography is a useful adjunct for the clinical evaluation of infectious endophthalmitis, especially in an eye with opaque media (Figure 6.5).

A patient with these symptoms and signs requires immediate anterior chamber tap and

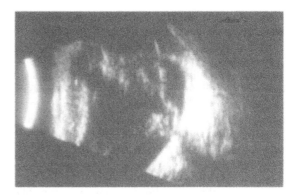

Figure 6.5

B-scan ultrasonography shows abnormal irregular high reflections in midvitreous as the result of severe vitritis and condensation of vitreous tissue. There is a high intensity on the prepapillary area and possible retinal detachment as seen behind the condensed vitreous.

vitreous biopsy (Chapter 8). Gram stain and semi-quantitative culture of aqueous and vitreous should be performed. Isolation of any bacterial colonies, on direct plating of four agar plates

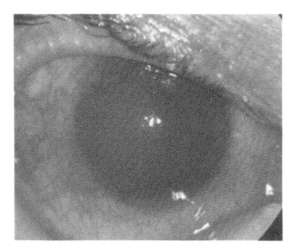

Figure 6.6

Conjunctival hyperemia, corneal edema, infiltration, and anterior chamber reaction without hypopyon 4 weeks after extracapsular cataract extraction. Gram stain and culture were negative.

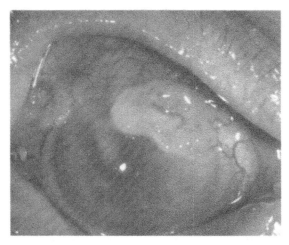

Figure 6.7

Acremonium (*Cephalosporium*) endophthalmitis diagnosed 1 year after extracapsular cataract surgery. The eye had been treated for persistent iritis for 6 months with topical corticosteroids.

cultured aerobically, microaerophilically, or anaerobically, should be deemed indicative of culture-positive endophthalmitis.

Patients who present within 6 weeks of cataract surgery with reduced visual acuity and signs of inflammation in the anterior chamber (Figure 6.6) that have been managed with corticosteroids may have been given the diagnosis of 'hypopyon uveitis.' They should be managed in the same manner as for acute endophthalmitis. If vitrectomy is not indicated, anterior chamber and vitreous taps will be required to confirm infection and to identify the microbe responsible, possibly including a polymerase chain reaction (PCR) test. Antibiotics should be instilled at the same time.

Patients presenting more than 6 weeks postoperatively with 'hypopyon uveitis' with inflammatory signs in the anterior chamber that have failed to respond to corticosteroids should be investigated for chronic infection (see below). The possibility should be considered that the inflammation results from chronic infection of the capsular sac with *P. acnes* or CNS; however, fungi may be involved as well with *Candida glabrata* producing a *Propionibacterium*-type clinical picture. The diagnosis can be confirmed even after 1 year by an anterior chamber or vitre-ous tap followed by Gram stain, culture, and a PCR test (see Chapter 3) and chronic infection section below).

Bacteria causing acute endophthalmitis include *S. aureus, Strep. pyogenes, Strep. pneumoniae, Enterococcus faecalis,* Enterobacteriaceae, *Moraxella* sp. and, after trauma, *Bacillus* spp. (commonly) and *Clostridium perfringens* (occasionally) – see section on trauma below. Causes of chronic endophthalmitis include CNS, *P. acnes*, diphtheroids, and occasionally streptococci. Expected antibiotic sensitivities are given in Chapter 5. Acute endophthalmitis occasionally follows squint surgery, when infection is usually due to *S. aureus* but may be due to *Haemophilus influenzae*. In pediatric cases, emergency examination under anesthesia is required with a vitreous tap and instillation of antibiotics.

Postoperative endophthalmitis caused by fungi usually follows cataract surgery (Figure 6.7). Such infection has been reported for at least the last 50 years (Table 6.1).[8–35] Fungal endophthalmitis is more common in tropical humid climates; outbreaks have occurred in temperate zones because of contaminated equipment. Cases of fungal endophthalmitis that developed after other ocular surgery are described in Table 6.2.[29,36,37]

Table 6.1 Fungus endophthalmitis following cataract surgery

Reference	Type of fungus (no. of infected patients)	Source	Age of patient (years)	Place
Lagnado et al, 2004[8]	Candida albicans (1)	Phaco/IOL	85	Nottingham, England
Spirn et al, 2003[9]	Trichosporon beigelii and Acremonium sp. (1)	Phaco/IOL. Systemic and ocular sarcoidosis. Pain and decreased vision after 8 days. Vitrectomy with intravitreal amphotericin 3 weeks after cataract surgery. LP with capsular plaque. Had further vitrectomy with removal of IOL and entire capsule; both were culture-positive for both pathogens. Responded to surgery and fluconazole. T. beigelii was resistant to amphotericin.	58	New Brunswick, USA
Garbino et al, 2002[10]	Paecilomyces lilacinus (1)	Phaco/IOL. Late-onset endophthalmitis resistant to amphotericin and itraconazole but responded well to voriconazole	61	Geneva, Switzerland
Narang et al, 2001[11]	Aspergillus flavus (16) Aspergillus fumigatus (3) Aspergillus niger (1) Acremonium kiliense (1) Candida albicans (3) Candida tropicalis (1) Candida guilliermondii (1) Fonsecaea pedrosoi (1)	12 ECCE/IOL; 1 ECCE; 1 Phaco/ IOL; 2 ICCE 1 ECCE/IOL; 1 ECCE; 1 Phaco, 1 ECCE 1, ECCE/IOL, 1 ECCE/IOL; 2 ICCE 1, ECCE/IOL, 1 Phaco/IOL, 1 Phaco/IOL	25–73	Chandigarh, India
Kaushik et al, 2001[12]	Curvularia lunata (1)	ECCE/IOL with secondary keratitis	40	Chandigarh, India
Huber et al, 2000[13]	Exophiala werneckii (1)	Phaco/IOL indolent endophthalmitis	NG	Salt Lake City, USA
Tabbara and al-Jabarti, 1998[14]	Aspergillus fumigatus (5)	Airborne contamination of hospital construction site during cataract surgery – ECCE/IOL. Onset 4–15 days postoperatively with endophthalmitis. Failed therapy with enucleation/evisceration in all cases	51–65	Jeddah, Saudi Arabia
Weissgold et al, 1998[15]	Fusarium solani (1) Acremonium kiliense (1)	Phaco/IOL. Endophthalmitis after 2 and 3 weeks. Delayed-onset keratitis after endophthalmitis	71, 81	Philadelphia, USA
Seal et al, 1998[16]	Aspergillus terreus (1)	ECCE/IOL – operation and infection in Pakistan	70	London, UK
Fridkin et al, 1996[17]	Acremonium kiliense (4)	Cataract surgery in a day-surgery center traced to an environmental reservoir – a humidifier that was fitted after the air filters, associated with being switched on in the morning producing an aerosol following a switched-off period	57, 73, 81, 88	Radnor, USA
Bartz-Schmidt et al, 1996[18]	Basidiomycetes (1)	ECCE/IOL with chronic endophthalmitis. Progressive infection over 1 year not responsive to intravitreal amphotericin and itraconazole	67	Cologne, Germany
Oxford et al, 1995[19]	Aspergillus sp. (1)	Phaco/IOL. Presented after 5 weeks. Failed therapy with vitrectomy and intravitreal amphotericin	94	San Francisco, USA
Verbraeken, 1995[20]	Aspergillus fumigatus (2) Aspergillus niger (1) Acremonium sp. (1) Candida albicans (2)	ICCE – Aspergillus fumigatus 1, Candida albicans 1; ICCE/IOL – Aspergillus fumigatus 1; Candida albicans 1; ECCE – Acremonium sp. 1; ECCE/IOL – Aspergillus niger 1	NG	Ghent, Belgium

cont.

Table 6.1 Fungus endophthalmitis following cataract surgery – *continued*

Reference	Type of fungus (no. of infected patients)	Source	Age of patient (years)	Place
Fekrat et al, 1995[21]	*Candida parapsilosis* (1)	Keratitis post-Phaco/IOL	68	Baltimore, USA
Ohkubo et al, 1994[22]	*Paecilomyces lilacinus* (1)	1 ECCE/IOL	NG	Japan
Das et al, 1993[23]	*Aspergillus terreus* (1)	ICCE. No IOL. Responded to vitrectomy and intravitreal amphotericin	50	Hyderabad, India
Bouchard et al, 1991[24]	*Pseudallescheria boydii* (1)	ECCE/IOL. Presented 5 weeks postoperatively. Responded to vitrectomy with intravitreal, IV, and topical amphotericin	80	Maywood, USA
Rao et al, 1991[25]	*Candida famata* (1)	ECCE/IOL. Presented 3 months postoperatively	74	Los Angeles, USA
Srinivasan et al, 1991[26]	*Penicillium* spp. (8) *Aspergillus fumigatus* (5) *Aspergillus niger* (3) *Phialaphora* sp. (1) *Humicola* sp. (1)	Post-cataract surgery = 10; other surgery = 1 (lensectomy); trauma 3; blood-borne (metastatic) = 2	>50	Pondicherry, India
Pulido et al, 1990[27]	*Histoplasma capsulatum*	ECCE/IOL. Diabetes mellitus. Hypopyon iritis, dense vitritis and vitreous wick. Failed therapy with IV and intravitreal amphotericin with enucleation	60	Iowa, USA
Orgel and Cohen, 1989[28]	Zygomycete (*Rhizopus* or *Absidia*) (1)	Phaco/IOL. Initial treatment with steroids for 10 weeks followed by vitrectomy, removal of IOL, and intravitreal amphotericin to give final vision of 20/60	50	Chapel Hill, USA
Pflugfelder et al, 1988[29]	*Candida parapsilosis* (2) *Aspergillus flavus* (1) *Acremonium* sp. (1) *Paecilomyces lilacinus* (1)	Repeat publication of the same cases as Driebe et al.[32]	76/80/ 78/80/ 67	Miami, USA
O'Day et al, 1987[30] and Stern et al, 1985[31]	*Candida parapsilosis* (23)	Multicenter outbreak due to a contaminated irrigating solution. Discrimination by enzyme profile and antimycotic susceptibility testing	62–82	Florida, TN & CA, USA
Driebe et al, 1986[32]	*Candida parapsilosis* (2) *Aspergillus flavus* (1) *Acremonium* sp. (1) *Paecilomyces lilacinus* (1)	5 out of 42 positive cultures were fungi in this retrospective review of all cases of ECCE and an IOL between 1974 and 1983	76/80/ 78/80/ 67	Miami, USA
Minogue et al, 1989[33]	*Paecilomyces lilacinus*	1 ECCE/IOL. Effective treatment given with multiple intravitreal injections of amphotericin	NG	USA
Pettit et al, 1980[34]	*Paecilomyces lilacinus* (13)	ICCE/IOL (10), ECCE/IOL (3). Contamination of neutralization solution for peroxide sterilization of IOLs. All cases presented within 6 weeks	61–92	Los Angeles & New Orleans, USA

cont.

Treatment of bacterial endophthalmitis with antibiotics

Historically, visual recovery following treatment for endophthalmitis has been poor,[38,39] possibly as the result of:

- Extreme sensitivity of the intraocular structures to inflammation (Chapter 1)
- Resistance of the organisms to antibiotics (Chapters 5 and 11)
- Poor host defense mechanisms (Chapter 2)
- Poor penetration of the antibiotics (Chapter 5).

Table 6.1 Fungus endophthalmitis following cataract surgery – *continued*

Reference	Type of fungus (no. of infected patients)	Source	Age of patient (years)	Place
Theodore, 1978[35]	*Acremonium* sp., *Aspergillus fumigatus*, *Aspergillus niger*, *Candida albicans*, *Candida lipolytica*, *Candida parakrusei*, *Curvularia* sp., *Hormodendrum* sp., *Hyalopus bogolepofii*, *Hyalosporus*, *Neurospora sitophila*, *Paecilomyces lilacinus*, *Penicillium* sp., *Pseudallescheria boydii*, *Scopulariopsis brevicaulis*, *Sporotrichum schenckii*, *Trichosporon cutaneum*, *Volutella cinerescens*, *Volutella* sp.	Review of all types of fungi cultured from post-cataract surgery endophthalmitis up to 1977	–	New York, USA

Phaco, phacoemulsification; IOL, intraocular lens; LP, light perception; ECCE, extracapsular cataract extraction; ICCE, intracapsular cataract extraction.

Table 6.2 Postoperative cases in which fungal endophthalmitis developed

Reference	Type of fungus (no. of infected patients)	Source	Age of patient (years)	Place
Kunimoto et al, 1999[36]	*Aspergillus* spp. (17) *Alternaria* sp. (1) *Bipolaris* sp. (1) *Helminthosporium* sp. (1) Unidentified hyaline fungus (1)	Single-center, prospective series of postoperative vitrectomy for endophthalmitis – type of surgery not recorded	Not given	Hyderabad, India
Scott et al, 1996[37]	*Paecilomyces* sp. (1) *Candida glabrata* (1)	Previous ocular surgery/secondary glaucoma requiring a filter	Not given	Miami, USA
Pflugfelder et al, 1988[29]	*Fusarium epispheria* (1)	3 years postsurgery	61	Miami, USA

As skills are developed to significantly alter the first three factors, increased intraocular penetration by antibiotics has been the focus of research in order to improve the outcome of endophthalmitis therapy. Even in 1960, Leopold and Apt[40] reflected this sentiment by stating that 'successful treatment of [endophthalmitis] depends on the prompt use of the appropriate antibiotic and chemotherapeutic agent and the proper choice of that route of administration which would insure the accessibility of the drug to the infected tissue and secure adequate concentrations.' Since that era when up to 50% of eyes with endophthalmitis were adequately treated with systemic chloramphenicol,[40] appropriate drugs and delivery methods, and other techniques to prevent

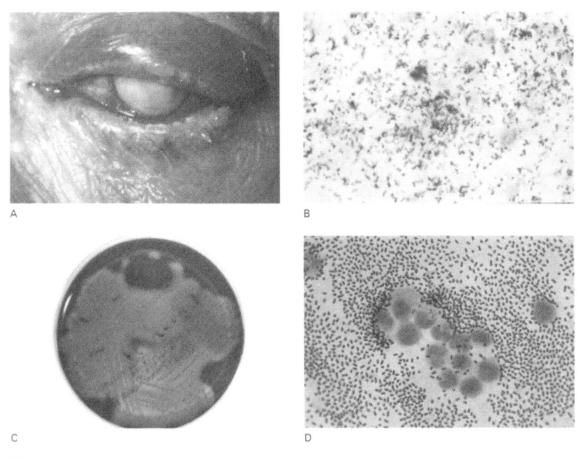

Figure 6.8

(A) Acute purulent endophthalmitis due to *Streptococcus pyogenes* at day 3 after extracapsular cataract surgery. Failed therapy with *intravenous* vancomycin. (B) Gram stain of vitreous for *S. pyogenes* from the eye shown in (A). (C) Vitreous culture on blood agar showing a pool of inhibition from intravenous vancomycin, at the site of plate inoculation, which had insufficient concentration to kill the bulk of the *S. pyogenes* cells in the vitreous. (D) Gram stain of *Streptococcus pneumoniae* (in pairs).

endophthalmitis, have been extensively investigated. The roles of adjuvant treatment such as steroids and indications for vitrectomy and vitreous tap/injection have been established (Chapter 8).

Improving antibiotic penetration into the eye is the most modifiable variable and has received the most attention. Systemic and topical administrations of antibiotics generally result in low and inconsistent intravitreal antibiotic levels (Figure 6.8A–C), except for chloramphenicol, which passes through the blood–brain barrier and is concentrated up to seven times, because it is lipid-soluble. Subconjunctival antibiotic administration may elicit adequate aqueous levels, but posterior segment concentration is generally inadequate.

The poor intraocular penetration after systemic administration is due to tight endothelial junctions that comprise the blood–retinal barrier (Chapter 5). Especially in the retinal pigment epithelium (RPE), structures called zonulae occludentes connecting the RPE and walls of the capillary endothelium prohibit penetration by antibiotics in the circulation into the vitreous space. Eventually, the inflammation cascade (Chapter 1) will overcome this blood–retinal barrier; however, irreversible retinal damage will usually have occurred by this stage.

Direct injection of antibiotics into the vitreous space, the most logical method to bypass this physiologic and anatomic barrier, can be carried out safely as an outpatient procedure. Intravitreal antibiotic injection was first attempted in the 1940s by von Sallmann et al, who successfully treated a rabbit model of staphylococcal endophthalmitis with intravitreal injection of penicillin.[41] In this study, they found that:

- Intravitreal injection of 25 mg sodium penicillin checked progression of infection in all instances when injected 6 or 12 hours after the inoculation.
- Damage to inner structures from a single penicillin injection was limited but repeated injection led to severe damage that was permanent in some cases.
- 10% solution of sodium sulfacetamide caused more inflammation with less effect on infection.

Leopold also found that intravitreal injection of 300 µg of penicillin stopped progression of 'ectogenous' vitreal infection resulting from *S. aureus*.[42] However, repeated subconjunctival and anterior chamber injections of penicillin only halted the progression of vitreous infection in 4 of 10 rabbit eyes.[43]

In a subsequent human treatment trial by von Sallmann,[44] four patients were treated with intravitreal antibiotic injection for endophthalmitis, resulting in two enucleations and stabilization in the other two cases. Useful vision was never recovered by any of the patients. One patient had no documentation of a pyogenic bacterium prior to treatment.

Intravitreal antibiotic injection was then abandoned for nearly two decades by these investigators and was not practiced in ophthalmology. In 1965, Pincus et al noted that 'directly administered antibiotics ... may be quite painful and irritating to the patient. In addition, it carries the hazard of introduction of new organisms or direct toxic damage to ocular tissues.'[45] A thorough toxicity study was never performed by the original investigators. If direct injection was required, subconjunctival penicillin G achieved bactericidal vitreous concentrations and intravitreal injection was thought to be unnecessary.[46]

Intravitreal antibiotic injection had been abandoned for 20 years when Peyman and others evaluated this route of administration in the 1970s. The therapeutic parameters for intravitreal injection of antibiotics were identified.

The clearances of various antibiotics and intravitreal toxicity studies were performed by using rabbit and nonhuman primate models of experimental endophthalmitis, produced by ocular injection of various organisms (Chapter 5). Retinal toxicity was determined using histopathologic examination and electroretinography (ERG) studies.[47] The disc sensitivity techniques of Kirby were used to obtain intravitreal concentrations of various drugs. Kawasaki and Ohnogi[48] reported that antibiotic-induced ERG changes in their *in vitro* model exhibited 'striking similarities' between the rabbit and human eye. They also stated that it would be reasonable to accept experimental results in rabbit eyes for proposed therapy in human eyes. The volume of the rabbit vitreous is 1.5 ml while that of the human vitreous measures 4 ml. The size differential also appears significant in reducing toxicity to the retina when using data obtained from rabbit eyes because it allows a margin of error in the larger human eye which can theoretically withstand a larger dose.

The results of animal experimentation formed the basis for human trials. Peyman's series in 1978 involved 26 eyes in 25 patients with endophthalmitis who were treated with intravitreal antibiotic with or without vitrectomy; 77% of the patients retained their eyes. Overall, 46% had visual acuity better than 20/100; 27% had vision ranging from light perception to 20/300, and 4% had no light perception.[49–51] Two factors influenced results in this series of endophthalmitis cases. The majority of eyes that achieved final visual acuity of 20/100 or better were treated within 36 hours after the onset of symptoms. Eyes infected with organisms elaborating significant amounts of exotoxins and proteolytic enzymes fared worse than other eyes. In the series reported by Vastine and co-workers[51] confirmed that the visual prognosis in eyes with endophthalmitis that have been treated with intravitreal antibiotics is related to these same factors: 1) interval between onset of symptoms and administration of intravitreal antibiotics, 2) exotoxins and proteolytic activity of the organisms isolated from the eye. Verbraeken reported on a large series of patients referred to his retinal unit and showed clearly that the virulence of the organism influenced the final visual acuity recovered from endophthalmitis.[20]

Bacterial endophthalmitis is treated today by a combination of intravitreal and systemic antibiotic therapy with either a vitreous tap or vitrectomy and the use of corticosteroids (refer to Chapter 8 for surgical and other details). Subconjunctival antibiotic therapy is a much less satisfactory alternative to the intravitreal route. An antibiotic combination is injected intravitreally and repeated as necessary according to the clinical response at intervals of 48–72 hours, depending on the persistence of the drugs selected within the eye (Chapters 5 and 8). Intravitreal antibiotic doses are scaled down to avoid retinal toxicity but the margin for error between chemotherapy and toxicity is narrow for the aminoglycosides (for gentamicin, 200 µg is effective but 400 µg can be toxic, causing macular infarction); thus, the total dose injected must be highly accurate.

A combination of intravitreal antibiotics should be instilled as vancomycin (1 mg) or cefazolin (2 mg) plus gentamicin (0.2 mg) or amikacin (0.4 mg); 0.1 ml of each of the two chosen antibiotics should be injected intravitreally after the tap or vitrectomy has been performed. Consideration should also be given to intravitreal injection of corticosteroids at the same time (Chapter 8).

The antibiotics should be supplied freshly diluted by the hospital pharmacy department; however, for cases of emergency only, a method for diluting the drugs in the operating room is given below (an alternative method suitable for use in the USA is given in Chapter 8). The procedure must use sterile equipment and be undertaken on a sterile surface; ideally, the hospital makes up sterile packs with bottles in advance for this purpose. All drugs should be mixed by inverting the bottle 25 times, avoiding frothing.

Some important 'do's' and 'do not's' are:

- **Never** return diluted drugs to the same or original vial for further dilution
- Do **not** use syringes more than once
- **Never** dilute at greater than 1 in 20
- Do **not** reuse bottles for further dilution

Gentamicin. *Dose for use = 200 µg* Method 1: Use a 'Minim' which contains 3000 µg/ml. Dilute to 2000 µg/ml by adding 2 ml of the Minim formulation to 1 ml of sterile normal (0.9%) saline (SNS) in a sterile bottle with lid. Mix well. Use 0.1 ml = 200 µg for injection. Method 2: Remove 0.5 ml, using a 1-ml syringe, from a vial containing 40 mg/ml unpreserved gentamicin and place in a sterile bottle with lid. Add 9.5 ml of SNS or BSS and mix well (= 2.0 mg/ml). Use 0.1 ml = 200 µg.

Amikacin. *Dose for use = 400 µg.* Reconstitute 1 vial of 500 mg and make up to 10 ml with SNS or BSS in a sterile bottle with lid. Mix well. Withdraw 0.8 ml, using a 1-ml syringe, and add to 9.2 ml of SNS or BSS in a sterile bottle with lid. Mix well (= 4.0 mg/ml). Use 0.1 ml = 400 µg.

Vancomycin. *Dose for use = 1000 µg.* Reconstitute one vial of 250 mg and make up to 10 ml with SNS or BSS in a sterile bottle with lid. Mix well. Withdraw 2 ml accurately and add to 3 ml of SNS or BSS in a sterile bottle with lid. Mix well (= 10 mg/ml). Use 0.1 ml = 1000 µg.

Cefazolin (or other cephalosporin). *Dose for use = 2000 µg.* Reconstitute one vial of 500 mg and make up to 10 ml with SNS or BSS in a sterile bottle with lid. Mix well. Withdraw 2 ml accurately and add to 3 ml of SNS or BSS in a sterile bottle with lid. Mix well (= 20 mg/ml). Use 0.1 ml = 2000 µg.

Clindamycin. *Dose for use = 1000 µg.* Transfer the contents of a 2-ml ampule containing 300 mg to a sterile bottle and add 1 ml SNS or BSS, replace lid, and mix well. Withdraw 1 ml, using a 1-ml syringe, and add to 9 ml of SNS or BSS in a sterile bottle with lid. Mix well (= 10 mg/ml). Use 0.1 ml = 1000 µg.

Amphotericin. *Dose for use = 5 µg.* Reconstitute a 50–mg vial with 10 ml water for injection. Withdraw 1 ml, using a 1-ml syringe, and add to 9 ml of water in a sterile bottle with lid for injection. Mix well. Withdraw 1 ml of this dilution, using a 1-ml syringe, and add to 9 ml of dextrose 5% in a sterile bottle with lid, to complete a dilution of 1/100. Mix well (= 50 µg/ml). Use 0.1 ml = 5 µg. (A dose of 10 µg has been used by some clinicians.)

Miconazole. *Dose for use = 10 µg.* Withdraw 1 ml, using a 1-ml syringe, from an ampule of intravenous miconazole containing 10 mg/ml and add to 9 ml SNS or BSS in a sterile bottle with lid. Mix well. Withdraw 1 ml, using a 1-ml syringe, and add to 9 ml SNS or BSS in a sterile bottle with lid. Mix well (= 100 µg/ml). Use 0.1ml = 10 µg.

The nontoxic doses of antibiotics have been described but should be reduced by 50% if given with a full vitrectomy (Chapter 8).

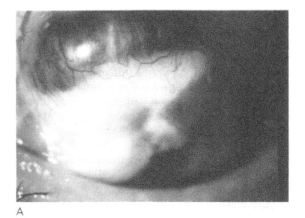

A

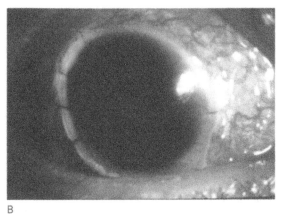

B

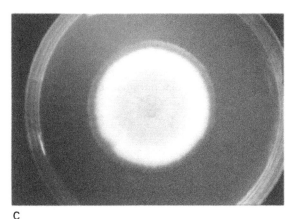

C

Figure 6.9

(A) *Aspergillus terreus* keratitis and a prolapsed iris after cataract surgery in India. (B) The same eye required a 10-mm graft and surgery to the iris. (C) *Aspergillus terreus* cultured from the anterior chamber of the eye in Figure 6.9(A).

Acute purulent endophthalmitis should be treated with additional systemic antibiotic therapy with the *same* drugs as used for intravitreal therapy. This regimen will maintain effective intravitreal levels of the drug for a longer period by reducing the diffusion gradient out of the eye. High doses are required and there is a need to be aware of the risks of systemic toxicity. Use of oral probenecid (dose 500 mg every 12 hours) retards outward transport of penicillins, cephalosporins, and ciprofloxacin across the retinal capillary endothelial cells, thus extending the half-life of the drug within the vitreous (Chapter 5). Probenecid also raises the plasma level by blocking secretion of these drugs by the proximal renal tubule.

Dexamethasone is often added to the intravitreal injection regimen (Chapter 8) (dose = 400 μg in 0.1 ml [use the commercial preparation containing 4 mg/ml]). Prednisolone can be added to the systemic regimen to reduce the vitreous inflammatory response and subsequent vitreous organization (oral prednisolone 60 mg daily on a reducing scale).

Antibiotic therapy is modified after 24–48 hours according to the clinical response and the antibiotic sensitivity profile of the cultured organism.

Gan et al have studied the efficacy of a low-dose regimen of intravitreal antibiotics in 17 patients with endophthalmitis.[52] This study design was based on the observation that vancomycin requires a prolonged time period rather than a high concentration to achieve a bactericidal effect. After injecting a dose of 0.2 mg of vancomycin and 0.05 mg gentamicin, the investigators performed a second vitreous biopsy 3 or 4 days later for culture and to measure antibiotic levels. Eleven patients had positive vitreous cultures, mostly with CNS; all of the second vitreous biopsies were sterile. Intravitreal vancomycin

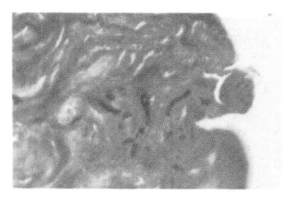

Figure 6.10

Gomori silver stain identifies hyphae of *Fusarium* sp. in tissue.

levels varied between 2.6 and 18 µg/ml (mean 10.3, SD 4.1) after 3 or 4 days, which is well above the MIC$_{90}$ for most Gram-positive bacteria. Concentrations of intravitreal gentamicin varied between 0.9 and 3.3 µg/ml (mean 1.6, SD 0.99) which are effective against Gram-negative bacteria. The authors concluded that these lower dosing levels were effective because of the sterile vitreous taps and that the drugs remained within the eye for over 1 week. However, these results can only be applied to endophthalmitis caused by CNS, which is a lower grade infection than highly virulent bacteria such as *Strep. pneumoniae* (Figure 6.8D).

Fungal endophthalmitis

Fungi may cause endogenous endophthalmitis (Chapter 9) or postoperative endophthalmitis

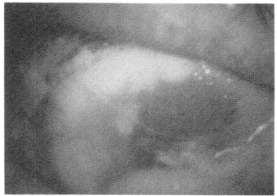

A

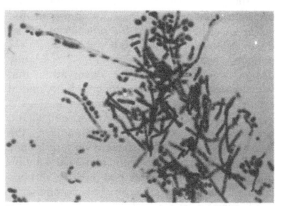

C

B

Figure 6.11

(A) *Trichosporon beigelii* iritis developed after extracapsular cataract surgery. (B) Microscopy of an iris specimen from the same eye as (A) demonstrates cells of *Trichosporon beigelii*. (C) Microscopy of *Trichosporum beigelii* plate culture from the same eye as (A).

Table 6.3 Fungal endophthalmitis associated with keratitis and scleritis

Reference	Type of fungus (no. of infected patients)	Source	Age of patient (years)	Place
Dursun et al, 2003[54]	Fusarium oxysporum (7) Fusarium solani (2) Fusarium sp. (1)	10/159 (6%) cases of Fusarium keratitis progressed to endophthalmitis	36–71	Ankara, Turkey
Leck et al, 2003[55]	Scedosporium apiospermum (Pseudallescheria boydii) (1)	Contact lens wearer and minor trauma in a wood	56	Southern England
Li-Shao-Wei et al, 2003[56]	Filamentous fungi (6)	Farming	NG	Shandong, China
Borderie et al, 1997[57]	Lasiodiplodia theobromae (1)	Keratitis treated with dexamethasone and gentamicin for 1 month	53	Paris, France
Okhravi et al, 1997[58]	Paecilomyces lilacinus (1)	Endogenous endophthalmitis with secondary keratitis requiring a PK. Case report and review of similar cases of endophthalmitis and keratitis due to P. lilacinus from 1975 to 1997	34	London, UK
Scott et al, 1996[37]	Fusarium solani (1) Fusarium oxyspurium (1)	Keratitis resulting in endophthalmitis	NG	Miami, USA
Jager et al, 1994[59]	Aspergillus niger (1)	Scleritis causing endophthalmitis	35	Leiden, Holland
Ksiazek et al, 1994[60]	Scedosporium apiospermum (Pseudallescheria boydii) (1)	Panophthalmitis secondary to keratitis. Diabetic	72	New York, USA
Pflugfelder et al, 1988[29]	Fusarium solani (1) Cylindrocarpon (1) Acremonium curvulum (1) Lasiodiplodia theobromae (1)	Deep keratitis (n = 4)	75, 68, 47, 62	Miami, USA
Slomovic et al, 1985[62]	Lasiodiplodia theobromae (1)	Keratitis progressed to scleritis and spontaneous perforation needing enucleation despite antimycotic antibiotics	62	Miami, USA

NG, not given; Pk, penetrating keratoplasty.

much more commonly in the tropical than temperate zones. Diagnosis may be delayed for a considerable period of time because pain and inflammation may be suppressed by the use of postoperative topical steroids. Fungal endophthalmitis typically demonstrates a subacute clinical presentation compared with bacterial endophthalmitis. Most commonly implicated fungi include *Candida* spp., *Aspergillus* spp. (Figure 6.9A-C), *Acremonium (Cephalosporium)* spp. (Figure 6.7), *Fusarium* spp. (Figure 6.10), volutella, neurospora, and *Trichosporon beigelii* (Figure 6.11A-C),[53] but the full range is given in Tables 6.1 and 6.2. The types of fungi causing

endophthalmitis secondary to keratitis and scleritis are described in Table 6.3.[29,37,54–61]

Patients with fungal endophthalmitis typically present with indolent inflammation, fibrinopurulent anterior chamber exudates, and vitreous reaction (snowballs, opacities). Symptoms tend to be mild but may be severe with subsequent loss of vision. Characteristically, fungal endophthalmitis demonstrates a longer latent period than bacterial endophthalmitis. However, there are a few exceptions depending on the virulence of the offending fungal organism, and fungal endophthalmitis should also be considered even when the presentation is acute. In contrast to bacterial endophthalmitis, where pain and redness characterize the majority of cases, fungal endophthalmitis may present without any ocular pain and with a relatively quiet external appearance. The majority of cases have infiltrates localized in the anterior chamber, anterior vitreous, or pupillary aperture. In one study, only 3 of 19 cases of exogenous fungal endophthalmitis presented with a diffuse intraocular inflammation as commonly observed in bacterial endophthalmitis.[29] Other investigators also noted that visual acuity at presentation tends to be better in fungal than in bacterial endophthalmitis. Cultures and PCR of aqueous and vitreous for bacteria and fungi are extremely important because of the variability in presentation of exogenous fungal endophthalmitis (Chapter 3).

Stern et al reported 15 cases of postoperative *Candida parapsilosis* endophthalmitis resulting from a contaminated irrigating solution.[31] After a vitreous tap or vitrectomy, the organism was identified in 11 of the 15 specimens. Treatment consisted of intravitreal amphotericin B and systemic amphotericin B and 5–fluorocytosine except in two clinical recurrences treated with intravitreal amphotericin B, removal of the lens, and oral ketoconazole. Eleven of the 14 pseudophakic patients retained the intraocular lens (IOL). Final visual acuities ranged from 20/25 to no light perception, with 8 of 15 patients having 20/60 or better visual acuities. Posterior capsulotomy and vitrectomy allowed more rapid clearance of amphotericin B and sequential intraocular injection of this drug within a short time period.

Fox et al reported 19 cases of delayed-onset pseudophakic endophthalmitis.[62] *Propionibacterium* spp., *Candida parapsilosis, S. epidermidis,* and *Corynebacterium* spp. were isolated in 12, 3, 3, and 1 eyes, respectively. The investigators noted that each infecting organism had specific clinical features which helped to establish a diagnosis. Dense vitreous infiltrates obscuring visualization were present in eyes infected with *S. epidermidis* and *Corynebacterium* sp. but not with *Propionibacterium* spp. In contrast, eyes infected with fungal organisms demonstrated localized white infiltrates in the anterior vitreous at some time during the infection. All patients demonstrated a transient response to corticosteroid therapy. Compared with acute endophthalmitis, visual acuity results were considerably better; 16 of the 19 patients had a visual acuity of 20/400 or better.

Exogenous or endogenous fungal endophthalmitis is invariably sight-threatening unless managed aggressively with surgery and antifungal chemotherapy. Although rare in the USA and Europe, where it is usually associated with surgical contamination, trauma, drug addiction, or immunocompromised individuals, fungal endophthalmitis can follow cataract and other surgery in rural settings of the developing world.

In Europe, the fungus responsible for endogenous infection is usually *Candida* spp. but the filamentous fungus *Fusarium* spp. can cause infection following corneal trauma with soil contamination (Chapters 7 and 9). The prevalence and type vary geographically: in India the most common causes are *Fusarium, Aspergillus,* and *Curvularia* spp. (Figure 6.12A-C), while *Candida* spp. are least common.

Because of the toxicity of the most effective antifungal agents, the relatively narrow activity spectrum of some agents, and the difficulties of clinical diagnosis, treatment is rarely instituted in the absence of direct evidence of a fungal etiology, based at least on the results of smears. Microscopy, culture, and molecular biology techniques are discussed in Chapter 3. Effective therapy requires mycological identification and, preferably, information about drug sensitivity. The most important mycelial fungus that is resistant to amphotericin is *Scedosporium apiospermum* (*Pseudallescheria boydii*; see Figure 3.12A and B), which should be treated with an imidazole. The number of drugs available for ocular use is limited not only by problems of local and systemic toxicity but by poor solubility or ocular penetration characteristics (Chapter 11).

Available drugs include the polyene antibiotics (amphotericin B, natamycin, and nystatin), the cytostatic 5–fluorocytosine (flucytosine, 5-FC), and the imidazoles (miconazole, ketoconazole, clotrimazole, econazole, fluconazole, itraconazole, and voriconazole). These drugs are all reviewed in Chapter 11.

Amphotericin B is the only fungicidal antibiotic, depending on the concentration achieved, and is active against a wide range of fungi including *Aspergillus* spp., most but not all strains of *Fusarium* spp. and *Candida* spp.; *Paecilomyces lilacinus* can be resistant.[63] Amphotericin B may be given topically as a drop (0.05–0.5%), subconjunctivally, intracamerally, and intravitreally (doses in Chapter 11). It is toxic by subconjunctival injection

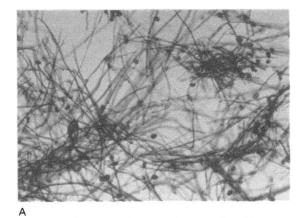

A

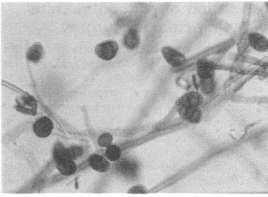

B

Figure 6.12

(A) Low-power view with cotton blue stain of a laboratory culture of *Curvularia* sp. shows hyphae and conidia. (B) High-power view demonstrates conidia of *Curvularia* sp. (C) *Curvularia* is grown on a plate culture.

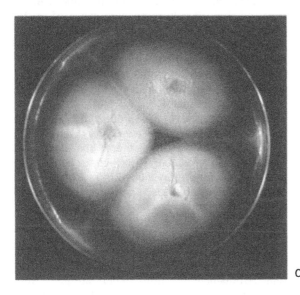

C

but the use of topical preparations at concentrations of 0.15% or less will minimize toxicity, which relates in part to the presence of deoxycholate in the parenteral preparation. Amphotericin is given parenterally by slow intravenous infusion in the management of endophthalmitis, often on a background of more widespread systemic infection, *in addition to* intravitreal therapy. Renal (low potassium) and hematologic status must be kept under surveillance; if toxicity occurs, the dose must be reduced.

For fungal endophthalmitis, amphotericin (5 µg) or miconazole (10 µg) is usually required intravitreally with a vitrectomy (Chapter 8). Amphotericin B can be administered intravenously combined with oral flucytosine (100–200 mg/kg per day) for severe *Candida* infection or oral ketoconazole (200–400 mg/day) or systemic voriconazole for other fungal infections. Careful monitoring is required. *Candida* endophthalmitis can be effectively treated with oral fluconazole or voriconazole combined with intravitreal amphotericin B; however, vitrectomy and fluconazole alone have been reported to be successful.

5-FC is only active against *Candida* spp. This drug is well absorbed by the oral route and achieves high blood and tissue levels; it has been used effectively in the treatment of *Candida* endophthalmitis, in combination with systemic or intravitreal amphotericin B to prevent the otherwise rapid emergence of resistant strains.

Prevention of endophthalmitis following cataract surgery

The incidence of postoperative endophthalmitis in a previously cataractous aging eye has dropped from 3.2% pre-1950 to 1.4% and later to 0.12% for surgery by the extracapsular cataract extraction (ECCE) method.[64] A recent retrospective, uncontrolled study has reported an incidence rate of 0.06% (20 cases out of 32,180 patients) with intracameral injection of 1 mg cefuroxime.[65] Most incidence studies have been reported from the USA and Canada rather than Europe. Circumstantial evidence from Belgium and France suggests that the true, rather than the reported, incidence of endophthalmitis after cataract surgery is closer to 0.3%.[20,66] In Manchester, UK, a retrospective study has reported an incidence of 0.3% while in a small prospective study in Glasgow, a rate of 0.2% was recorded.[67] In Canada, recently reported rates were 0.22% for ECCE, and 0.3% or 0.179% for phacoemulsification.[68] A 'true' incidence figure of 0.25% following phacoemulsification was reported in a poster presentation at the 2002 annual meeting of the Association for Research in Vision and Ophthalmology (ARVO).[69] There is, therefore, an urgent need to establish the true incidence of postoperative (phacoemulsification) cataract surgery endophthalmitis in both Europe and the USA and whether intraocular or topical antibiotic prophylaxis, or the combination, can prevent this damaging complication.

Current standards of practice for cataract surgery in the aging population involve the full range of choice from withholding antibiotics to their application pre-, intra-, and postoperatively, delivered either intra- or extraocularly. There is considerable debate over the possible effectiveness of antibiotic prophylaxis. No large definitive study has been performed in either Europe or the USA; therefore, all results of prophylaxis studies are anecdotal. Questionnaire surveys of antibiotic use in relation to cataract surgery have been used

in Germany and the USA in the last 2 years; however, only 66% of surgeons polled returned their questionnaire in each survey.[70,71] Both surveys did suggest, however, that subconjunctival antibiotics commonly given in the European Union (EU) after surgery did not significantly reduce the incidence of endophthalmitis, further corroborated by others.[72] The use of intraocular antibiotics such as vancomycin (20 mg/l), gentamicin (8 mg/l), or both during surgery, given as a supplement to the irrigation fluid, produced the lowest (unproven) incidence rates of infection, similarly experienced by others.[73] These findings are not supported by other studies, or by laboratory tests (see p.121). In addition, Aaberg et al reported that 23 culture-positive cases of acute onset postoperative endophthalmitis had received prophylactic subconjunctival antibiotics at the end of surgery; 14 isolates were sensitive to the antibiotic used, and 9 were resistant.[73] The use of subconjunctival prophylactic antibiotics is discussed in Chapter 4.

The problem with interpreting all of these incidence rates is also reviewed and discussed in Chapter 4. However, as there has been no reliable, large, prospective, well-controlled study, these figures for prophylaxis by intraocular antibiotics were described as 'unreliable' in a recent review of evidence-based medicine on this subject.[3]

Several advances in sterile technique for cataract surgery have been made over the last 5 years, including the introduction of small-incision phacoemulsification (ultrasonic) surgery and foldable plastic intraocular lenses (IOLs) inserted through sterile injectors.[74] Although a decrease in incidence of endophthalmitis after the use of these techniques has been reported,[68,75] postoperative endophthalmitis continues to occur.

In patients with atopic allergic blepharitis, the surgeon should be wary of endophthalmitis because up to 70% of their lid margins can be heavily colonized by *S. aureus*;[76] appropriate prophylaxis against *S. aureus* is needed.

Bacterial contamination of the anterior chamber during cataract surgery

Research has shown that the addition of vancomycin (20 mg/l) and gentamicin (8 mg/l) to the irrigation fluid reduces the number of bacteria culture-positive anterior chamber aspiration samples from 20% in saline-based controls to 2.7% in those receiving the infusion-based antibiotics.[77] Reducing the bacterial inoculum in the anterior chamber can be expected to reduce the infection rate but there is a considerable body of opinion against the use of vancomycin for this type of prophylaxis, because vancomycin must be kept in reserve to treat infections caused by methicillin-resistant *S. aureus* (MRSA), as it is the only effective antibiotic to do so in MRSA endophthalmitis or septicemias. The US Centers for Disease Control have deplored the prophylactic use of vancomycin for cataract surgery in this way and advised ophthalmologists not to use vancomycin for routine prophylaxis of endophthalmitis following cataract surgery.

Sherwood et al in 1989 cultured bacteria from the conjunctival sac of 90 eyes, and from the anterior chamber aspirate of 29 (30%) of them.[78] The authors also demonstrated a flow of fluorescein through the cataract wound into the anterior chamber and suggested that this flow was a likely source of postoperative endophthalmitis in some cases. In 1991, Dickey et al cultured the anterior chamber aspirate of 30 patients undergoing ECCE and found a contamination rate of 43% with CNS as the most common organism.[79] Similar findings were also made by Egger et al in 1994, with 71% of conjunctival smears contaminated with CNS and 27% of anterior chamber aspirates being culture-positive intraoperatively.[80] Egger et al have repeated the study in patients undergoing phacoemulsification with contamination results of 14%, with CNS and corynebacteria being the most common isolates. Mistlberger et al also found that preoperative neomycin drops had no effect on contamination of the anterior chamber, although they did not use a lipophilic quinolone antibiotic and did apply povidone-iodine to the eye before surgery.[81] Mendivil Soto and Mendivil also found that the use of topical povidone-iodine 5% for 5 and 10 minutes before surgery failed to give a statistical reduction in positive intraocular cultures at the end of surgery.[5]

In practice, because of this bacterial contamination, many ophthalmologists in both Europe and the USA are adding either vancomycin or gentamicin or both to the irrigation fluid and claiming a low incidence rate of postoperative endophthalmitis.[70,71] Gimbel has reported from Canada a series of 12,000 cataract operations adding vancomycin and gentamicin to the irrigation fluid without a single case of postoperative endophthalmitis.[82] Others, however, continue to practice phacoemulsification surgery with povidone-iodine antisepsis preoperatively and only make use of postoperative antibiotic drops to prevent wound infection; they also claim low rates of postoperative infection.

Investigators from Canada have found a possible difference between a clear cornea approach and use of a scleral tunnel,[68] which could influence the results of antibiotic prophylaxis. Similar findings, but with statistical significance incriminating the clear cornea incision as being more risky for endophthalmitis, have been reported recently from Japan.[75] A meta-analysis, presented recently, has similar findings as well, but this type of analysis can be biased (Chapter 4).[83]

Antibiotic prophylaxis

A reduction in the incidence of endophthalmitis after cataract surgery may be achieved by reducing the bacterial inoculum on the conjunctiva and cornea with 5% povidone-iodine and aseptic surgery and placing a high dose of an antibiotic, such as cefuroxime (1 mg in 0.1 ml), into the 0.2–0.5 ml of the aphakic anterior chamber. A concentration of at least 3000 µg/ml is produced, giving a level that is 400 times the MIC_{90} of most but not all bacteria, MRSA, and *E. faecalis*[84] being particular exceptions.

Phacoemulsification surgery has reduced wound size and bacterial contamination of the anterior chamber.[77–81] In addition, the insertion of the foldable plastic IOLs through a sterile injector has reduced expected bacterial contamination and has been suggested, but not statistically proven, to reduce postoperative endophthalmitis rates from 1.21% for directly placed IOLs to 0.3% for foldable IOLs.[74] This study, a retrospective review of cases in one hospital setting over 10 years, recommended a multicenter trial, for which data are being collected in the European Society of Cataract and Refractive Surgeons (ESCRS) study. Despite these new techniques, the incidence of postoperative phacoemulsification endophthalmitis, although low at approximately 0.25%, still remains a concern because of its potentially devastating consequences.[69]

The ESCRS study, taking place between January 2004 and December 2005 in 30,000 patients in 18 operating centers in 8 European countries, will assess the beneficial effect of prophylaxis for phacoemulsification surgery with a high-dose intracameral bactericidal antibiotic (cefuroxime as 1 mg in 0.1 ml) in comparison with a high dose of a topical quinolone antibiotic (levofloxacin 0.5%), a combination of both regimens, and placebo controls. All patients will also receive 5% povidone-iodine antiseptic prophylaxis before surgery and postoperative levofloxacin 0.5% for 6 days from the first postoperative day, 18 hours after surgery, to prevent postoperative wound infection.

The rationale for this study design is as follows. The current incidence rates of infective endophthalmitis where no intraocular antibiotics are used are up to 0.5%, but in other studies where such antibiotics are used, incidence rates range from 0.2% to 0.02% (Chapter 4). These latter studies, however, have not been standardized or controlled. In particular, the center that developed the technique of injecting an antibiotic (cefuroxime) into the anterior chamber postoperatively reports an incidence rate of 0.06%, but this Swedish study was retrospective, without placebo controls, and the result, while interesting, remains unconfirmed.[65] However, it does suggest that it may be possible to reduce the incidence of infective endophthalmitis to provide an almost zero level of infection (less than 1 per 2000 operations or 0.05%) for safe cataract surgery. The comparison in the ESCRS study of four groups each of 7500

patients will ensure that a reduction in incidence from 0.25% to 0.08% will be detected with 80% statistical power using 5% significance level tests. The ESCRS study has a classic Fisher 2 × 2 factorial design, similar to the Endophthalmitis Vitrectomy Study (Chapters 4 and 8) with full randomization in blocks of 12; all data are collected electronically at the time of surgery and follow-up.

Possible confounding variables influencing infection rates will include surgeon practice, including experience; site of incision (clear cornea or scleral tunnel, reviewed in Chapter 4); complications of surgery (posterior capsule damage and vitreous leak); type of patient (diabetic or immunosuppressed); type of intraocular lens (acrylic or silicone); and type of operating room hygiene, which means that patients must be fully randomized in a multicenter setting to remove these causes of bias. Strict randomization and masking prevent bias in patient selection and management. Randomization coding, prepared *in advance of the start of the study* in blocks of 12, forces immediate random allocation of a patient on presentation for surgery through a unique trial number to a treatment group that cannot be altered by the trial clinician. The randomization code is built into the local computer program. The 2 × 2 Fisher factorial design, including a placebo control group masked for the administration of vehicle-only drops perioperatively and without the injection of cefuroxime, permits either a powerful assessment of each intervention on its own, in the absence of interaction between them; or alternatively the reliable detection and assessment of such interaction. Sources of error that must be avoided include misallocation of interventions, poor compliance with drop administration, misdiagnosis of outcome (endophthalmitis), and poor follow-up.

A recent evidence-based update of bacterial endophthalmitis prophylaxis for cataract surgery has considered all the evidence from retrospective studies, limited noncontrolled prospective studies, and questionnaire surveys for antibiotic prophylaxis.[3] The authors have concluded that good quality, reliable scientific evidence is lacking to justify the use of antibiotic prophylaxis in cataract surgery. They have only found reliable evidence to support the prophylactic use of 5% povidone-iodine in BSS immediately prior to surgery.[1] However, this approach also has its problems, particularly in only being able to review the evidence that exists, which is considered in Chapter 4. The conclusion that 'no' evidence for prophylactic antibiotics should mean that they can be withdrawn totally appears to be dangerous. Such results have been put into practice by others and found to give the opposite effect to that which had been predicted, contributing instead to an increased number of cases of postoperative endophthalmitis (refer to 'no' evidence versus evidence section in Chapter 4). Great care is needed in interpreting data from different studies that are not randomized, placebo-controlled, or prospective.

Choice of antibiotic

Vancomycin

Vancomycin is the ideal bactericidal antibiotic, effective against all Gram-positive bacteria likely to cause postoperative endophthalmitis including *E. faecalis*[84] (Chapter 11); however, it is also the antibiotic of 'last resort' for treating endophthalmitis caused by MRSA. The use of vancomycin as prophylaxis against endophthalmitis for all cases of cataract surgery within a large hospital may not be advisable.

Mendivil Soto and Mendivil found a statistically significant reduction (p = 0.032) in intraocular culture rates at the end of surgery when vancomycin 20 mg/l was added to the irrigating fluid in cataract surgery; however, this finding has not been confirmed by others.[5] Feys et al found no effect on intraocular contamination with bacteria as evaluated by anterior chamber taps.[85] Ferro et al found a reduction in intraocular contamination rates but it was not statistically significant,[86] while Gritz et al found that exposure of bacteria to vancomycin for 2 hours, as performed when it is added to the irrigation fluid for cataract surgery, had no effective antibacterial action.[87] Vancomycin is time-dependent for its action, requiring a longer exposure period than the beta-lactams of up to 4 hours, in contrast to the aminoglycosides and quinolones which demonstrate an increase in bactericidal activity at higher concentrations with a shorter time interval.[88]

Cefuroxime

The second-generation cephalosporin cefuroxime was chosen in Sweden as a good alternative antibiotic to the aminoglycosides (gentamicin) and vancomycin, lacking their toxicity. This drug is highly effective against staphylococci (except MRSA), streptococci (except *E. faecalis*),[84] and *P. acnes* and diphtheroids that cause late-onset saccular bag endophthalmitis. In contrast gentamicin is effective against staphylococci and many strains of MRSA but is not effective against streptococci, including *E. faecalis*,[84] and *P. acnes*. Cefuroxime has good activity against Gram-negative bacteria that occasionally cause postoperative endophthalmitis with the exception of activity against *Pseudomonas aeruginosa*. However, this bacterium does not usually cause endophthalmitis unless there has been a breakdown in the aseptic technique with contamination of equipment, most particularly of reusable solutions. Good basic hygiene and use of disposable solutions and tubing with sterilization is thus still imperative for aseptic surgery. Cefuroxime has been successfully used as an intracameral injection (1 mg in 0.1 ml) at the end of cataract surgery in over 50,000 patients in Sweden[65] and is not toxic to the anterior chamber or corneal endothelium.[89] Cefuroxime has not been approved for ocular use in the UK.

Cefuroxime is an ideal antibiotic for prophylaxis of normal lid and conjunctival bacterial flora that are responsible for 85% of cases of postoperative endophthalmitis.[65] MRSA has not been a problem with the use of cefuroxime in Sweden, with no cases of postoperative endophthalmitis caused by this strain; however, 5 cases out of 32,180 patients occurred with enterococci. Because cataract surgery is mainly practiced on community-based rather than hospital-based patients, in whom MRSA is found in a very small percentage as lid flora, the lack of effect of cefuroxime against MRSA is not expected to be problematic. Additional prophylaxis against the enterococci will be gained by the use of povidone-iodine as the preoperative antiseptic in all patient groups. It is imperative, however, that all surgical equipment must be sterile.

Others have investigated cefuroxime for prophylaxis of endophthalmitis by the topical and subconjunctival routes;[90] it has been shown to best penetrate into the anterior chamber by the subconjunctival route with 125 mg when mean levels in the anterior chamber of 20 µg/ml are gained; however, there is a delay of 60 minutes before this is reached, in contrast to the intracameral injection of 1000 µg (1 mg) when an immediate concentration is gained of at least 3000 µg/ml. These data are important as the MIC_{90} for the CNS is 8 µg/ml. The MIC_{90} values for the other expected bacteria causing postoperative endophthalmitis include *S. aureus* at 1–4 µg/ml, *Strep. pneumoniae* at 0.125 µg/ml, coliforms (excluding *Ps. aeruginosa* which is resistant) 4 µg/ml, and *P. acnes* (and aerobic diphtheroids) 0.1 µg/ml. These figures explain why subconjunctival cefuroxime does not achieve sufficient levels to be successful, ideally at least ×4 MIC_{90} should be gained, whereas the intracameral route provides high levels without any delay. At the concentration achieved by the intracameral route, there is highly effective bactericidal prophylaxis against most pathogens causing endophthalmitis after cataract surgery.

Toxicity must be considered for any antibiotic used as prophylaxis. Cefuroxime has been found to be nontoxic for the endothelium and the anterior chamber by investigators testing low levels administered by the topical and subconjunctival routes[90] as well as those giving high levels by the intracameral route,[89] with no evidence of endothelial cell loss caused by the drug; in addition, there was no disturbance of the blood–aqueous barrier. It should be diluted in normal saline (0.9%) and not in water for injection to maintain the correct osmolality in the anterior chamber. The Swedish study also found no evidence that cefuroxime causes cystoid macular edema, which can occur with vancomycin. The possibility of an anaphylactic reaction must be considered. In the Swedish study, 5183 patients were screened in 1997 for allergy to cefuroxime and only 3 had a positive response to a skin test. After 1997, two more patients had a positive response; of the five patients demonstrating allergy on prick testing, four had cefuroxime instilled in the anterior chamber after being given an oral antihistamine. The risk for systemic anaphylaxis caused by an intracameral injection of cefuroxime is probably as small as that seen with a subcutaneous injection of allergen in the course of a desensitization program, i.e. 0.06%.[91] The Swedish study showed that type-1 hypersensitivity to cefuroxime is extremely rare.

Levofloxacin

Levofloxacin is a synthetic antibacterial agent of the fluoroquinolone class. Levofloxacin is the

L-isomer of the racemic drug substance ofloxacin. The antibacterial activity of ofloxacin resides primarily in the L-isomer. As a fluoroquinolone antibacterial agent, levofloxacin acts on the DNA–DNA–gyrase complex and topoisomerase IV in bacteria. This antibiotic is effective in 0.5% (5 mg/ml) eye drops to treat infections caused by staphylococci (except MRSA), streptococci (note: intermediate susceptibility of *Enterococcus* [*Streptococcus*] *faecalis* at 2–4 µg/ml for the MIC_{90}), corynebacteria, propionibacteria, and Gram-negative bacteria including *Ps. aeruginosa*. Environmental contaminants such as *Alcaligenes* spp. may be sensitive as well. Levofloxacin 0.5% was recently licensed for use in 11 EU countries including Austria, Denmark, Finland, Germany, Holland, Iceland, Italy, Luxembourg, Portugal, the UK, and Sweden by Santen Gmbh (Germany) to treat bacterial infections of the conjunctiva and cornea. Levofloxacin is marketed in the USA with the trade name Oftaquix.

In vitro testing has shown levofloxacin to be highly effective against ocular bacterial isolates that can cause endophthalmitis.[92] Because most postoperative infection is derived from the patient's own bacterial flora,[1] and this flora is sensitive to levofloxacin, there is the distinct possibility that pre- and perioperative use will reduce the rate of postoperative endophthalmitis. Some surgeons already rely on topical levofloxacin 0.5% as their sole antibiotic prophylaxis for cataract surgery. This will be achieved by both the bactericidal effect of levofloxacin 0.5% on the conjunctiva, given as two doses each of one drop on the hospital ward between 60 and 15 minutes before surgery (it has a bactericidal effect within 15 minutes), as well as from its absorption into the anterior chamber from a pulsed dose given three times every 5 minutes immediately following surgery. In addition, this pulsed dose will have an ongoing bactericidal effect on the conjunctiva for at least 12 hours, as described in Chapter 5.

Some surgeons administer a quinolone antibiotic such as ofloxacin or ciprofloxacin by the oral route to patients for 2 days before surgery; however, this use is considered both excessive and impractical. Antibiotic prophylaxis should be given as a short-course high-dose application *at the time of surgery* combined with postoperative antibiotic drops (levofloxacin 0.5% or others) given four times daily for 6 days, starting at the first postoperative day to reduce the chance of wound infection.

Levofloxacin will be absorbed into the anterior chamber because of its lipophilicity; levofloxacin levels in the anterior chamber will reach MIC_{90} levels for most bacteria, including streptococci. Details on actual levels attained in the conjunctiva and anterior chamber with topical drop application are given in Chapter 5.

Little toxicity has been associated with the use of levofloxacin which, in common with other quinolones, is remarkably free of side effects. However, adverse reactions at the time of instillation of the drops in 1–10% of patients can include ocular burning (1.6%), decreased vision (1.2%), and mucous strand (1.2%). Uncommon adverse reactions in 0.1–1% of patients can include lid matting (0.9%), chemosis (0.7%), conjunctival papillary reaction (0.7%), lid edema (0.5%), ocular discomfort (0.5%), ocular itching (0.5%), ocular pain (0.5%), conjunctival injection (0.2%), conjunctival follicles (0.2%), ocular dryness (0.2%), lid erythema (0.2%), and photophobia (0.2%).

Other reactions observed in the clinical studies have included headache (0.9%) and rhinitis (0.5%). Corneal precipitates, similar to those produced by ciprofloxacin, were not observed in clinical studies with levofloxacin. In Japan 30 million doses have been prescribed; only two cases with an anaphylactoid reaction occurred, which caused localized swelling of the face and neck soon after the drops were applied, but systemic symptoms with life-threatening anaphylactic shock did not occur.

The topical drop method with levofloxacin 0.5% is used for prophylaxis by some surgeons as it is a noninvasive technique that maintains sterility.

Combination of cefuroxime and levofloxacin

The combination of cefuroxime and levofloxacin has not been tried before in these circumstances. However, both are bactericidal antibiotics acting on different targets, inhibition of the cell wall and DNA polymerase activity, respectively; thus there should be an additive effect with possible synergy. The ESCRS study design will permit detection of any such beneficial interaction. While the combination has little additional effect against the Gram-positive bacteria, there is considerable additional effect against the Gram-negative bacteria, particularly by the levofloxacin component, for pseudomonads and cefuroxime-resistant environmental Gram-negative bacteria, which could help prevent an outbreak resulting from contamination of 'sterile' equipment or solutions. The outcome of the ESCRS study will be able to establish if there is any benefit in prophylaxis in using the combination of cefuroxime and levofloxacin.

Intracameral injection at the end of cataract surgery

Injection of a known quantity of antibiotic into the eye has a considerable advantage compared with the addition of an antibiotic to the irrigation fluid. With the latter technique, the quantity of antibiotic delivered to the anterior chamber depends on the amount of fluid used for irrigation, which in turn depends on the length of the surgery. Also, a lower dose of antibiotic is infused into the eye than an injected bolus dose. Adding antibiotics to the irrigation fluid can also be inaccurate and it involves the danger of introducing environmental bacteria to the sterile infusate which may be used as a multidose bottle for patients on one operating room list. This is a possible source of an outbreak of contamination, albeit limited to the patients having surgery in one operating room. For these reasons, the sterile bolus injection of an antibiotic is preferred. If using vancomycin or cefuroxime, the dose to give is 1 mg in 0.1 ml saline, instilled into the anterior chamber.

Chronic postoperative endophthalmitis, usually following cataract surgery

Postoperative bacterial endophthalmitis that presents more than 6 weeks after the surgery is arbitrarily classified as chronic endophthalmitis. Most commonly cultured organisms include *P. acnes*, CNS (Figure 6.13A, B),[93,94] *Corynebacterium* spp. (Figure 6.14A, B),[62,95] *Actinomyces neuii*,[96] and fungi including *Candida* spp., *Aspergillus* spp. (see Figure 6.9), and *Fusarium*

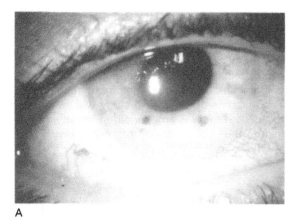
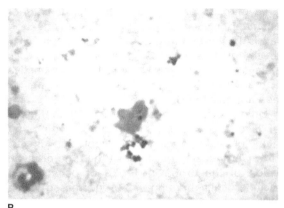

A   B

Figure 6.13

(A) Chronic endophthalmitis caused by coagulase-negative staphylococcus (CNS) which was treated with corticosteroids. (B) Gram stain of CNS in vitreous from the eye shown in Figure 6.13(A).

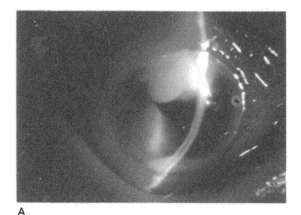
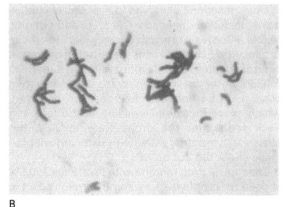

A   B

Figure 6.14

(A) Postoperative endophthalmitis due to *Corynebacterium macginleyi*. (B) Gram stain of *Corynebacteria*.

spp. (Figure 6.15A, B). In addition, *Streptococcus* spp., *Actinomyces* spp.,[97] *Nocardia asteroides*, *Achromobacter* spp., and *Xanthomas maltophilia* have also been reported.[88] Dense vitreous infiltrates obscuring visualization can be present in eyes infected with CNS and *Corynebacterium* spp. but not with *Propionibacterium* spp.

P. acnes organisms are anaerobic, Grampositive or Gram-variable rods found in 10–70%

of routine conjunctival cultures, from a depot in the lacrimal sac, and sequestered as white plaques on the posterior capsule (saccular or capsule bag endophthalmitis). It is also found in the mucosa of the mouth, intestines, urethra, and vagina. In one study, 65% of the preoperative conjunctival swabs were positive for growth, with corynebacteria, CNS, and *P. acnes* being the most frequently cultured.[88] Webster et al reported that

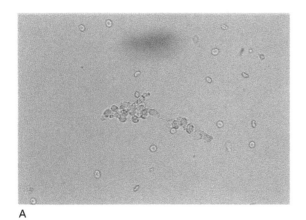

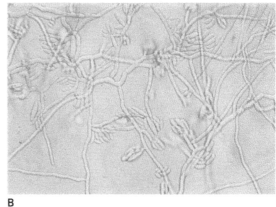

A   B

Figure 6.15

(A) Wet preparation of aqueous showing branching hyphae and conidia. (B) Branching septate hyphae of *Fusarium* sp.

P. acnes possesses a cell wall that is uniformly resistant to degradation by polymorphonuclear (PMN) lymphocytes, and was variably degraded by monocytes.[98] Such resistance may account for its chronic nature.

This syndrome of indolent, chronic granulomatous uveitis was described in 1986; *P. acnes* was proven by electron microscopy to be a cause.[99] This organism is difficult to recover in cultures of intraocular specimens because of its fastidious nature and slow growth. In fact, the generation doubling time for *P. acnes* is 5.1 hours as opposed to 24 minutes for *S. aureus*.[99] Consequently, anaerobic culture medium should not be discarded but observed for at least 2 weeks when this organism is suspected. Clark et al demonstrated that the mean time to culture positivity is 8 days;[100] in another study, Meisler and Mandelbaum showed the time to culture positivity to be 4.7 days.[101] Molecular biology with PCR can provide positive results within 6 hours (see Chapter 3).

Clinical presentation of *P. acnes* can take several forms, either individually or in combination:

- Solitary nodule with a granulomatous reaction on the corneal endothelial surface.
- Hypopyon and white-appearing plaque on the posterior lens capsule which may enlarge over time. The term 'saccular' endophthalmitis denotes chronic uveitis associated with thickening of the lens capsule around the plastic IOL.
- Beaded fibrin strands in the anterior chamber.

P. acnes can be freed from the posterior capsule after Nd:YAG capsulotomy to cause chronic, delayed-onset endophthalmitis. *P. acnes* endophthalmitis has been reported in several clinical scenarios:

- In pseudophakic eyes following Nd:YAG laser capsulotomy. It has been postulated that the organism, which was introduced into the eye at the time of surgery, is sequestered in the posterior capsule and protected from the inflammatory response. Nd:YAG laser capsulotomy releases the organism into the eye triggering either an antigenic response to the extracellular organism or an inflammatory response to the variety of exoenzymes contained by the organism.[102] In addition to *P. acnes*, CNS have also been isolated from the vitreous.[103]
- Intracapsular cataract extraction and anterior chamber intraocular lens implantation in the presence of a posterior corneal plaque. Histopathologic studies have demonstrated that the organism is sequestered in the retrocorneal plaque.
- After Nd:YAG iridotomy.[104]

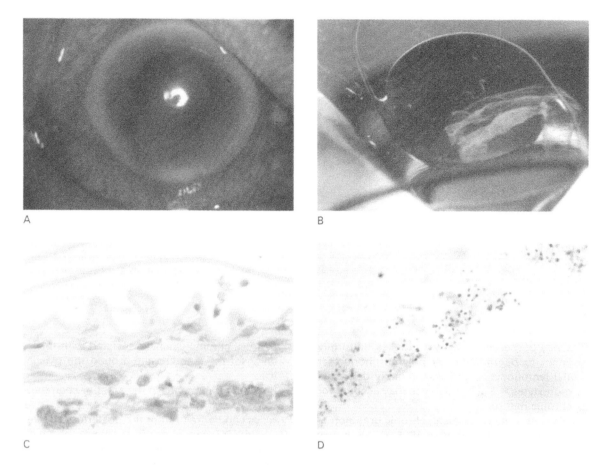

A

B

C

D

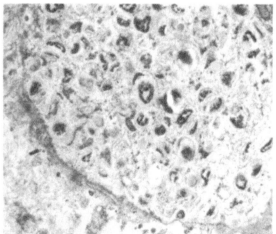

E

Figure 6.16

(A) Chronic capsular endophthalmitis 9 months after cataract surgery suppressed with corticosteroids. (B) Intraocular lens removed from eye shown in (A) together with capsule fragment. (C) Macrophages seen in a paraffin-embedded section of the capsule fragment (B). Hematoxylin and eosin stain. (D) Gram 'positive' staining showing cocco-bacilli inside macrophages in the capsule fragment (B) (paraffin-embedded section). (E) Electron micrograph of cocco-bacilli inside macrophages from the capsule fragment (B).

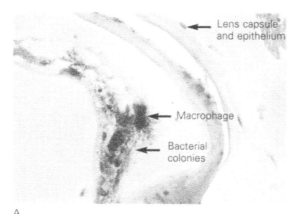

A

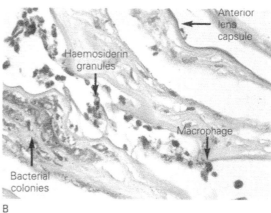

B

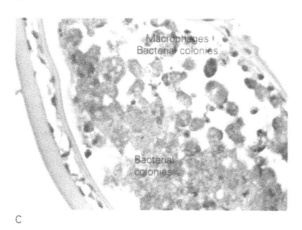

C

Figure 6.17

(A-C) Hematoxylin and eosin stain of the capsule fragment removed surgically from three patients with chronic 'saccular' endophthalmitis showing macrophages and bacterial colonies.

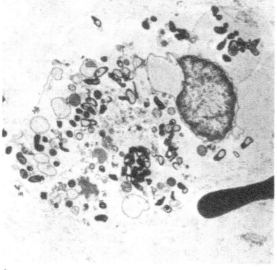

A

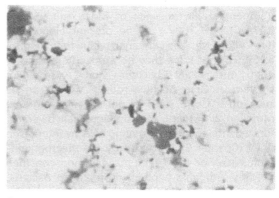

B

Figure 6.18

(A) Electron micrograph shows *Propionibacterium acnes* in a macrophage. *P. acnes* was cultured from an eye with late-onset chronic plaque-type endophthalmitis. (B) Gram stain of *P. acnes*.

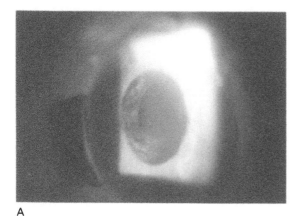

A

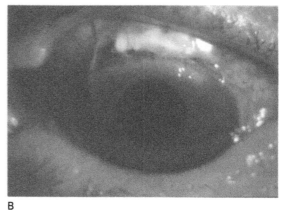

B

Figure 6.19

(A) Chronic saccular endophthalmitis showing white plaque before treatment with oral clarithromycin 500 mg b.i.d. (B) The same eye after successful treatment with clarithromycin.

A similarity exists between phacoantigenic uveitis and *Propionibacterium* endophthalmitis (Figure 6.16A-E) in both clinical course and histopathological findings from the anterior chamber. Both demonstrate giant cells, foamy macrophages, and epithelioid cells. Meisler and Mandelbaum proposed that the organism may have adjuvant-like properties with lens material.[101] This interaction results in immunopotentiation with subsequent exacerbation of intraocular inflammation.

Macrophages are found lining the capsule fragment in the absence of PMN cells (Figure 6.17A-C).[105,106] They may be present alone with intracellular bacteria contained within them (Figure 6.18A, B)[105] or there may be a mixed situation of both intracellular bacteria and extracellular clusters of Gram-positive rods,[106] which can be seen on a Gram stain of the capsule fragment removed at surgery. Macrophages can be transformed into antigen-presenting cells by interleukin (IL)-1 (Chapter 2), produced by the macrophages themselves or by B lymphocytes, and can then process antigenic peptides from these bacteria, enzymatically degrading them to oligopeptides with an unfolded secondary structure. These peptides are expressed at their surface bound to major histocompatibility complex class II molecules for presentation to Th1 lymphocytes to stimulate a cell-mediated immune response, not normally present in the anterior chamber because

of its immune deviation (Chapter 2). This immunologic response is suppressed by corticosteroids, but recurs when the steroids are withdrawn, or disappears with surgical removal of the capsule. This situation represents antigen-mediated cell-mediated immunity with inflammation rather than infection with PMNs. Because the bacteria in the capsule are the ultimate source of the antigens, they must be removed surgically or with effective antibiotic therapy (Figure 6.19A, B) to stop the inflammatory process.

Management

Zambrano et al suggested that milder cases of chronic postoperative endophthalmitis be initially treated with intraocular vancomycin alone (1 mg/0.1 ml), and that more severe cases be treated with intraocular vancomycin or vitrectomy plus intraocular vancomycin.[107] However, several investigators have noted a high recurrence rate of chronic *Propionibacterium* endophthalmitis managed initially with intravitreal antibiotics but a high cure rate following removal of the capsule.[108,109] Therefore, these investigators suggested that the chronic use of steroids to suppress inflammation be limited to eyes presenting with good vision and mild inflammation. In eyes unresponsive to steroids or where

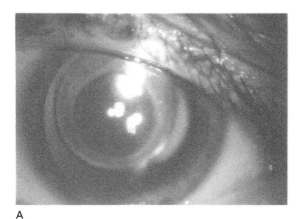
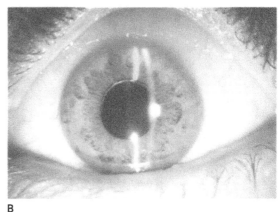

A   B

Figure 6.20

(A-B) Saccular plaque-type endophthalmitis before (A) and after (B) effective clarithromycin therapy.

the presentation is more severe, removal of the plaque with or without the entire posterior capsule was recommended. The extent of capsulectomy is dependent on the amount of the involved capsule that can be visualized. When the extent of the capsular involvement could be determined, pars plana vitrectomy to remove only the involved portion of the posterior capsule along with the plaques was recommended. The entire capsule was removed through a limbal approach when there was recurrent endophthalmitis following partial capsulotomy or if the complete extent of capsule involvement could not be visualized. In such cases, the intraocular lens had to be removed but replaced at a later date with an anterior chamber lens in some cases because of the reduced likelihood of aggravating the inflammation. At the end of this procedure, the investigators recommend injecting intravitreal vancomycin (1 mg).

P. acnes is sensitive to a variety of antimicrobial agents including penicillin, cefoxitin, cefuroxime (very sensitive), clindamycin, erythromycin, and the fluoroquinolones. The problem, however, is for the antibiotic to penetrate into the anterior chamber in a sufficiently high concentration to reach the bacteria contained within the macrophages and capsule fragment. Other authors have demonstrated that the initial choice of treatment, often vancomycin or a cephalosporin, influences the number of recurrences but

not the final visual outcome. The problem with these two latter types of antibiotics is that they do not penetrate effectively into cells (Chapter 5). The new erythromycin-derivative drugs, azithromycin and clarithromycin, are far superior because they are concentrated 200-fold into cells including macrophages, as well as penetrating into the tissues of the eye in effective concentrations when given orally (500 mg b.i.d.) (Chapters 5 and 11). Increased experience with the use of clarithromycin in particular has demonstrated its ability to effectively kill bacteria within the capsular plaque, as described above, without the need for surgery.[110,111] In addition, clarithromycin has been used for management of chronic endophthalmitis in a tertiary referral hospital as an additional drug; those patients who received it had a much better response.[112] Figures 6.19A, B and 6.20A, B show two patients with chronic 'capsular' or 'saccular' endophthalmitis who responded to oral clarithromycin without requiring surgical removal of the capsule and IOL. Patients should be given a trial of therapy with clarithromycin before contemplating surgical removal of the capsule.

Fox et al reported 19 cases of delayed-onset pseudophakic endophthalmitis.[62] The investigators noted that each infecting organism had specific clinical features which helped to establish a diagnosis. Dense vitreous infiltrates obscuring visualization were present in eyes infected with *S.*

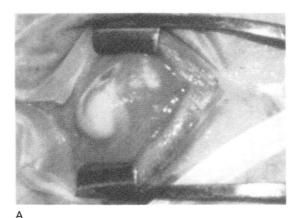

A

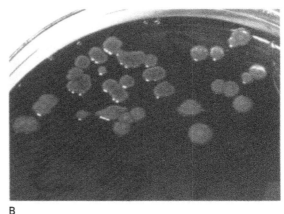

B

Figure 6.21

(A) *Pseudomonas aeruginosa* endophthalmitis and panophthalmitis after a corneal infection secondary to contact lens wear and keratitis. (B) *P. aeruginosa* colonies on blood agar.

epidermidis and *Corynebacterium* spp. but not *Propionibacterium* spp. In contrast, eyes infected with fungal organisms demonstrated localized white infiltrates in the anterior vitreous at some time during the infection. All patients demonstrated a transient response to corticosteroid therapy. Compared with acute endophthalmitis, visual acuity results were considerably better. Sixteen of the 19 patients had a visual acuity of 20/400 or better.

A variety of other organisms have been reported to cause chronic, delayed-onset postoperative endophthalmitis. Bacteria responsible for this infection include *S. epidermidis*, *Corynebacterium* spp., and *Xanthomas maltophilia*.[113] Gram-negative organisms are generally more virulent and cause more severe ocular damage with worse visual outcome.

Chen and Roy reported five cases of endophthalmitis which demonstrated chronic and recurrent presentation after cataract surgery using a bacteria-contaminated viscoelastic solution.[114] The causative organism was *Bacillus circulans*, which in contrast to other *Bacillus* spp., does not generally produce the same by-products and toxins damaging to the eye. The authors speculated that the lens capsule in affected eyes may sequester the bacteria and afford protection. Subsequently, four of the five eyes required eventual IOL and capsule removal before becoming quiescent.

Late-onset, polymicrobial endophthalmitis is another possibility. Ray and Hainsworth reported a patient with CNS endophthalmitis 41 months after uncomplicated cataract extraction with placement of an IOL; resolution followed intravitreal antibiotics.[115] The patient developed an indolent endophthalmitis 26 months later, caused by *P. acnes,* that required removal of the IOL and capsule. This case illustrates that endophthalmitis may be caused by multiple organisms at different times in the same eye. Similarly, there can be polymicrobial infection when one, two, or three types of bacteria can be isolated at the same time.[116] This situation requires aggressive management with removal of the entire capsular bag and the IOL, particularly if there is recurrent inflammation, after which the eye settles quickly.[109] The patient should also be given a trial of therapy with clarithromycin.

Endophthalmitis associated with severe keratitis

Scott et al described 14 patients with endophthalmitis associated with severe keratitis; 13 had documented keratitis before endophthalmitis developed.[37] A frequent history of corticosteroid use, systemic conditions associated with relative immune dysfunction, lack of an intact posterior

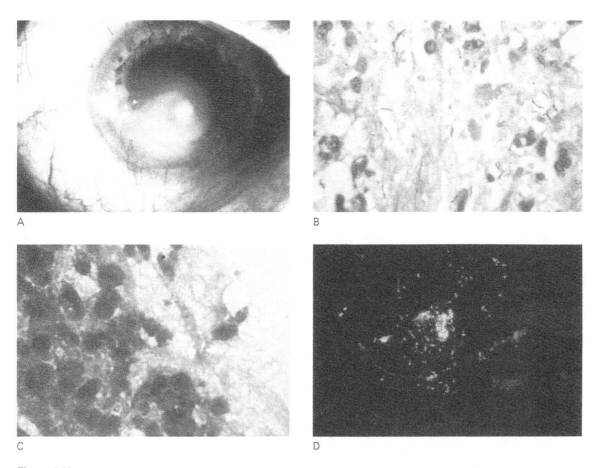

A

B

C

D

Figure 6.22

(A) *Nocardia* keratitis, later becoming fulminant endophthalmitis (B) A corneal specimen from the same eye (Figure 6.22(A)) shows *Nocardia* sp. in the cornea. (Modified Ziehl-Neelsen stain). (C) Vitreous sample of the same eye shows *Nocardia* sp. (Modified Ziehl-Neelsen stain). (D) Vitreous sample of the same eye shows *Nocardia* sp. (Acridine orange stain).

capsule, dry eye, wound abnormalities and/or corneal perforation were found. Three cases were due to *S. aureus;* two to *Capnocytophaga* spp. (an anaerobe); and one each to *Strep. pneumoniae, Strep. viridans, Haemophilus influenzae, Proteus mirabilis, Klebsiella oxytoca, Ps. aeruginosa* (Figure 6.21A, B), and *Mycobacterium chelonae*.[117] Four cases had a fungal etiology; two resulted from *Fusarium* spp. (*F. solani, F. oxysporum*), and one each from *Candida glabrata* and *Paecilomyces* sp. One case had a mixed infection of three different bacteria.

Endophthalmitis can also follow keratitis caused by *Nocardia* spp.,[118] often associated as a secondary infection of Sjögren's syndrome.

Nocardia can stain poorly with the Gram stain, or as weakly Gram-positive beaded rods that may be missed. They are weakly acid, nonalcohol fast, and should be stained with the modified Ziehl-Neelsen stain (Chapter 3) although they also stain well with acridine orange (Figure 6.22A-D). *Nocardia* spp. require a minimum incubation period of 72 hours on blood agar plates to give tiny colonies which are missed altogether if agar plate disposal occurs after 48 hours when a false-negative report is made.[119] When endophthalmitis is recognized, surgery and antibiotic treatment with amikacin and a quinolone antibiotic are required; however, the infection is often progressive, eventually requiring enucleation.[118,120]

Dursun et al described 10 cases of endophthalmitis in Turkey arising from keratitis caused by fungi (seven *F. oxysporum*, two *F. solani*, and one *Fusarium* sp.). They followed up 159 cases of fungal keratitis of which 10 (6%) progressed to endophthalmitis.[54] Other cases are listed in Table 6.3 which is notable because all cases were caused by mycelial fungi and none by *Candida* spp.

References

1. Speaker MG, Menikoff JA. Prophylaxis of endophthalmitis with topical povidone iodine, *Ophthalmology* (1991) **98**:1769–75.
2. Apt L, Isenberg S, Yoshimori R et al. Chemical preparation of the eye in ophthalmic surgery: III. Effect of povidone-iodine on the conjunctiva, *Arch Ophthalmol* (1984) **102**:728–9.
3. Ciulla TA, Starr MB, Masket S. Bacterial endophthalmitis prophylaxis for cataract surgery. An evidence-based update, *Ophthalmology* (2002) **109**:13–24.
4. Apt L, Isenberg SJ, Yoshimori R et al. The effect of povidone-iodine solution applied at the conclusion of ophthalmic surgery, *Am J Ophthalmol* (1995) **119**:701–5.
5. Mendivil Soto, Mendivil MP. The effect of povidone-iodine, intraocular vancomycin, or both on aqueous humor cultures at the time of cataract surgery, *Am J Ophthalmol* (2001) **131**:293–300.
6. Alp BN, Elibol O, Sargon MF et al. The effect of povidone iodine on the corneal endothelium, *Cornea* (2000) **19**:546–50.
7. Zamora JL. Chemical and microbiologic characteristics and toxicity of povidone iodine solutions, *Am J Surg* (1986) **151**:400–6.
8. Lagnado R, Gupta R, Osborne et al. A case of postoperative Candida endophthalmitis, *Eye* (2004) (in press).
9. Spirn MJ, Roth DB, Yarian DL et al. Postoperative fungal endophthalmitis caused by *Trichosporon beigelii* resistant to amphotericin B, *Retina* (2003) **23**:404–5.
10. Garbino J, Ondrusova A, Baligvo E et al. Successful treatment of *Paecilomyces lilacinus* endophthalmitis with voriconazole, *Scand J Infect Dis* (2002) **34**:701–3. [Erratum appears in *Scand J Infect Dis* (2003) **35**:79.]
11. Narang S, Gupta A, Gupta V et al. Fungal endophthalmitis following cataract surgery: clinical presentation, microbiological spectrum, and outcome, *Am J Ophthalmol* (2001) **132**:609–17.
12. Kaushik S, Ram J, Chakrabarty A et al. *Curvularia*

lunata endophthalmitis with secondary keratitis, *Am J Ophthalmol* (2001) **131**:140–2.
13. Huber CE, LaBerge T, Schwiesow T et al. *Exophiala werneckii* endophthalmitis following cataract surgery in an immunocompetent individual, *Ophthalmic Surg Lasers* (2000) **31**:417–22.
14. Tabbara KF, al-Jabarti AL. Hospital construction-associated outbreak of ocular aspergillosis after cataract surgery, *Ophthalmology* (1998) **105**:522–6.
15. Weissgold DJ, Orlin SE, Sulewski ME et al. Delayed-onset fungal keratitis after endophthalmitis, *Ophthalmology* (1998) **105**:258–62.
16. Seal DV, Bron AJ, Hay J. *Ocular Infection – Investigation and Treatment in Practice* (Martin Dunitz: London, 1998).
17. Fridkin S, Kremer FB, Bland LA et al. *Acremonium kiliense* endophthalmitis that occurred after cataract extraction in an ambulatory surgical center and was traced to an environmental reservoir, *Clin Infect Dis* (1996) **22**:222–7.
18. Bartz-Schmidt KU, Tintelnot K, Steffen M et al. Chronic basidiomycetous endophthalmitis after extracapsular cataract extraction and intraocular lens implantation, *Graefes Arch Clin Exp Ophthalmol* (1996) **234**:591–3.
19. Oxford KW, Abbott RL, Fung WE et al. *Aspergillus* endophthalmitis after sutureless cataract surgery, *Am J Ophthalmol* (1995) **120**:534–5.
20. Verbraeken H. Treatment of postoperative endophthalmitis, *Ophthalmologica* (1995) **209**:165–71.
21. Fekrat S, Haller JA, Green WR et al. Pseudophakic *Candida parapsilosis* endophthalmitis with a consecutive keratitis, *Cornea* (1995) **14**:212–6.
22. Ohkubo S, Toriaski M, Higashide T et al. Endophthalmitis caused by *Paecilomyces lilacinus* after cataract surgery: a case report, *Nippon Ganka Gakkai Zasshi* (1994) **98**:103–10.
23. Das T, Vyas P, Sharma S. *Aspergillus terreus* postoperative endophthalmitis, *Br J Ophthalmol* (1993) **77**:386–7.
24. Bouchard CS, Chacko B, Cupples HP et al. Surgical treatment for a case of postoperative *Pseudallescheria boydii* endophthalmitis, *Ophthalmic Surg* (1991) **22**:98–101.
25. Rao NA, Nerenberg AV, Forster DJ. *Torulopsis candida* (*Candida famata*) endophthalmitis simulating *Propionibacterium acnes* syndrome, *Arch Ophthalmol* (1991) **109**:1718–21.
26. Srinivasan R, Kanungo R, Goyal JL. Spectrum of oculomycosis in South India, *Acta Ophthalmol (Copenh)* (1991) **69**:744–9.
27. Pulido JS, Folberg R, Carter KD et al. *Histoplasma capsulatum* endophthalmitis after cataract extraction, *Ophthalmology* (1990) 97: 217–20.
28. Orgel IK, Cohen KL. Postoperative Zygomycetes endophthalmitis, *Ophthalmic Surg* (1989) **20**: 584–7.

29. Pflugfelder SC, Flynn HW Jr, Zwickey TA et al. Exogenous fungal endophthalmitis, *Ophthalmology* 1988; **95**:19–30.

30. O'Day DM, Head WS, Robinson RD et al. An outbreak of *Candida parapsilosis* endophthalmitis: analysis of strains by enzyme profile and antifungal susceptibility. Clinical findings and management of 15 causative cases, *Br J Ophthalmol* (1987) **71**:126–9.

31. Stern WH, Tamura E, Jacobs RA. Epidemic postsurgical *Candida parapsilosis* endophthalmitis, *Ophthalmology* (1985) **92**:1701–9.

32. Driebe WT, Mandelbaum S, Forster RK et al. Pseudophakic endophthalmitis. Diagnosis and management, *Ophthalmology* (1986) **93**:422–8.

33. Minogue MJ, Playfair TJ, Gregory-Roberts JC et al. Cure of *Paecilomyces* endophthalmitis with multiple intravitreal injections of amphotericin B. Case report, *Arch Ophthalmol* (1989) **107**:1281.

34. Pettit TH, Olson RJ, Foos RY et al. Fungal endophthalmitis following intraocular lens implantation. A surgical epidemic, *Arch Ophthalmol* (1980) **98**: 1025–39.

35. Theodore FH. Etiology and diagnosis of fungal postoperative endophthalmitis, *Ophthalmology* (1978) **85**:327–40.

36. Kunimoto DY, Das T, Sharma S et al. Microbiologic spectrum and susceptibility of isolates: Part I. Postoperative endophthalmitis, *Am J Ophthalmol* (1999) **128**:240–2.

37. Scott IU, Flynn HW Jr, Feuer W et al. Endophthalmitis associated with microbial keratitis, *Ophthalmology* (1996) **103**:1864–70.

38. Neveu M, Elliot AJ. Prophylaxis and treatment of endophthalmitis, *Am J Ophthalmol* (1959) **48**: 368–73.

39. Burns RP. Postoperative infections in an ophthalmologic hospital with comments upon bacteriophage typing of staphylococci as a preventive tool, *Am J Ophthalmol* (1959) **48**:519–26.

40. Leopold IH, Apt L. Postoperative intraocular infections, *Am J Ophthalmol* (1960) **50**:1225–47.

41. Von Sallmann L, Meyer K, DiGrandi J. Experimental study on penicillin treatment of ectogenous infection of vitreous, *Arch Ophthalmol* (1944) **32**: 179–89.

42. Leopold IH. Intravitreal penetration of penicillin and penicillin therapy of infection of the vitreous, *Arch Ophthalmol* (1945) **33**:211–16.

43. Von Sallmann L, Meyer K. Penetration of penicillin into the eye, *Arch Ophthalmol* (1944) **31**:1–7.

44. Von Sallmann L. Penicillin therapy of infections of the vitreous, *Arch Ophthalmol* (1945) **33**:455–62.

45. Pincus J, Deiter P, Sears ML. Experiences with five cases of postoperative endophthalmitis, *Am J Ophthalmol* (1965) **59**:403–9.

46. Sorsby A, Ungar J. Distribution of penicillin in the eye after injections of 1,000,000 units by the subconjunctival, retrobulbar and intramuscular routes, *Br J Ophthalmol* (1948) **32**:864–78.

47. Peyman GA, Schulman JA. *Intravitreal Surgery: Principles and Practice*. 2nd edn (Appleton & Lange: Norwalk, CT, 1994) 851–922.

48. Kawasaki K, Ohnogi J. Nontoxic concentration of antibiotics for intravitreal use – evaluated by human *in-vitro* ERG, *Doc Ophthalmol* (1989) **70**: 301–8.

49. Peyman GA, Vastine DW, Raichand M. Symposium: Postoperative endophthalmitis: experimental aspects and their clinical application, *Ophthalmology* (1978) **85**:374–85.

50. Peyman GA, Sanders DR. *Advances in Uveal Surgery, Vitreous Surgery, and the Treatment of Endophthalmitis* (Appleton-Century-Crofts: New York, 1975) 184–208.

51. Vastine DW, Peyman GA, Guth SB. Visual prognosis in bacterial endophthalmitis treated with intravitreal antibiotics. *Ophthalmic Surg* (1979) **10**:76–83.

52. Gan IM, van Dissel JT, Beekhuis WH et al. Intravitreal vancomycin and gentamicin concentrations in patients with postoperative endophthalmitis, *Br J Ophthalmol* (2001) **85**: 1289–93.

53. Sunaric-Megevand G, Pournaras CJ. Current approach to postoperative endophthalmitis, *Br J Ophthalmol* (1997) **81**:1006–15.

54. Dursun D, Fernandez V, Miller D et al. Advanced *Fusarium* keratitis progressing to endophthalmitis, *Cornea* (2003) **22**:300–3.

55. Leck A, Matheson M, Tuft S et al. *Scedosporium apiospermum* keratomycosis with secondary endophthalmitis, *Eye* (2003) **17**:841–3.

56. Li-Shao-Wei, Xie Li Xin, Jin Xiu Ming et al. A retrospective medical history analysis of the patients with severe fungal keratitis, *Zhonghua Yan Ke Za Zhi* (2003) **39**:274–7.

57. Borderie VM, Bourcier TM, Poirot JL et al. Endophthalmitis after *Lasiodiplodia theobromae* corneal abscess, *Graefes Arch Clin Exp Ophthalmol* (1997) **235**: 259–61.

58. Okhravi N, Dart JKG, Towler HM et al. *Paecilomyces lilacinus* endophthalmitis with secondary keratitis: a case report and literature review, *Arch Ophthalmol* (1997) **115**:1320–4.

59. Jager MJ, Chodosh J, Huang AJW et al. *Aspergillus niger* as an unusual cause of scleritis and endophthalmitis, *Br J Ophthalmol* (1994) **78**:584–6.

60. Ksiazek SM, Morris DA, Mandelbaum S et al. Fungal panophthalmitis secondary to *Scedosporium apiospermum* (*Pseudallescheria boydii*) keratitis, *Am J Ophthalmol* (1994) **118**: 531–3.

61. Slomovic MR, Forster RK, Gelender H. *Lasiodiplodia theobromae* panophthalmitis, *Can J Ophthalmol* (1985) **20**:225–8.

62. Fox GM, Joondeph BC, Flynn HW Jr et al. Delayed-

onset pseudophakic endophthalmitis, *Am J Ophthalmol* (1991) **111**: 163–73.

63. Scott IU, Flynn HW Jr, Miller D et al. Exogenous endophthalmitis caused by amphotericin B-resistant *Paecilomyces lilacinus*: treatment options and visual outcomes. *Arch Ophthalmol* (2001) **119**:916–9.

64. Javitt JC, Vitale S, Canner JK et al. National outcomes of cataract extraction. Endophthalmitis following inpatient surgery, *Arch Ophthalmol* (1991) **109**:1085–9.

65. Montan PG, Wejde G, Koranyi G et al. Prophylactic intracameral cefuroxime. Efficacy in preventing endophthalmitis following cataract surgery, *J Cataract Refract Surg* (2002) **28**: 977–82.

66. Fisch A, Salvanet A, Prazuck T et al. Epidemiology of infective endophthalmitis in France, *Lancet* (1991) **338**:1373–6.

67. Ramsay AL, Diaper CJM, Saba SN et al. Simultaneous bilateral cataract extraction, *J Cataract Refract Surg* (1999) **25**:753–62.

68. Colleaux KM, Hamilton WK. Effect of prophylactic antibiotics and incision type on the incidence of endophthalmitis after cataract surgery, *Can J Ophthalmol* (2000) **35**:373–8.

69. Jensen MK, Fiscella RG. Comparison of endophthalmitis rates over four years associated with topical ofloxacin vs. ciprofloxacin, Proceedings of the Annual Meeting of the Association for Research in Vision and Ophthalmology (ARVO), Ft Lauderdale, FL, USA, 2002; abstract no. 4429.

70. Schmitz S, Dick HB, Krummenauer F et al. Endophthalmitis in cataract surgery. Results of a German survey, *Ophthalmology* (1999) **106**:1869–77.

71. Masket S. Questionnaire survey of cataract surgery practice in the USA. Presented to the annual meeting of the ASCRS, 1998.

72. Liesegang TJ. Prophylactic antibiotics in cataract operations, *Mayo Clin Proc* (1997) **72**:149–59.

73. Aaberg TM Jr, Flynn HW Jr, Schiffman J et al. Nosocomial acute-onset postoperative endophthalmitis survey, *Ophthalmology* (1998) **105**: 1004–10.

74. Mayer E, Cadman D, Ewings P et al. A 10 year retrospective study of cataract surgery and endophthalmitis in a single eye unit: injectable lenses lower the incidence of endophthalmitis, *Br J Ophthalmol* (2003) **87**:867–9.

75. Nagaki Y, Hayasaka S, Kadoi C et al. Bacterial endophthalmitis after small-incision cataract surgery. Effect of incision placement and intraocular lens type, *J Cataract Refract Surg* (2003) **29**:20–6.

76. Tuft S J, Ramakrishnan M, Seal DV, Kemeney DM, Buckley RJ. Role of *Staphylococcus aureus* in chronic allergic conjunctivitis, *Ophthalmology* (1992) **99**:180–4.

77. Beigi B, Westlake W, Chang B et al. The effect of intracameral, per-operative antibiotics on microbial contamination of anterior chamber aspirates during phacoemulsification, *Eye* (1998) **12**:390–4.

78. Sherwood DR, Rich WJ, Jacob JS et al. Bacterial contamination of intraocular and extraocular fluids during extracapsular cataract surgery, *Eye* (1989) **3**:308–12.

79. Dickey JB, Thompson KD, Jay WM. Anterior chamber aspirate cultures after uncomplicated cataract surgery, *Am J Ophthalmol* (1991) **112**:278–82.

80. Egger SF, Huber-Spitzy V, Skorpik C et al. Different techniques of extracapsular extraction: bacterial contamination during surgery, *Graefes Arch Clin Exp Ophthalmol* (1994) **232**:308–11.

81. Mistlberger A, Ruckhofer J, Raithel E et al. Anterior chamber contamination during cataract surgery with intraocular lens implantation, *J Cataract Refract Surg* (1997) **23**: 1064–9.

82. Gimbel HV, Sun R, DeBrof BM. Prophylactic intracameral antibiotics during cataract surgery: the incidence of endophthalmitis and corneal endothelial cell loss, *Eur J Implant Ref Surg* (1994) **6**:280–5.

83. Taban M. Clear cornea incisions implicated in endophthalmitis: a meta-analysis. Presented at the American Academy of Ophthalmology, Anaheim, CA, 2003, and at the Association for Research in Vision and Ophthalmology (ARVO), Ft. Lauderdale, FL, 2004; abstract number 505.

84. Scott IU, Loo RH, Flynn HW Jr et al. Endophthalmitis caused by *Enterococcus faecalis*: antibiotic selection and treatment outcomes. *Ophthalmology* (2003) **110**:1573–7.

85. Feys J, Salvanet-Bouccara A, Emond J et al. Vancomycin prophylaxis and intraocular contamination during cataract surgery, *J Cataract Refract Surg* (1997) **23**:894–7.

86. Ferro JF, de-Pablos M, Logrono MJ et al. Postoperative contamination after using vancomycin and gentamicin during phacoemulsification, *Arch Ophthalmol* (1997) **115**:165–70.

87. Gritz DC, Cevallos AV, Smolin G et al. Antibiotic supplementation of intraocular irrigating solutions. An *in vitro* model of antibacterial action, *Ophthalmology* (1996) **103**:1204–9.

88. Kresloff MS, Castellarin AA, Zarbin MA. Endophthalmitis, *Surv Ophthalmol* (1998) **43**: 193–224.

89. Montan PG, Wejde G, Setterquist H et al. Prophylactic intracameral cefuroxime. Evaluations of safety and kinetics in cataract surgery, *J Cataract Refract Surg* (2002) **28**: 982–7.

90. Jenkins CDG, Tuft SJ, Sheraidah G et al. Comparative intraocular penetration of topical and injected cefuroxime, *Br J Ophthalmol* (1996) **80**:685–8.

91. Ragusa FV, Passalacqua G, Gambardella R et al. Nonfatal systemic reactions to subcutaneous

immunotherapy: a 10-year experience, *J Invest Allergol Clin Immunol* (1997) **7**:151–4

92. Graves A, Henry M, O'Brien T et al. *In vitro* susceptibilities of bacterial ocular isolates to fluoroquinolones, *Cornea* (2001) **20**:301–5. [Erratum appears in *Cornea* (2001) **20**:546.]

93. Ormerod LD, Ho DD, Becker LE et al. Endophthalmitis caused by the coagulase-negative staphylococci. 1. Disease spectrum and outcome, *Ophthalmology* (1993) **100**:715–23.

94. Ormerod LD, Becker LE, Cruise RJ et al. Endophthalmitis caused by the coagulase-negative staphylococci. 2. Factors influencing presentation after cataract surgery, *Ophthalmology* (1993) **100**:724–9.

95. Ferrer C, Ruiz-Moreno JM, Rodriguez AR et al. Postoperative *Corynebacterium macginleyi* endophthalmitis, *J Cataract Refract Surg* (2004) (in press).

96. Raman SV, Evans N, Shreshta B et al. Chronic *Actinomyces neuii* postoperative endophthalmitis, *J Cataract Refract Surg* (2004) (in press).

97. Roussel TJ, Olson ER, Rice T et al. Chronic postoperative endophthalmitis associated with *Actinomyces* species, *Arch Ophthalmol* (1991) **109**:60–2.

98. Webster GF, Seyden JJ, Musson RA et al. Susceptibility of *Propionibacterium acnes* to killing and degradation by human neutrophils and monocytes *in vitro*, *Infect Immun* (1985) **49**:116–21.

99. Meisler DM, Palestine AG, Vastine DW et al. Chronic *Propionibacterium* endophthalmitis after extracapsular cataract extraction and intraocular lens implantation, *Am J Ophthalmol* (1986) **102**:733–9.

100. Clark WL, Kaiser PK, Flynn HW Jr et al. Treatment strategies and visual acuity outcomes in chronic postoperative *Propionibacterium acnes* endophthalmitis, *Ophthalmology* (1999) **106**:1665–70.

101. Meisler DM, Mandelbaum S. *Propionibacterium*-associated endophthalmitis after extracapsular cataract extraction. Review of reported cases, *Ophthalmology* (1989) **96**:54–61.

102. Carlson AN, Koch DD Endophthalmitis following Nd:YAG laser posterior capsulotomy, *Ophthalmic Surg* (1988) **19**:168–70.

103. Neuteboom GH, de Vries-Knoppert WA. Endophthalmitis after Nd:YAG laser capsulotomy, *Doc Ophthalmol* (1988) **70**:175–8.

104. Margo CE, Lessner A, Goldey SH et al. Lens-induced endophthalmitis after Nd:YAG laser iridotomy, *Am J Ophthalmol* (1992) **113**:97–8.

105. Warheker PT, Gupta SR, Mansfield DC et al. Postoperative saccular endophthalmitis caused by macrophage-associated staphylococci, *Eye* (1998) **12**: 1019–21.

106. Abreu JA, Cordoves L, Mesa CG et al. Chronic pseudophakic endophthalmitis versus saccular endophthalmitis, *J Cataract Refract Surg* (1997) **23**:1122–5.

107. Zambrano W, Flynn HW Jr, Pflugfelder SC et al. Management options for *Propionibacterium acnes* endophthalmitis, *Ophthalmology* (1989) **96**:1100–5.

108. Winward KE, Pflugfelder SC, Flynn HW Jr et al. Postoperative *Propionibacterium* endophthalmitis. Treatment strategies and long-term results, *Ophthalmology* (1993) **100**:447–51.

109. Aldave AJ, Stein JD, Deramo VA et al. Treatment strategies for postoperative *Propionibacterium acnes* endophthalmitis, *Ophthalmology* (1999) **106**:2395–401.

110. Warheker PT, Gupta SR, Mansfield DC et al. Successful treatment of saccular endophthalmitis with clarithromycin, *Eye* (1998) **12**: 1017–19.

111. Karia N, Aylward GW. Postoperative *Propionibacterium acnes* endophthalmitis, *Ophthalmology* (2001) **108**:634.

112. Okhravi N, Guest S, Matheson MM et al. Assessment of the effect of oral clarithromycin on visual outcome following presumed bacterial endophthalmitis, *Curr Eye Res* (2000) **21**:691–702.

113. Patton N. Post-traumatic endophthalmitis caused by *Xanthomonas maltophilia*, *Eye* (2001) **15**:801–2.

114. Chen JC, Roy M. Epidemic *Bacillus* endophthalmitis after cataract surgery II: chronic and recurrent presentation and outcome, *Ophthalmology* (2000) **107**:1038–41.

115. Ray CJ, Hainsworth DP. Delayed onset of polymicrobial postsurgical endophthalmitis, *Retina* (2000) **20**:411–12.

116. Rogers NK, Fox PD, Noble BA et al. Aggressive management of an epidemic of chronic pseudophakic endophthalmitis: results and literature survey, *Br J Ophthalmol* (1994) **78**:115–19.

117. Scott IU, Lieb DF, Flynn HW Jr et al. Endophthalmitis caused by *Mycobacterium chelonae*: selection of antibiotics and outcomes of treatment. *Arch Ophthalmol* (2003) **121**:573–6.

118. Heathcote JG, McCartney AC, Rice NS et al. Endophthalmitis caused by exogenous nocardial infection in a patient with Sjögren's syndrome, *Can J Ophthalmol* (1990) **25**:29–33.

119. Ficker L, Kirkness C, McCartney A et al. Microbial keratitis – the false negative, *Eye* (1991) **5**:549–59.

120. Ferry AP, Font RL, Weinberg RS et al. Nocardial endophthalmitis: report of two cases studied histopathologically, *Br J Ophthalmol* (1988) **72**:55–61.

7

Other causes of exogenous endophthalmitis

Endophthalmitis after filtering procedure

Epidemiology

Endophthalmitis may develop in the period immediately following a filtration procedure or may occur months or years later. In early-onset cases, the causative organism is probably directly inoculated into the eye at the time of surgery, with *Staphylococcus epidermidis* (a coagulase-negative staphylococcus [CNS]) as the most common isolate.[1] An intraocular infection developing soon after glaucoma surgery is directly related to the surgical procedure with the presence of a bleb (Figures 7.1 and 7.2) as an incidental factor and may be treated accordingly.

In late-onset endophthalmitis, the most prevalent organisms are streptococci followed by *Haemophilus influenzae*. In 36 cases of bleb-associated endophthalmitis, Mandelbaum and Forster noted that *Streptococcus* spp. and *H. influenzae* were cultured from 57% and 23% of eyes, respectively (Figure 7.3).[2] In this study, endophthalmitis developed from 4 months to 66 years after surgery. Additionally, *Staphylococcus aureus* and *Pseudomonas aeruginosa* were isolated from two eyes, respectively, while an additional eye was infected with *Moraxella non-liquefaciens* and another eye with *Fusarium* sp.

Greenfield et al also noted a similar spectrum of organisms in an evaluation of late-onset endophthalmitis after filtration surgery with mitomycin.[3] Nine of 13 (69.2%) eyes were culture-positive, with *Streptococcus sanguis* and

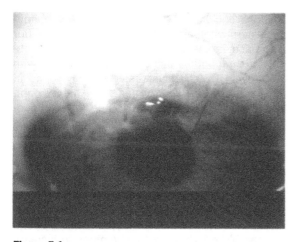

Figure 7.1

Bleb at graft site predisposing to endophthalmitis.

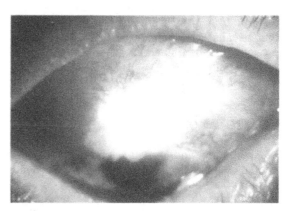

Figure 7.2

Infected bleb.

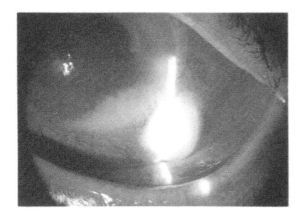

Figure 7.3

Bleb-related endophthalmitis.

H. influenzae comprising 42% of the isolates. Ciulla et al identified 27 cases of late-onset endophthalmitis after glaucoma filtering surgery.[1] *Streptococcus* spp. and Gram-negative bacteria were isolated in 42% of culture-positive eyes.

However, in a 10-year review of late bleb-related endophthalmitis, Waheed et al found a different infecting microbiological spectrum.[4] The authors found that the majority of infections were caused by staphylococci followed by streptococci. Specifically, Waheed et al found *S. aureus* (13/42), *S. epidermidis* (12/42), streptococci (8/42), and *H. influenzae* (2/42). A final visual acuity of 20/400 or better was achieved in 32 of 49 cases (65%).

Waheed et al also reported three cases of bleb-related ocular infection in children after trabeculectomy with mitomycin C.[5] CNS were cultured from all eyes and the investigators noted that because children are such poor historians, parents must be trained to recognize the signs of endophthalmitis.

Source of organism

Mandelbaum and Forster obtained external ocular cultures from 36 patients with delayed-onset endophthalmitis associated with conjunctival filtering blebs.[2] Eighteen of 26 patients cultured in this series demonstrated growth of organisms from the lid, conjunctiva, and intraocular fluid. Yet, only five of these cases demon-strated a correlation between organisms grown from the external culture and those cultured from intraocular fluids. Additionally, swabs were taken from the external surface of the bleb in five eyes with positive intraocular cultures and only one eye demonstrated the same organism from the vitreous and the swab. The report of another series of three patients did not find any correlation between eyelid and conjunctival cultures and intraocular cultures. These results suggest that the use of long-term prophylactic topical antibiotics after filtration surgery is only indicated in eyes with thin-walled or chronic leaking blebs. Extraocular cultures and intraocular cultures do not correlate highly. The infecting organisms may invade the eye during the perioperative period.

The etiology of the infecting organism due to migration from the external ocular structure appears in doubt. Rather, the organisms may have been sequestered at the time of surgery or in the perioperative period. The long latent interval after surgery before infection develops and the high incidence of infection with causative organisms which are not part of the normal ocular flora suggest that the infections are caused by migration through the filtering bleb of organisms which transiently colonize on the conjunctiva or arise from bloodstream spread. This latter route particularly favors streptococci.

Risk factors

A higher incidence of bleb-related endophthalmitis occurs when an inferior rather than a superior approach is used. In a series of cases of bleb-related endophthalmitis after trabeculectomy with mitomycin C, intraocular infection developed in 8% of procedures performed from below compared with 1.1% of procedures performed superiorly.[6] The cumulative risk of endophthalmitis developing from inferiorly compared with superiorly located blebs was 7.7. Another series found that late-onset endophthalmitis occurred in 13% of inferiorly performed procedures compared with 1.6% of procedures performed superiorly.[3]

Several factors appear to contribute to the higher risk for endophthalmitis in eyes with inferiorly located blebs.[6] These factors combine to increase intraocular access through the bleb to potential pathogens present in the tear lake and lid margin.

- The upper eyelid covers and protects superiorly located blebs. In contrast, the lower eyelid is less effective in performing this function and frequently leaves the bleb exposed.
- In addition, the blinking and eye movement of the lower eyelid causes chronic mechanical irritation of the inferior bleb. This mechanical trauma weakens and subsequently breaks down the structural integrity of the bleb.

The characteristics of filtration blebs also influence the incidence of endophthalmitis:

- Eyes with thin-walled cystic blebs appear to be more susceptible to intraocular infection than eyes with thick-walled spongy blebs. The use of antimetabolites promotes the formation of thinner, avascular blebs with denuded epithelium and underlying stromal damage.
- The physical barrier effect of the bleb, along with the conjunctiva's ability to initiate an immune response, appear to be compromised by these morphological changes. The result is an increased susceptibility of these eyes to infection.

Lehmann et al[7] and Beck et al[8] demonstrated the increased risk of developing posttrabeculectomy endophthalmitis when using an antifibrotic agent.[7,8] Lehmann et al also identified previous development of blebitis and diabetes mellitus as additional risk factors.[7] Beck et al found additional risk factors including poor lid hygiene, inadequate patient follow-up, recent trauma, the chronic use of antibiotics and steroids, concurrent eyelid disease, and dementia.[8] Beck also observed phacoanaphylaxis associated with a chronic uveitis histopathologically in all four eyes with late-onset endophthalmitis. This inflammatory response was speculated to contribute to the poor outcome in these eyes. Others have identified contact lens wear and upper respiratory tract infections as factors predisposing to late-onset bleb endophthalmitis. Mandelbaum and Forster also suggested chronic bleb leaks as a risk factor.[2]

Prognosis

Ayyala et al cautioned that the term 'blebitis' should be used to describe a limited form of infec-
tion and inflammation confined to the bleb and the peribleb area, with or without anterior chamber involvement.[9] In contrast, the more classic form of endophthalmitis is the virulent form of bleb-related infection. These patients present with rapidly worsening visual acuity, redness, and pain with diffuse conjunctival congestion, opalescent blebs (with or without epithelial defects) with intense fibrin and/or a hypopyon in the anterior chamber, and a florid vitritis. Blebitis is a limited form of bleb-related infection with limited inflammation and infection involving only the bleb.

Brown et al described blebitis as a syndrome characterized by a prodrome of red eyes, pain, and blurred vision lasting 3 or more days in some of the 14 patients in his series.[10] The bleb in all patients appeared to contain inflammatory material with a whitened milky appearance. The anterior chamber reaction was considered too extreme for a diagnosis of conjunctivitis with six patients presenting with hypopyon. The vitreous was not involved in 13 of 14 eyes. A positive Seidel test was present in 9 of 13 patients. In contrast, in the series of culture-proven late-onset endophthalmitis described by Mandelbaum and Forster, bleb leakage was much less frequent.[2]

Patients with late bleb-related endophthalmitis characteristically present with an abrupt onset of ocular pain, decreased vision, and redness associated with varying degrees of intraocular inflammation in an eye which has previously been quiet. The signs and symptoms characterizing bleb-associated endophthalmitis tend to be rapidly progressive. Blebitis has been documented to progress to culture-proven endophthalmitis.[11] Subsequently, eyes with blebitis require frequent observation so that intravitreal antibiotics can be administered in a timely manner should vitreous involvement be observed.

Blebitis

In the series provided by Brown et al, patients were hospitalized and treated with intravenous cefazolin and topical fortified gentamicin and cefazolin given every 30 minutes on an alternating dosage schedule.[10] Upon discharge, patients were placed on a tapering schedule of topical cefazolin and oral cephradine for 5 days. A rapid improvement in ocular symptoms and signs occurred soon after therapy was initiated. Within hours, vision in most patients returned to pre-infection levels. The investigators considered blebitis to be a precursor of late-onset bleb-associated endophthalmitis. In another series, all patients were treated with a topical fortified antibiotic, with seven patients also receiving topical steroids. The infection resolved in nine eyes using this treatment regimen, with prompt return of preinfection visual acuity in five eyes.

Endophthalmitis

The visual prognosis in late-onset bleb endoph-thalmitis is generally poor. In contrast to the Endophthalmitis Vitrectomy Study (EVS) in which 85% of patients had visual acuities better than 5/200 at 9–12 months after treatment of endophthalmitis, 31–68% of late-onset bleb endophthalmitis eyes had visual acuity worse than 20/400.[11,12]

Mandelbaum et al reported a final visual acuity worse than 20/400 in 68% of eyes,[12] while Phillips et al reported this level of visual acuity in only 43% of patients.[13] Mandelbaum et al indicated that the poor visual results correlated with the virulence of the pathogenic organisms and the advanced extent of intraocular inflammation. Ten of 16 eyes infected with streptococci for which follow-up data were available lost all light percep-tion, while two additional eyes retained light perception but developed irreparable tractional retinal detachments. Only 3 of 16 eyes with strep-tococcal endophthalmitis retained visual acuity of better than 20/400. Light perception was lost in both eyes infected with *Ps. aeruginosa*. In the *H. influenzae* group, one eye retained 20/25 vision. In another eye, vision declined from 20/30 to 20/300. Four eyes were left with count fingers or light perception vision while an additional eye lost light perception. In contrast, visual results were better in the culture-negative cases. Kangas et al reported a final visual acuity of 20/400 or better in only 15 of 32 eyes (47%).[14] Lehmann et al also reported a poor visual result with a post-Snellen visual acuity of 20/40 or better and control of intraocular pressure (IOP) without treatment being achieved in just 3 of 23 eyes.[7]

Initial treatment of late-onset postfiltration endophthalmitis must include topical and intra-vitreal broad-spectrum antibiotics that cover *Streptococcus* spp., *S. aureus*, CNS, and Gram-negative bacteria. We use vancomycin and amikacin but ceftazidime may be substituted for amikacin. When the infectious process involves the vitreous, we routinely perform a pars plana vitrectomy. Antibiotic selection may need to be modified when cultures of vitreous aspirates obtained during vitrectomy or by tap identify the causative organism. The results of the EVS are not directly applicable to late-onset endophthalmitis following glaucoma filtration surgery because of a unique spectrum of organisms and a different pathogenesis.[15] In addition, antibiotic resistance varies from one locality to another, and within each locality. For example, 40% of *S. aureus* isolates in hospitalized or nursing home patients can be resistant to methicillin (MRSA) and all cephalosporins, plus sometimes aminoglycosides and quinolones as well, as opposed to commu-nity-based patients where the incidence of MRSA is very low (at most 1%). Consideration should be given to use of intravitreal corticosteroids (Chapter 8), especially for streptococcal infections.

Posttraumatic endophthalmitis

Epidemiology

Posttraumatic endophthalmitis comprises a minority of cases of exogenous endophthalmitis with the majority of cases occurring from postsur-gical causes. Reports indicate that penetrating trauma accounts for 13–25% of all cases of endophthalmitis (Figure 7.4A–C).[16,17] After pene-trating trauma, the reported incidence of endoph-thalmitis varies from 2.8% to 22%.[18,19] Duch-Samper et al found endophthalmitis developed less frequently following purely corneal trauma (2.1%) compared with patients with posterior pole involvement (7%).[20] Eyes with traumatic endoph-thalmitis have a poorer visual prognosis than eyes with postoperative endophthalmitis.[21]

Eight percent of cases of intraocular foreign bodies (IOFBs) develop an endophthalmitis and half of these lose most vision, making antibiotic prophylaxis essential for most trauma injuries with an IOFB,[22] as discussed below.

Most reports identify *S. epidermidis* as the most commonly isolated organism in posttraumatic endophthalmitis; it is incriminated in 25% of cases.

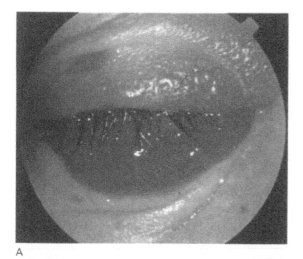

A

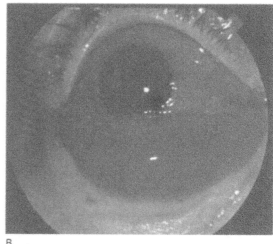

B

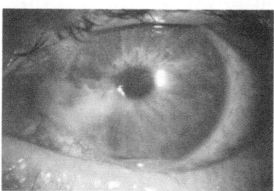

C

Figure 7.4

(A and B) Severe acute endophthalmitis after corneal foreign body trauma. Lid edema, severe chemosis and hyperemia, anterior chamber reaction, and hypopyon were seen. Severe endophthalmitis and panophthalmitis caused by *Staphylococcus aureus*. (C) Endophthalmitis with hypopyon following penetrating corneal trauma.

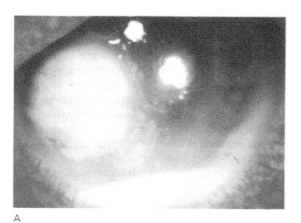

A

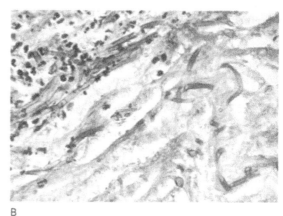

B

Figure 7.5

(A) Severe keratitis with hypopyon that progressed to endophthalmitis as the result of infection with *Fusarium* sp. in an English farmer. (B) Periodic acid–Schiff stain for hyphae of *Fusarium* sp. in the cornea of the same eye as in (A).

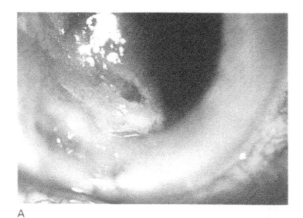

A

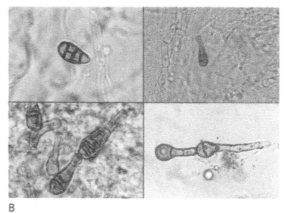

B

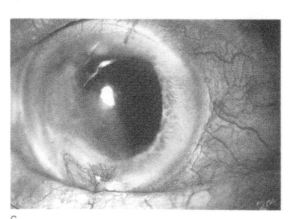

C

Figure 7.6

(A) Corneal injury with a lemon tree branch caused keratitis and endophthalmitis from *Alternaria infectoria* in an agricultural worker. (B) Light photomicrographs showing typical conidia of *A. infectoria* with transverse and longitudinal septa. Conidia are brown, smooth-walled with a rounded base and beaked apex. Conidium has typical long secondary conidiophores (false beaks) which are one-third larger than the length of the conidium. (C) The eye shown in (A) 3 months after treatment.

The characteristics of this organism are discussed in the sections on postoperative endophthalmitis (Chapter 6) and microbiology (Chapter 3). The second most common etiological agent is usually *Bacillus* spp. with 20% prevalence, followed by streptococci in 12% of eyes. However, there have been reports citing a different prevalence – staphylococci (26.5%), streptococci (20.6%), and *Bacillus* spp. (14.7%). *S. aureus* accounts for 6% and Gram-negative bacteria for 14% of eyes. Among the Gram-negative bacteria, *Proteus mirabilis*, *Pseudomonas* spp., and *Klebsiella pneumoniae* are the most commonly isolated. Fungus involvement is uncommon, but a fungus is isolated in 8% of eyes. *Fusarium* spp. (Figure 7.5), *Aspergillus flavus*, *Paecilomyces lilacinus*, *Candida* spp., *Alternaria infectoria* (Figure 7.6) and others have been recorded (Table 7.1).[23–47]

Endophthalmitis following ocular trauma occurs much less frequently in pediatric patients than in adults. The incidence of reported posttraumatic pediatric endophthalmitis varies from 2.8% to 29%. A retrospective study performed by Alfaro et al on pediatric posttraumatic endophthalmitis demonstrated that streptococci were present in 56% of eyes compared with staphylococci (22%) and *Bacillus cereus* (13%).[33] A review of other pediatric endophthalmitis cases supports the finding that the primary offending organism in this age group involves streptococci;[35] however, *H. influenzae* is also an important pathogen for children, causing endophthalmitis after intraocular surgery and filtering bleb placement.[48]

Risk factors

An increased risk of intraocular infection following penetrating trauma has been associated in

Table 7.1 Posttraumatic fungal endophthalmitis

Reference	Type of fungus (no. of infected patients)	Source	Age of patient (years)	Place
Ferrer et al, 2003[23]	Alternaria infectoria (1)	Corneal injury with a lemon tree branch. Posttraumatic cataract. Phaco-steroids. Responded to intravitreal and IV amphotericin and oral fluconazole.	66	Alicante, Spain
Lieb et al, 2003[24]	Phialophora richardsiae (1)	Metallic IOFB into middle of vitreous. Returned after 10 weeks with acute onset painful loss of vision following cataract surgery. Vitrectomy with removal of cocoon of fibrinous membranes around the IOFB. Given intravitreal amphotericin and ketoconazole but failed therapy because of delay in diagnosis	36	Miami, FL, USA
Domniz et al, 2001[25]	Paecilomyces lilacinus (1)	Posttrauma and foreign body in the cornea. Successful outcome	30	Chatswood, Australia
Scott et al, 2001[26]	Paecilomyces lilacinus (1)	Posttrauma. P. lilacinus resistant to amphotericin	29	Miami, FL, USA
Pintor et al, 2001[27]	Paecilomyces lilacinus (1)	Posttrauma	21	Spain
Kunimoto et al. 1999[28]	Aspergillus spp.(9) Fusarium spp.(2) Acremonium sp.(1) Bipolaris sp.(1) Cladosporium sp.(1) Humicola sp. (1) Unidentified dematiaceous fungus (5)	20 fungus isolations out of 182 eyes with posttraumatic endophthalmitis. 113/182 eyes were culture-positive with 139 isolates of which 20 (14%) were fungal; 23 (20%) of 113 eyes were polymicrobial and 3 (2.7%) were trimicrobial. 6/20 (30%) of fungal infections also contained a bacterial pathogen; thus empiric antibacterial treatment should be given as well	NG	Hyderabad, India
Houtmann et al, 1998[29]	Absidia corymbifera (1)	Posttrauma	35	France
Gariano and Kalina 1997[30]	Scopulariopsis brevicaulis (1)	Posttrauma, failed therapy	42	Seattle, WA, USA
Carney et al, 1996[31]	Pseudallescheria boydii (1)	Nail injury. Good response to vitrectomy and intravitreal miconazole	11	Richmond, VA, USA
Thompson et al, 1995[32]	Aspergillus sp.(1) Candida sp.(1)	Increased risk of endophthalmitis with a sharp injury (13/205 including bacterial cases) compared with a blunt one (0/44). Increased risk with lens disruption. Prognosis poor with virulent organisms	NG	Miami, FL, USA
Alfaro et al, 1995[33]	Candida albicans (1)	Corneal laceration – review of infection in 12 cases of which only 1 was fungal. Mixed infection with CNS and streptococci	6	Bethesda, MD, USA
Das et al, 1994[34]	Helminthosporium (1)	Tree branch injury 6 weeks after ECCE/IOL in a patient with diabetes	60	Hyderabad, India
Alfaro et al, 1994[35]	Candida albicans (mixed bacterial) (2)	Corneal laceration (2)	NG	Bethesda, MD, USA
Al-Rajhi et al, 1993[36]	Scytalidium dimidiatum (1)	Penetrating injury by a thorn	46	Riyadh, Saudi Arabia
Srdic et al, 1993[37]	Fusarium moniliforme (2)	Metallic foreign body penetrated to vitreous in both patients – Pseudomonas sp. also isolated	NG	Belgrade, Serbia
D'Mellow et al, 1991[38]	Paecilomyces sp.(1)	Primary intralenticular infection. Bulldozing paddock with prickly pears prior to inflammation. Small corneal laceration	20	Queensland, Australia

continued

Table 7.1 Posttraumatic fungal endophthalmitis – *continued*

Reference	Type of fungus (no. of infected patients)	Source	Age of patient (years)	Place
Witherspoon et al, 1990[39]	*Sporothrix schenkii* (1)	Penetrating injury with vegetable matter. Review of 17 previous known cases of which 1 was due to trauma. Final vision 20/50 but others all enucleated	13	Birmingham, AL, USA
Boldt et al, 1989[40]	*Cladosporium* sp.(1) *Penicillium* sp.and *Streptomyces* sp.(1)	Hammering on a combine harvester, eye struck with fencing wire	49, 30	Iowa, USA
Pflugfelder et al, 1988[41]	*Aspergillus flavus* (1) *Fusarium solani* (1) *Tubercularia vulgaris* (1) *Cylindrocarpon tonkinese* (1) *Acremonium* sp. (1) *Paecilomyces lilacinus* (1)	Corneal perforation with a 'sewer snake'. Corneal laceration with a nail. Corneal perforation with a thorn. Corneal perforation with a thorn. Ruptured cataract surgery wound. Corneal–scleral laceration with a nail	75, 42, 21, 16, 82, 33	Miami, FL, USA
Affeldt et al, 1987[21]	*Fusarium solani* (2) *Aspergillus flavus* (1) *Cylindrocarpon tonkinese* (1) *Tubercularia vulgaris* (1)	Nail/thorn injury, metal fragment, tree branch, thorn injury	42, 68, 75, 16, 21	Miami, FL, USA
Brinton et al, 1984[42]	Review of cases – *Fusarium* spp.(3), *Candida* spp. (1)	7% of posttraumatic endophthalmitis due to fungi	NG	Wisconsin, USA
Rowsey et al, 1982[19]	*Fusarium* spp. (2)	Posttraumatic endophthalmitis	NG	USA
Eschete et al, 1981[43]	*Penicillium chrysogenum* (1)	Report of first recognized case following trauma. Hammer injury with metallic IOFB in the posterior lens. Acute pain and hypopyon. Therapy with amphotericin eradicated the fungus	32	Shreveport, LA, USA
Peyman et al, 1980[44]	*Candida* sp. (1)	Posttraumatic endophthalmitis	10	Chicago, IL, USA
Forster et al, 1980[45]	*Fusarium* sp. (1)	Posttraumatic endophthalmitis	NG	Miami, FL, USA
Savir et al, 1978[46]	*Penicillium* sp. (1)	Broken drill bit penetrated into the anterior chamber. Hypopyon and nonreactive pupil developed after 4 days with CF vision. Anterior chamber tap yielded fungus. Poor response to subconjunctival and topical amphotericin. Responded to 5–fluorocytosine 1500 mg q.d.s. orally, final vision 6/6	57	Tel Aviv, Israel
Rodrigues and McCleod, 1975[47]	*Paecilomyces viridis*	Corneal laceration by a nail while hammering in a barn. 12–mm oblique laceration and iris tear	17	Philadelphia, PA, USA

CF, counting fingers; CNS, coagulase-negative staphylococci; ECCE, extracapsular cataract extraction; IOFB, intraocular foreign body; IOL, intraocular lens; NG, not given.

previous reports with a retained IOFB (Figure 7.7), delayed timing of the primary repair, a rural setting, and lens disruption.[40,49] In a retrospective study involving 258 consecutive patients with penetrating ocular trauma, risk factors for endophthalmitis resulting from trauma were investigated.[32] Factors such as scleral wounds, hyphema, uveal prolapse, retinal detachment, and IOFBs were investigated. Endophthalmitis did not occur in eyes that had blunt injuries. In those eyes with a lacerating injury, only disruption of the crystalline lens was identified as an indepen-

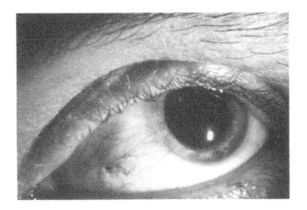

Figure 7.7

Metallic intrascleral foreign body.

dent risk factor for endophthalmitis. No other risk factors were statistically significant.

Mieler et al noted that endophthalmitis developed in 7–13.5% of eyes following penetrating injuries with a retained IOFB.[50] When the foreign body was contaminated with particulate material from a rural setting, the incidence of endophthalmitis in one series was 26%. The National Eye Trauma Study (NETS) found a statistically significant increased incidence of endophthalmitis with IOFB especially if surgical repair occurred more than 24 hours after the injury.[51] Further review of 492 eyes with IOFBs from the NETS Registry concluded that a 24–hour delay in primary repair places individuals over 50 years of age at increased risk for developing infectious endophthalmitis.[52]

Boldt et al in a 10-year retrospective study found an increased incidence of endophthalmitis following rural trauma compared with nonrural injuries (30% vs 11%, respectively).[40] The investigators suggested that the higher incidence in a rural environment might be attributed to a higher virulence of organisms, greater initial intraocular inoculum, and more extensive ocular lacerations. In contrast to previous reports from urban centers, which showed a low incidence of mixed microbial infection, more than two organisms were cultured in 42% of cases of rural endophthalmitis. In this study, the incidence of *Bacillus* spp. endophthalmitis was extremely high (46%). These data suggest that endophthalmitis occurring after a traumatic injury in a rural environment

differs from the same disease occurring in a nonrural setting, particularly with the type of infecting pathogens. In one case with a different cause, bacterial endophthalmitis resulted after a penetrating injury caused by a cat's claw; *Ps. aeruginosa* was cultured from the vitreous sample obtained during a vitrectomy. *Rochalimaea henselae* might have been suspected in this eye; however, Gram-negative *Ps. aeruginosa* was the causative bacterium. [53]

Bacillus and *Clostridium* endophthalmitis

The characteristics of staphylococcal endophthalmitis (caused by *S. aureus* or CNS) have been discussed in the above section on postoperative endophthalmitis. In this section, *Bacillus* spp. and *Clostridium* spp. will be considered.

B. cereus endophthalmitis was first reported in 1952 by Davenport and Smith; this bacterium has been recognized as an increasingly important cause of posttraumatic endophthalmitis.[54,55] The most common *Bacillus* spp. isolate incriminated in posttraumatic endophthalmitis is *B. cereus* (Figures 7.8–7.10). *Bacillus* spp. have been estimated to be the causative organism in 25–46% of cases of culture-positive posttraumatic endophthalmitis.[40] *Bacillus* spp. are considered the second most common pathogen responsible for posttraumatic endophthalmitis.

Bacillus spp. are ubiquitous spore-forming bacteria found in air, dust, dirt, decaying organic matter, and water. They are aerobic or facultative anaerobic, Gram-positive, spore-forming rods. Their virulence is caused by several exotoxins (loop fluid-inducing/necrotic toxin skin test, cereolysin) and enterotoxins (phospholipase C). *Bacillus* spp. also produce beta-lactamases that render resistance to all cephalosporins and penicillins. Chapter 3 discusses these organisms in more detail.

Endophthalmitis caused by *Bacillus* spp. may be associated with systemic findings including fever, mild leucocytosis, and malaise. According to O'Day et al the only other organism capable of causing similar systemic manifestations in this setting is *Clostridium perfringens*, which is discussed later.[54] Progressive corneal destruction including the formation of ring corneal abscesses

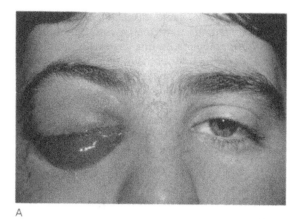

A

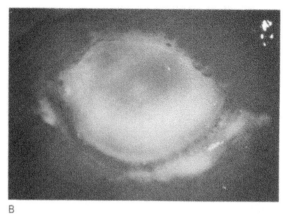

B

Figure 7.8

(A and B) Intraocular foreign body and endophthalmitis caused by *Bacillus cereus*.

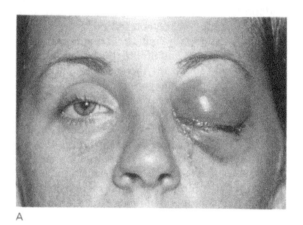

A

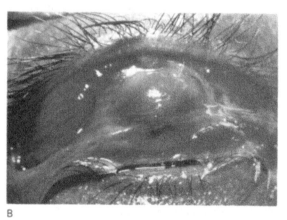

B

Figure 7.9

(A and B) Intraocular foreign body and endophthalmitis caused by *Bacillus cereus*.

within 48 hours of onset may be seen, although it has also been described in endophthalmitis caused by *Proteus* spp. and *Pseudomonas* spp.[54] These developments are often preceded by periorbital edema, peripheral corneal edema, chemosis, and proptosis. The endophthalmitis frequently runs a rapidly destructive course. Visual prognosis is poor, with a significant number of affected eyes failing to retain even light perception vision.

The incidence of *Bacillus* endophthalmitis tends to be higher in rural environments. Intuitively, the nature of a rural injury is different, given the prevalence of farming equipment and animals. In this setting, the injury would involve a different constituent of contaminants. Van Bijsterveld and Richards obtained seven positive conjunctival cultures for *Bacillus* spp. from 40 eyes in individuals with occupational exposure to dust, soil, and hay.[56] The result suggests that colonization of the

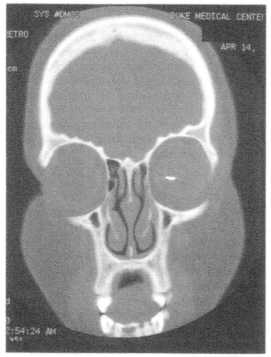

A

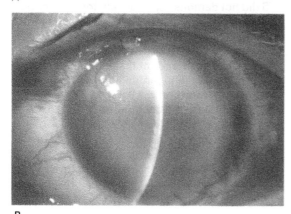

B

Figure 7.10

(A and B) Intraocular foreign body and endophthalmitis caused by *Bacillus cereus*.

external ocular flora with *Bacillus* species may also be a contributing factor. A combination of these two mechanisms likely accounts for the finding that *Bacillus* spp. are more prevalent in rural settings.

Prognosis

Several investigators have noted[42,56] that prognostic factors following traumatic endophthalmitis include:

- virulence of the offending organisms
- nature and severity of the injury
- duration between the onset of endophthalmitis and initiation of treatment
- treatment modality
- retinal breaks or retinal detachment associated with endophthalmitis which adversely affect the final outcome.

As mentioned previously, posttraumatic endophthalmitis is frequently caused by more virulent organisms such as *B. cereus* (25–46%)[37] and Gram-negative bacteria (10–20%).[57] As a result, although the initial signs of postoperative and posttraumatic endophthalmitis may be comparable, the prognosis is worse with trauma. Eighty-five percent of the EVS patients with postoperative endophthalmitis achieved a final visual acuity of 20/400 or better; however, studies of patients with posttraumatic endophthalmitis obtained this visual acuity in only 22–42% of cases.[21,45] In another study, 54% achieved visual acuity of 20/400 or greater; endophthalmitis caused by CNS had the best visual outcome, with 7/11 (64%) of patients obtaining visual acuity of 20/400 or better.[52]

The use of intravitreal antibiotics, microsurgical techniques, earlier establishment of a diagnosis, and identification of offending organisms through simultaneous aqueous and vitreous taps have improved the visual outcome of posttraumatic endophthalmitis. However, the overall prognosis remains poor.

Several other factors contribute to the dire prognosis associated with posttraumatic endophthalmitis.

- Presentation of endophthalmitis may be masked by the inflammation resulting from the trauma.
- Damage to the sclera and vitreous and intraocular hemorrhage accompanying trauma may delay the determination as to whether pain and external signs are caused by trauma or endophthalmitis.

- Underlying injury can either obscure the signs of endophthalmitis or simulate the early appearance of endophthalmitis, further delaying the diagnosis.
- The virulence of the infecting organisms and presence of a polymicrobial infection also adversely affect the outcome.
- Damage from the trauma, especially when retinal detachment is present, may cause permanent structural alteration, limiting final visual recovery.

However, some authors have noted good visual outcome after traumatic endophthalmitis. Mieler et al[50] as well as Mittra and Mieler[56] found that bacterial cultures of removed intraocular material were positive in 7 of 27 eyes with retained IOFBs undergoing surgical repair. Despite the presence of positive cultures, no eye developed signs or symptoms of intraocular infection. Visual acuity of 20/70 or better was maintained in all seven eyes with an average follow-up of 10 months. The authors attributed the failure of endophthalmitis to develop in this series of eyes sustaining trauma to prompt surgical intervention after presentation, the use of intravitreal antibiotics, and the use of supplemental intravenous, subconjunctival, and topical antibiotics. Because the foreign body in several eyes was removed by an external magnet, the investigators could not evaluate the role of vitrectomy in preventing endophthalmitis.

A recent series also suggests that certain eyes with B. cereus endophthalmitis can recover good vision and maintain ocular integrity.[57,58] Five patients with penetrating ocular injury (four cases with an IOFB) developed B. cereus endophthalmitis. Endophthalmitis was diagnosed preoperatively and intraoperatively in three and two patients, respectively. The time from presentation to surgery was less than 3 hours in four patients and 16 hours in the remaining patient. All patients had intravitreal antibiotics consisting of vancomycin with aminoglycoside or ceftazidime in four of five eyes (Bacillus spp. are sensitive to vancomycin but resistant to all cephalosporins). Postoperatively, three eyes developed retinal detachment which was successfully repaired. Final visual acuities were 20/25 (two eyes), 20/30, and 20/200 (two eyes). Reasons advanced for these favorable results include early recognition and prompt surgical management of the endophthalmitis, the early use of intravitreal antibiotics that were extremely efficacious against B. cereus in four of five eyes, infection with less virulent strains of B. cereus, and lack of surgical trauma to vital areas of the eye. Other case reports have suggested that useful vision can be preserved in eyes with posttraumatic B. cereus endophthalmitis[59,60] but this experience is not universal. Hemady et al reported that 5 of 10 eyes with Bacillus endophthalmitis required enucleation; only two eyes with endophthalmitis following elective surgery retained useful vision.[61]

Treatment

We recommend an aggressive approach to traumatic endophthalmitis as do Mittra and Mieler, rather than generalizing the EVS findings to the posttraumatic setting.[56] This usually involves immediate vitrectomy, with Gram stain and cultures, debridement of necrotic tissue, and removal of any IOFB. Antibiotic therapy is recommended via systemic, subconjunctival, intravitreal, and topical routes (Chapter 8). Although the EVS did not demonstrate a benefit for intravenous antibiotic use in postoperative endophthalmitis, we consider systemic intravenous or oral antibiotic use as the adjunctive 'standard of care' in trauma-associated endophthalmitis, because the eye is inflamed and antibiotics will penetrate (Chapter 5).[51] Mittra and Mieler recommend the use of intravitreal vancomycin (1.0 mg) and ceftazidime (2.25 mg);[56] they do not use gentamicin because of possible macular toxicity in the inflamed disorganized eye. Ceftazidime should not be used alone as Bacillus spp. are resistant to it. The same antibiotic can be given intravenously as given by the intravitreal route (Chapter 5).

Prophylaxis

Because 8% of posttraumatic eyes with an IOFB develop a devastating endophthalmitis, 66% of which are expected to lose all light perception, we recommend that prophylactic intravitreal antibiotics are usually used, although this is still controversial.[22,56] The benefit of preventing endophthalmitis conflicts with possible toxicity of the intravitreal antibiotics. It is probably best to avoid gentamicin and to use vancomycin (1.0 mg) against Gram-positive bacteria and ceftazidime (2.25 mg) against Gram-negative bacteria or clindamycin (1.0 mg) as an alternative against Gram-positive bacteria. Some species of bacillus may be resistant to clindamycin. Subconjunctival vancomycin (25 mg) and clindamycin (34 mg) may also be needed along with systemic and topical therapy. Drug concentrations should be reduced by 50% if a full vitrectomy is performed.

Conflicting data exist regarding the efficacy of different antimicrobial agents in treating posttraumatic *Bacillus* endophthalmitis. O'Day et al reported four patients with gentamicin-sensitive *B. cereus* endophthalmitis who failed treatment with periocular, systemic, and intravitreal administration of gentamicin.[54] These eyes required eventual evisceration. The investigators noted that clindamycin was more effective than gentamicin. The greatest benefit in treating the infection was obtained from the combined administration of both clindamycin and gentamicin, which demonstrated synergy. On the other hand, in vitro testing by Kervick et al demonstrated that 22% of tested *Bacillus* isolates from ocular infections were resistant to clindamycin while all isolates were sensitive to vancomycin and gentamicin.[62] Clindamycin has an advantage in inhibiting production of toxins at subinhibitory levels.

Weber et al tested the in vitro susceptibility of 89 strains of *Bacillus* spp. isolated from clinical blood cultures to selected antimicrobial agents.[63] Susceptibility testing using disk diffusion methods showed that 100%, 100%, 98%, and 72% of *B. cereus* strains were susceptible to vancomycin, imipenem, ciprofloxacin, and clindamycin, respectively. Similar testing demonstrated that the susceptibility of non *B. cereus* strains to vancomycin, imipenem, ciprofloxacin, and clindamycin was 100%, 97%, 100%, and 40%, respectively. In this study, the investigators suggested that vancomycin is the drug of choice for treatment of *Bacillus* infections but that two drugs should always be used simultaneously.

Alfaro et al evaluated the efficacy of different intravitreal antibiotics in an experimental swine model of posttraumatic *Bacillus* endophthalmitis.[64] The results demonstrated a significant efficacy for vancomycin and imipenem when given early in the course of the infection in limiting the intraocular inflammation and tissue destruction. In contrast, eyes treated with 100 μg of intravitreal ciprofloxacin responded similarly to both the control eyes and eyes treated with normal saline. In contrast, intravitreal ciprofloxacin appeared to have little or no effect on the course of the endophthalmitis and should not be used.

Two experimental models of posttraumatic *B. cereus* endophthalmitis have demonstrated that overwhelming host inflammatory response plays a major role in causing intraocular damage.[65] Significant infiltration of the vitreous cavity and subretinal space by polymorphonuclear leukocytes with abscess formation and retinal necrosis rapidly causes destruction of the eye. **The investigators suggested a possible role for intravitreal corticosteroids in providing optimal therapy for B. cereus endophthalmitis.**

The reasons for better outcomes in the management of IOFBs include improved localization of posterior segment IOFBs with computerized tomography, more frequent intravitreal surgery with better vitrectomy techniques, and the use of the intraocular magnet.[66] Other aggressive surgical procedures for traumatic injuries include cataract extraction, posterior chamber intraocular lens (IOL), and complete vitrectomy in a one-stage procedure that has been reported to give reasonable retention of vision with 50% of eyes achieving at least 20/40 vision.[67]

Clostridium spp.

Endophthalmitis resulting from *Clostridium* spp. causes gas gangrene panophthalmitis. This type of endophthalmitis is rare and invariably follows penetrating injury to the globe, often with mud or dirt, frequently in the presence of a metallic IOFB.[35,68–71] This kind of *Clostridium* infection is typical of hammer-, farmyard-, or bomb blast-associated injury. Cases resulting from endogenous spread have also been reported.[70–74] Systemic reactions are frequently associated with the ocular infection and include fever and leukocytosis and less frequently prostration and glycosuria. O'Day et al noted that *Bacillus* species are the only other organisms capable of causing a panophthalmitis associated with fever and leukocytosis.[54]

Duke-Elder summarized the signs and symptoms of gas gangrene panophthalmitis as including a rapid onset and progression to significant ocular disruption and blindness within 24–48 hours after ocular injury.[75] This intraocular infection is associated with significant pain caused in part by a rise in IOP and significant swelling of the eyelids. A coffee-colored discharge is present as the result of the hemolytic action of toxins produced by *Clostridium* spp. on blood along with air bubbles in the anterior chamber. *Bacillus* spp. are also capable of producing intraocular gas. The visual outcome is usually total disruption of the eye, frequently leading to enucleation or evisceration. The infection has not been reported to spread beyond the orbit following either of these surgical procedures.

Clostridium spp. are ubiquitous throughout nature, are found in soil, and are present in the normal intestinal flora of humans. All species are Gram-positive bacilli and obligate anaerobes. *Cl. perfringens (welchii)* is known to produce at least 10 toxins including the destructive exotoxins hyaluronidase and collagenase. Four *Clostridium* spp. (*Cl. perfringens, Cl. novyi, Cl. septicum*, and *Cl. histolyticum*) that cause gas gangrene in man have been identified. With rare exceptions, gas gangrene panophthalmitis has been caused most frequently by *Cl. perfringens*. A single case has been reported caused by *Cl. bifermentans* following trauma[76] and three endogenous cases caused by *Cl. septicum*.[77–79]

Wiles and Ide reported a successful outcome in a case of traumatic *Cl. perfringens* endophthalmitis treated with early lensectomy followed by vitrectomy, which removed both the foci of infection and enterotoxins.[80] After treatment with intravenous and intravitreal antibiotics, this 14–year-old boy recovered 20/40 visual acuity 18 months later. A second report described an individual who underwent vitrectomy and intravitreal injection of antibiotics within 8 hours after injury with a manure-contaminated nail followed by a 10–day course of intravenous antibiotic.[81] Cultures of the vitreous isolated *Cl. perfringens*. After 6 months, the visual acuity was 20/25.

A high degree of suspicion leading to prompt intervention must be maintained in eyes sustaining penetrating injuries with soil-contaminated foreign bodies because of the fulminant nature of an intraocular infection caused by *Clostridium* or *Bacillus* spp. Treatment consists of vitrectomy in conjunction with intravitreal and systemic (intravenous) administration of antibiotics. Penicillin is the drug of choice in *Clostridium* infection,

combined with clindamycin and/or metronidazole, which also are active against it. Vancomycin may be substituted for clindamycin to provide more effective coverage for *Bacillus* spp. infection, which can also occur in this clinical setting. Ceftazidime should also be given intravitreally in case the infection is polymicrobial with Gram-negative bacteria.

Endophthalmitis after conventional retinal detachment surgery

There are several reports of endophthalmitis developing after scleral buckling procedures[82–84] and removal of scleral buckles in the literature.[85] Bacon and associates found that the incidence of endophthalmitis after explant surgery with or without drainage of subretinal fluid was 0.19%.[84] An intraocular component, the external drainage of subretinal fluid and the intraocular injection of gas or air, is now part of conventional retinal surgery. These procedures along with the inadvertent perforation of the sclera during buckle suturing may permit direct entry of organisms into the globe. Scleral perforation is not a prerequisite for the development of endophthalmitis.

Folk et al demonstrated the development of progressive scleral abscesses in 14 eyes in animal studies following use of scleral buckles contaminated with *S. aureus*.[86] Nine of these 14 eyes had vitreous cultures positive for *S. aureus*, demonstrating penetration of the sclera by this organism. Extrapolating these results to humans, the investigators suggested that development of endophthalmitis in the absence of scleral perforation could happen by a similar mechanism.

Endophthalmitis has also been reported following pneumatic retinopexy.[87–89] The causative organism was identified as *S. epidermidis* (a CNS), a normal inhabitant of the external ocular flora which probably entered the eye through the scleral injection site. A culture taken of the gas passed through a Millipore filter excluded contamination of the gas or a defect in the filter as a cause of the endophthalmitis in one case. One of the authors has personal experience of endophthalmitis involving pneumatic retinopexy, which developed due to *Salmonella* sp. Extensive investigation could not find the source.

Endophthalmitis after pars plana vitrectomy

Endophthalmitis is an extremely rare complication after pars plana vitrectomy. The reported incidence of endophthalmitis after vitrectomy has ranged from 0.07% to 0.14%.[90,91]

We are aware of only a total of 32 reported cases in which both visual acuity and culture results were available. Visual results in most eyes were extremely poor. The visual outcome is influenced by the virulence of the offending organism, as highly virulent organisms in a site not readily accessible to antimicrobial treatment can rapidly initiate a devastating inflammatory response. Review of the 32 reported cases of postvitrectomy endophthalmitis reveals that ambulatory vision (5/200) was not retained by an eye infected with any organism other than *S. epidermidis*.

The largest series of patients with postvitrectomy endophthalmitis involved 18 cases.[90] Based on data from four of the medical centers in this series, the incidence of endophthalmitis was 0.07% (9 of 12,216 eyes). Positive intraocular cultures were obtained in all the infected eyes, with the final visual outcome directly related to the pathogenicity of the isolated organisms in patients without mixed infections. Only five patients (28%) in this series retained a final visual acuity of 20/50 or better. These five eyes (71%) were part of a group of seven eyes infected with *S. epidermidis*. The remaining eyes had final visual acuities ranging from hand motion to light perception. Two additional patients in this series, with mixed infections caused by streptococci and *S. epidermidis*, retained final visual acuity of 20/400.

Several risk factors have been identified:

- Diabetes. Despite performing vitrectomy on only 34% of patients with diabetes, Cohen et al found that 61% of patients who developed endophthalmitis were diabetic.[92] This finding is similar to a second report describing four cases of postvitrectomy endophthalmitis; the incidence of endophthalmitis in patients without diabetes was 0.07% versus 0.22% in patients with diabetes.[91]

- Previous intraocular surgery. The scarred and poorly vascularized tissue resulting from previous surgery limits the antimicrobial response to infections. Furthermore, foreign bodies such as exoplants and sutures may act as a nidus for infection and prevent effective phagocytosis of the bacteria.[45]
- The duration and complexity of the procedure. The continuous net outflow of fluid from an eye during vitrectomy normally denies pathogens access to the vitreous cavity during the procedure. In a long or complex procedure, repeated reintroduction of instruments into the eye increases the risk of intraocular microbial contamination. Procedures lasting 2 hours or more may increase the risk of intraocular infection.

The poor visual results in postvitrectomy and endophthalmitis appear to be related to additional factors:[90]

- Many of these eyes already have advanced vitreoretinal disease.
- Patients at the time of surgery may have extremely poor visual acuity, which compromises their ability to recognize a decline in postoperative vision. Therefore, the diagnosis of endophthalmitis may be delayed because the signs and symptoms of endophthalmitis including ocular pain and intraocular inflammation may be masked by surgically induced uveitis and significant vitreous haze caused by residual intravitreal blood.
- Corneal haziness and fibrin formation are not an uncommon finding in vitrectomized eyes, especially when a variety of other intraocular procedures have been performed.

Endophthalmitis after refractive keratotomy

Refractive keratotomy for correction of astigmatism is a commonly performed ophthalmic surgical procedure. The Keratorefractive Society conducted a survey of complications following radial keratotomy and found four cases of endophthalmitis (0.00636%) among the 62,814 cases accumulated.[94]

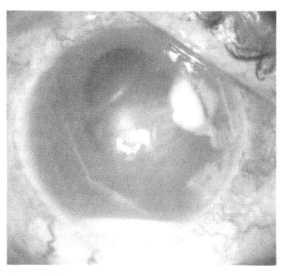

Figure 7.11

Keratitis and endophthalmitis caused by *Staphylococcus aureus* after radial keratotomy.

McLeod et al reported four cases of endophthalmitis following radial and other forms of keratotomy.[93] Microperforations occurred in three of the four eyes, serving as the portal of entry for the pathogen to enter the eye. These three cases were similar to other reported cases of endophthalmitis following radial keratotomy (Figure 7.11).[94–97] The fourth patient in this series, unlike previously reported cases, developed endophthalmitis although no perforation was noted at the time of surgery. Postoperatively, the patient developed severe keratitis of an incision base causing extreme corneal thinning and necrosis. Eventually, corneal perforation occurred. Intraocular cultures demonstrated *Pseudomonas* spp. that were probably introduced into the eye at the time of perforation.

This case caused the investigators to recommend that when keratitis develops in an incision, these eyes must be treated as an impending endophthalmitis. The cornea must be scraped for tissue samples for Gram stain and culture. Topical broad-spectrum antibiotics should be started to increase the likelihood of successfully treating the keratitis and avoid the development of endophthalmitis before the tissue culture results are available. The investigators also suggested initi-

ating therapy with oral ciprofloxacin as an adjunct to topical antimicrobial agents; ciprofloxacin is better replaced today with levofloxacin (Chapter 5). Serial examinations at 12–hour intervals were also recommended in all eyes developing postoperative infectious keratitis following radial keratotomy. Because of the possibility of endophthalmitis developing bilaterally, the investigators also caution against performing simultaneous bilateral radial keratotomy.

Endophthalmitis following penetrating keratoplasty

Endophthalmitis following penetrating keratoplasty (PK) is usually a devastating complication. The rate of bacterial endophthalmitis complicating PK has been reported as 0.1–0.8% in 1991;[98] until 1993, only 45 cases of bacterial endophthalmitis were reported in the literature worldwide.

In the US National Outcomes of Penetrating Keratoplasty study, the 6-month risk of rehospitalization for endophthalmitis following surgery was 0.77%.[98] The likelihood of rehospitalization for endophthalmitis in this study, which used a national database, was greatest immediately postoperatively, but the risk of developing endophthalmitis persisted for many months following keratoplasty. In contrast, a relatively small risk for endophthalmitis developing 1 or more years after surgery has been reported.[99] The investigators suggest that the late rehospitalizations for intraocular infections were either the result of an infection with slow-growing infectious agents such as *Propionibacterium acnes* or suture infection, suture removal, wound dehiscence, and initial misdiagnosis of an infection as sterile when an infectious etiology was involved.

This report demonstrated a lower risk of endophthalmitis in keratoplasty performed in phakic eyes than in pseudophakic and aphakic eyes. Additionally, the risk of rehospitalization for endophthalmitis in the first 6 months postoperatively was increased 1.5 times in eyes in which a vitrectomy was performed at the time of corneal transplantation compared with eyes requiring only PK. These results highlight the importance of maintaining the integrity of the vitreous or the posterior capsule at the time of surgery. The study

Table 7.2 Fungal endophthalmitis following penetrating keratoplasty

Reference	Type of fungus (no. of infected patients)	Source	Age of patient (years)	Place
Merchant et al, 2001[101]	Candida albicans (1)	Contaminated donor eye	Donor 68, patient 58	Karachi, Pakistan
Cameron et al, 1998[102]	Candida glabrata (1)	Endophthalmitis cluster from contaminated donor corneas. Culture of the donor rim recommended. Rim of this case grew Enterococcus faecalis, Klebsiella oxytoca, and C. glabrata. Also had three cases of endophthalmitis after PK due to E. faecalis	46	Riyadh, Saudi Arabia
Kloess et al, 1993[100]	Candida albicans (1)	Mixed infection with streptococci. Cultured from donor rim	82	Atlanta, GA, USA
Cameron et al, 1991[103]	Candida albicans (1) Aspergillus flavus (1)	PK for keratoconus ×2, bullous keratopathy. Found a higher infection rate (1.25%) in donor corneas from Sri Lanka than from the USA (0.14%), with 3 bacterial and 3 fungal cases out of 3000 PK operations	17, 22, 80	Riyadh, Saudi Arabia
Pflugfelder et al, 1988[41]	Fusarium solani (2) Fusarium oxysporum (1)	Keratoplasty – ? source	58, 58, 60	Miami, FL, USA
Insler and Urso, 1987[104]	Candida albicans (2)	Contaminated organ donor – two grafts	78, 66	New Orleans, LA, USA

PK, penetrating keratoplasty.

also determined that the risk of rehospitalization for endophthalmitis after PK was approximately five times greater than for cataract surgery.

Kloess et al reviewed 55 cases of previously reported endophthalmitis postkeratoplasty, noting that 36 eyes had a final visual acuity of counting fingers or less and 17 of the eyes became either phthisical or required removal.[100] A fungal etiology was found to be a rare cause of postkeratoplasty endophthalmitis but is well recognized due to *C. albicans*, *Fusarium* spp., and *Aspergillus* spp. (Table 7.2).[100–104]

In a retrospective review, Kloess et al found four cases of endophthalmitis complicating 1010 consecutive PKs.[100] All eyes in the series had extremely poor visual outcomes; three of the four became phthisical and the remaining eye retained only light perception vision before the patient died. The offending organism was bacterial in three eyes and fungal in the fourth eye.

In this study, donor rim cultures which were taken from 932 eyes demonstrated positive cultures

in 14% of cases. Three of the four eyes developing endophthalmitis demonstrated the same organism on intraocular and donor rim cultures. This finding led the investigators to speculate that the donor rim was the usual source of the offending organism. Furthermore, streptococci accounted for 50–59% of the contamination source.[105] Unfortunately, these organisms are resistant to gentamicin, which is the sole antibiotic present in this storage medium; this situation has required improvement for a long time. Other studies confirmed these findings,[106] although Antonios et al found that the most common organisms isolated were *Propionibacterium* spp. 26%, diphtheroids 24%, *S. epidermidis* 22%, and fungi 9%.[107] A statistically significant increase (p<0.005) was found in the percentage of contaminated donor rims with a preservation time of more than 5 days. The risk of developing endophthalmitis was 12 times greater with a positive donor rim culture.

Speaker et al, utilizing techniques of molecular epidemiology, demonstrated the role of the external ocular flora in the pathogenesis of acute postoperative endophthalmitis.[108] In one case of postkeratoplasty endophthalmitis, the donor rim cultures were negative but the same organism was isolated from the patient's external flora and infected eye. Cameron et al reported four cases of endophthalmitis developing within a 1-week period after PK procedures.[102] All donor corneas were from the same eye bank. The causative organism was cultured from the recipient eye and the corresponding donor rim in all four instances: *Enterococcus faecalis* endophthalmitis in three patients and *Candida (Torulopsis) glabrata* endophthalmitis in one patient (see Table 7.2).[41,101–104] The investigators noted that an acute onset after corneal transplantation may result from the patient's external flora, organisms introduced at the time of surgery from donor tissue, a breakdown in aseptic surgical technique, or contaminated sutures, irrigating solution, or IOLs. Late-onset endophthalmitis may result from wound dehiscence, migration of infection from a suture abscess or corneal ulcer, infection with lens virulent organisms, or endogenous spread of bacteria from a transient source or an established infection.

Donor material must be collected in the most sterile manner possible; ideally donor corneas should not cross national boundaries but should be used locally. The method used to collect and store the donor eye influences the bacterial contamination rate. Ideally, the donor eye should always be cultured the day before PK surgery is performed to avoid serious contamination with pathogens such as *Ps. aeruginosa*, which can cause a fulminating endophthalmitis postPK in both recipients from one contaminated donor. In addition, fungi and streptococci, which are resistant to gentamicin in the storage medium, can contaminate the donor material and cause endophthalmitis. Cameron et al have recorded two episodes of increased rates of endophthalmitis following PK with donor material from one US eye bank and one Sri Lankan eye bank.[102,103] In the former case, after PK, four patients developed endophthalmitis, with *E. faecalis* in three and *C. glabrata* in one patient; this outbreak stopped when another US source of donor material was obtained.[102] In the latter case, a postoperative endophthalmitis rate of 1.25% occurred with donor material from a Sri Lankan eye bank, compared with a rate of 0.14% in those patients receiving US eye bank tissue.[103] Another report that involved export of donor eyes for PK from Sri Lanka to Hong Kong described endophthalmitis following this procedure caused by *Proteus* sp. which required triple surgery to recover useful vision.[109] *Citrobacter diversus*, another Gram-negative rod, has been reported as a cause of endophthalmitis postPK.[110]

Endophthalmitis following keratoprosthesis

Nouri et al reported 13 cases of bacterial endophthalmitis in 108 eyes after placement of a keratoprosthesis.[111] These cases occurred 2–46 months postoperatively. The preoperative diagnosis was found to be the most important risk factor predisposing eyes to develop endophthalmitis. In Stevens–Johnson syndrome and ocular cicatricial pemphigoid, the incidences of endophthalmitis were 39% and 19%, respectively, compared with 7% in ocular burn cases. The offending organisms in all cases were either streptococci or staphylococci. Visual results were poor; 9 of 10 eyes infected with either streptococci or *S. aureus* lost all vision. The two eyes infected with *S. epidermidis* and an additional eye infected with *Strep. mitis* retained some useful vision when treatment was initiated within 6 hours of the onset of symptoms.

Endophthalmitis complicating secondary lens implantation

A series reporting the incidence of hospital-linked endophthalmitis demonstrated that the incidence of endophthalmitis was approximately four times greater after secondary IOL implantation (0.30%) compared with extracapsular cataract extraction with or without IOL implantation (0.072%).[99] A case-control study of endophthalmitis after secondary lens implantation demonstrated that patients with diabetes were also more likely to develop endophthalmitis.[112] Compared with the four case controls with posterior lenses fixated in the ciliary sulcus, the three posterior chamber lenses in patients developing endophthalmitis were fixated with transscleral sutures. The suture tracts afforded an intraocular path of entry for bacteria. Eyelid abnormalities were also present preoperatively in 50% of patients developing endophthalmitis compared with 2.9% of control patients. The external eye is the likely source of the majority of intraocular pathogens. Eyelid abnormalities may predispose to heavier colonization of the external ocular surface, creating more favorable conditions for the development of endophthalmitis. In addition, the lids of atopic individuals have a higher colonization rate (up to 70%) with *S. aureus* compared with only 10% in the nonatope.[113]

Wound defect has been reported as a factor predisposing to the development of endophthalmitis. Significantly, 50% of cases had wound abnormalities compared with 2.9% of control eyes. Additionally, case subjects were more likely than controls to have had an IOL inserted through a superior incision rather than a temporal incision. A superior incision involves reopening the old cataract wound, which in many instances may affect wound closure, resulting in wound defects.

Ninety percent of infected eyes had positive cultures with *S. epidermidis* isolated in 50% of cases. *S. epidermidis* is also the most commonly isolated organism in endophthalmitis following other intraocular surgery.[4] Ninety percent of eyes achieved a visual acuity of 20/100 or better; 60% of eyes demonstrated vision of 20/60 or better.

All infected individuals presented with decreased visual acuity and marked anterior chamber inflammation. Conjunctival injection was present in 90% of eyes. Mild ocular discomfort or tenderness was present in 50% of eyes; however, moderate or severe ocular pain was noted in only 20% of eyes. Corneal edema or hypopyon was present in 50% and 40% of eyes, respectively.[99]

Endophthalmitis following strabismus surgery

Endophthalmitis following pediatric strabismus surgery is extremely rare. Recchia et al reported a retrospective study of six cases over a 15-year period at two institutions.[114] The offending organisms identified by vitreous cultures were *Strep. pneumoniae, S. aureus,* and *H. influenzae.* At a median interval of 3 days postoperatively, children presented with the systemic findings of lethargy and asymmetric eye redness, with or without swelling or fever. Only two of the six

children were old enough to verbalize complaints of pain or visual loss. Examination revealed a blunting of the red reflex compared with the uninvolved eye; three of six eyes had hypopyon. Children were often taken to the pediatrician rather than an ophthalmologist. The endophthalmitis was uniformly severe in all cases, with eyes either being enucleated or becoming phthisical. These poor results occurred despite treatment in all cases including pars plana vitrectomy and intravitreal antibiotic injections.

Two eyes on histopathological examination failed to reveal global perforation by scleral sutures, which is one mechanism postulated to cause endophthalmitis. The authors speculated that a scleral abscess may develop in thin sclera, resulting in endophthalmitis through contiguous spread. Alternatively, sepsis may have developed with seeding of organisms to the eye.

Endophthalmitis following pterygium surgery

Endophthalmitis following pterygium surgery has been described as the result of the fungus *Scedosporium prolificans.*[115] Scleral necrosis occurred after the surgery when the infection began. *Scedosporium* is resistant to amphotericin, requiring treatment with imidazoles (Chapter 11), but often requires a combination of surgical debridement and imidazole drugs to bring the infection under control.

References

1. Ciulla TA, Beck AD, Topping TM et al. Blebitis, early endophthalmitis, and late endophthalmitis after glaucoma-filtering surgery, *Ophthalmology* (1997) **104**:986–95.

2. Mandelbaum S, Forster RK. Endophthalmitis associated with filtering blebs, *Int Ophthalmol Clin* (1987) **27**:107–11.

3. Greenfield DS, Suner IJ, Miller MP et al. Endophthalmitis after filtering surgery with mitomycin, *Arch Ophthalmol* (1996) **114**:943–9.

4. Waheed S, Ritterband DC, Greenfield DS et al. New patterns of infecting organisms in late bleb-related endophthalmitis: a ten year review, *Eye* (1998) **12**:910–15.

5. Waheed S, Ritterband DC, Greenfield DS et al. Bleb-related ocular infection in children after trabeculectomy with mitomycin C, *Ophthalmology* (1997) **104**: 2117–20.

6. Higginbotham EJ, Stevens RK, Musch DC et al. Bleb-related endophthalmitis after trabeculectomy with mitomycin C, *Ophthalmology* (1996) **103**: 650–6.

7. Lehmann OJ, Bunce C, Matheson MM et al. Risk factors for development of post-trabeculectomy endophthalmitis, *Br J Ophthalmol* (2000) **84**: 1349–53.

8. Beck AD, Grossniklaus HE, Hubbard B et al. Pathologic findings in late endophthalmitis after glaucoma filtering surgery, *Ophthalmology* (2000) **107**:2111–14.

9. Ayyala RS, Bellows AR, Thomas JV et al. Bleb infections: clinically different courses of 'blebitis' and endophthalmitis, *J Ophthalmic Nurs Technol* (1997) **16**:292–300.

10. Brown RH, Yang LH, Stanley DW et al. Treatment of bleb infection after glaucoma surgery, *Arch Ophthalmol* (1994) **112**:57–61.

11. Seal DV. New patterns of infecting organisms in late bleb-related endophthalmitis, *Eye* (1998) **12**:903–4.

12. Mandelbaum S, Forster RK, Gelender H et al. Late onset endophthalmitis associated with filtering blebs, *Ophthalmology* (1985) **92**:964–72.

13. Phillips WB II, Wong TP, Bergren RL et al. Late onset endophthalmitis associated with filtering blebs, *Ophthalmic Surg* (1994) **25**:88–91.

14. Kangas TA, Greenfield DS, Flynn HW Jr et al. Delayed-onset endophthalmitis associated with conjunctival filtering bleb, *Ophthalmology* (1997) **104**:745–52.

15. Kresloff MS, Castellarin AA, Zarbin MA. Endophthalmitis, *Surv Ophthalmol* (1998) **43**: 193–224.

16. Shrader SK, Band JD, Lauter CB et al. The clinical spectrum of endophthalmitis: incidence, predisposing factors, and features influencing outcome, *J Infect Dis* (1990) **162**:115–20.

17. Forster RK. Endophthalmitis. In: Duane TD, ed. *Clinical Ophthalmology*, vol 4 (Harper & Row: New York, 1985) 1–29.

18. Fisch A, Salvanet A, Prazuck T et al. Epidemiology of infective endophthalmitis in France, *Lancet* (1991) **338**:1373–6.

19. Rowsey JJ, Newsom DL, Sexton DJ et al. Endophthalmitis: current approaches, *Ophthalmology* (1982) **89**:1055–66.

20. Duch-Samper AM, Menezo JL, Hurtado-Sarrio M. Endophthalmitis following penetrating eye injuries, *Acta Ophthalmol Scand* (1997) **75**:104–6.

21. Affeldt JC, Flynn HW Jr, Forster RK et al. Microbial endophthalmitis resulting from ocular trauma, *Ophthalmology* (1987) **94**:407–13.

22. Seal DV, Kirkness CM. Criteria for intravitreal antibiotics during surgical removal of intraocular foreign bodies, *Eye* (1992) **6**:465–8.

23. Ferrer C, Montero J, Alió J et al. Rapid molecular diagnosis of posttraumatic keratitis and endophthalmitis caused by *Alternaria infectoria*, *J Clin Microbiol* (2003) **41**: 3358–60.

24. Lieb DF, Smiddy WE, Miller D et al. Case report: fungal endophthalmitis caused by *Phialophora richardsiae*, *Retina* (2003) **23**:406–7.

25. Domniz Y, Lawless M, Sutton GL et al. Successful treatment of *Paecilomyces lilacinus* endophthalmitis after foreign body trauma to the cornea, *Cornea* (2001) **20**:109–11.

26. Scott IU, Flynn HW Jr, Miller D et al. Exogenous endophthalmitis caused by amphotericin B-resistant *Paecilomyces lilacinus*: treatment options and visual outcomes, *Arch Ophthalmol* (2001) **119**: 916–19.

27. Pintor E, Martin M, Garcia P et al. Endophthalmitis due to *Paecilomyces lilacinus* after non-surgical penetrating trauma, *Enferm Infec Microbiol Clin* (2001) **19**:347–8.

28. Kunimoto DY, Das T, Sharma S et al. Microbiologic spectrum and susceptibility of isolates: Part II. Posttraumatic endophthalmitis, *Am J Ophthalmol* (1999) **128**:242–4.

29. Houtmann I, Bacin F, Amara-Allieu S et al. A case of post-traumatic *Absidia corymbifera* fungal endophthalmitis, *J Fr Opthalmol* (1998) **21**:764–8.

30. Gariano RF, Kalina RE. Posttraumatic fungal endophthalmitis resulting from *Scopulariopsis brevicaulis*, *Retina* (1997) **17**:256–8.

31. Carney MD, Tabassian A, Guerry RK. *Pseudo-Allescheria boydii* endophthalmitis, *Retina* (1996) **16**:263–4.

32. Thompson WS, Rubsamen PE, Flynn HW Jr et al. Endophthalmitis after penetrating trauma. Risk factors and visual acuity outcomes, *Ophthalmology* (1995) **102**:1696–701.

33. Alfaro DV, Roth DB, Laughlin RM et al. Paediatric post-traumatic endophthalmitis, *Br J Ophthalmol* (1995) **79**:888–91.

34. Das T, Gopinathan U, Sharma S. Exogenous *Helminthosporium* endophthalmitis, *Br J Ophthalmol* (1994) **78**:492–3.

35. Alfaro DV, Roth DB, Liggett PE. Posttraumatic endophthalmitis. Causative organisms, treatment, and prevention, *Retina* (1994) **14**:206–22.

36. Al-Rajhi AA, Awad AH, Al-Hedaithy SSA et al. *Scytalidium dimidiatum* fungal endophthalmitis, *Br J Ophthalmol* (1993) **77**: 388–90.

37. Srdic N, Radulovic S, Nonkovic Z et al. Two cases of exogenous endophthalmitis due to *Fusarium moniliforme* and *Pseudomonas* species as associated aetiological agents, *Mycoses* (1993) **36**: 441–4.

38. D'Mellow G, Hirst LW, Whitby M et al. Intralenticular infections, *Ophthalmology* (1991) **98**:1376–8.

39. Witherspoon CD, Kuhn F, Owens SD et al. Endophthalmitis due to *Sporothrix schenckii* after penetrating ocular injury, *Ann Ophthalmol* (1990) **22**:385–8.

40. Boldt HC, Pulido JS, Blodi CF et al. Rural endophthalmitis, *Ophthalmology* (1989) **96**:1722–6.

41. Pflugfelder SC, Flynn HW Jr, Zwickey WW et al. Exogenous fungal endophthalmitis, *Ophthalmology* (1988) **95**:19–30.

42. Brinton GS, Topping TM, Hyndiuk RA et al. Posttraumatic endophthalmitis, *Arch Ophthalmol* (1984) **102**:547–50.

43. Eschete ML, King JW, West BC et al. *Penicillium chrysogenum* endophthalmitis, *Mycopathologica* (1981) **74**:125–7.

44. Peyman GA, Raichand M, Bennett TO. Management of endophthalmitis with pars plana vitrectomy, *Br J Ophthalmol* (1980) **64**:472–5.

45. Forster RK, Abbott RL, Gelender H. Management of infectious endophthalmitis, *Ophthalmology* (1980) **87**:313–19.

46. Savir H, Henig E, Lehrer N. Exogenous mycotic infections of the eye and adnexa, *Ann Ophthalmol* (1978) **10**:1013–18.

47. Rodrigues MM, MacLeod D. Exogenous fungal endophthalmitis caused by *Paecilomyces*, *Am J Ophthalmol* (1975) **79**:687–90.

48. Pach JM. Traumatic *Haemophilus influenzae* endophthalmitis, *Am J Ophthalmol* (1988) **106**:497–8.

49. Reynolds DS, Flynn HW Jr. Endophthalmitis after penetrating ocular trauma, *Curr Opin Ophthalmol* (1997) **8**:32–8.

50. Mieler WF, Ellis MK, Williams DF et al. Retained intraocular foreign bodies and endophthalmitis, *Ophthalmology* (1990) **97**:1532–8.

51. Aaberg TM Jr, Sternberg P. Trauma: principles and techniques of treatment. In: Ryan SJ, ed. *Retina*. Vol 3. (Mosby Year Book, St Louis: 2001) 2400–26.

52. Thompson JT, Parver LM, Enger CL et al. Infectious endophthalmitis after penetrating injuries with retained intraocular foreign bodies. National Eye Trauma System, *Ophthalmology* (1993) **100**: 1468–74.

53. Doi M, Ikeda T, Yasuhara T et al. A case of bacterial endophthalmitis following perforating injury caused by a cat claw, *Ophthalmic Surg Lasers* (1999) **30**:315–16.

54. O'Day DM, Smith RS, Gregg CR et al. The problem of *Bacillus* species infection with special emphasis on the virulence of *Bacillus cereus*, *Ophthalmology* (1981) **88**:833–8.

55. Van Bijsterveld OP, Richards RD. Bacillus infections of the cornea, *Arch Ophthalmol* (1965) **74**:91–5.

56. Mittra RA, Mieler WF. Controversies in the manage-

57. Parrish CM, O'Day DM. Traumatic endophthalmitis, *Int Ophthalmol Clin* (1987) **27**:112–19.

58. Foster RE, Martinez JA, Murray TG et al. Useful visual outcomes after treatment of *Bacillus cereus* endophthalmitis, *Ophthalmology* (1996) **103**: 390–7.

59. Barletta JP, Small KW. Successful visual recovery in delayed onset *Bacillus cereus* endophthalmitis, *Ophthalmic Surg Lasers* (1996) **27**:70–2.

60. Beer PM, Ludwig IH, Packer AJ. Complete visual recovery after *Bacillus cereus* endophthalmitis in a child, *Am J Ophthalmol* (1990) **110**:212–13.

61. Hemady R, Zaltas M, Paton B et al. *Bacillus*-induced endophthalmitis: new series of 10 cases and review of the literature, *Br J Ophthalmol* (1990) **74**:26–9. [Erratum appears in *Br J Ophthalmol* (1991) **75**:255.]

62. Kervick GN, Flynn HW Jr, Alfonso E et al. Antibiotic therapy for *Bacillus* species infections, *Am J Ophthalmol* (1990) **110**:683–7.

63. Weber DJ, Saviteer SM, Rutala WA et al. In vitro susceptibility of *Bacillus* spp. to selected antimicrobial agents, *Antimicrob Agents Chemother* (1988) **32**:642–5.

64. Alfaro DV III, Hudson SJ, Steele JJ et al. Experimental posttraumatic *Bacillus cereus* endophthalmitis in a swine model. Efficacy of intravitreal ciprofloxacin, vancomycin, and imipenem, *Retina* (1996) **16**:317–23.

65. Alfaro DV, Davis J, Kim SL et al. Experimental *Bacillus cereus* post-traumatic endophthalmitis and treatment with ciprofloxacin, *Br J Ophthalmol* (1996) **80**:755–8.

66. De Souza S, Howcroft MJ. Management of posterior segment intraocular foreign bodies: 14 years' experience, *Can J Ophthalmol* (1999) **34**:23–9.

67. Soheilian M, Ahmadieh H, Afghan MH et al. Posterior segment triple surgery after traumatic eye injuries, *Ophthalmic Surg* (1995) **26**:338–42.

68. Walsh TJ. Clostridial ocular infections – case report of gas gangrene panophthalmitis, *Br J Ophthalmol* (1965) **49**:472–7.

69. Levitt JM, Stam J. *Clostridium perfringens* panophthalmitis, *Arch Ophthalmol* (1970) **84**:227–8.

70. Obertynski H, Dyson C. *Clostridium perfringens* panophthalmitis, *Can J Ophthalmol* (1974) **9**:258–9.

71. Crock GW, Heriot WJ, Janakiraman P et al. Gas gangrene infection of the eyes and orbits, *Br J Ophthalmol* (1985) **69**:143–8.

72. La Cour M, Norgaard A, Prouse JU et al. Gas gangrene panophthalmitis: a case from Greenland, *Acta Ophthalmol* (1994) **72**:524–8.

73. Frantz JF, Lemp MA, Font RL et al. Acute endogenous panophthalmitis caused by *Clostridium perfringens*, *Am J Ophthalmol* (1974) **78**:295–303.

74. Leavelle RB. Gas gangrene panophthalmitis, *Arch Ophthalmol* (1955) **53**:634–2.

75. Duke-Elder S. Mechanical injuries, *System of Ophthalmology*, vol XIV, part 1 (Henry Kimpton: London, 1972) 405–7.

76. Rehany U, Dorenboim Y, Fefler E et al. *Clostridium bifermentans* panophthalmitis after penetrating eye injury, *Ophthalmology* (1994) **101**: 839–42.

77. Insler MS, Karcioglu ZA, Naugle T Jr. *Clostridium septicum* panophthalmitis with systemic complications, *Br J Ophthalmol* (1985) **69**:774–7.

78. Green MT, Font RL, Campbell JV et al. Endogenous *Clostridium* panophthalmitis, *Ophthalmology* (1987) **94**:435–8.

79. Cannistra AJ, Albert DM, Frambach DA et al. Sudden visual loss associated with clostridial bacteremia, *Br J Ophthalmol* (1988) **72**:380–5.

80. Wiles SB, Ide CH. *Clostridium perfringens* endophthalmitis, *Am J Ophthalmol* (1991) **111**:654–6.

81. Kelly LD, Steahly SP. Successful prophylaxis of *Clostridium perfringens* endophthalmitis, *Arch Ophthalmol* (1991) **109**:1199.

82. McMeel JW, Naegele DF, Pollalis S et al. Acute and subacute infections following scleral buckling operations, *Ophthalmology* (1978) **85**:341–9.

83. Ho PC, McMeel JW. Bacterial endophthalmitis after retinal surgery, *Retina* (1983) **3**:99–102.

84. Bacon AS, Davison CR, Patel BC et al. Infective endophthalmitis following vitreoretinal surgery, *Eye* (1993) **7**:529–34.

85. Hugkulstone CE, Rubasingham AS. Endophthalmitis after removal of an encircling bond, *Br J Ophthalmol* (1991) **75**:178.

86. Folk JC, Cutkomp J, Koontz FP. Bacterial scleral abscesses after retinal buckling operations. Pathogenesis, management, and laboratory investigations, *Ophthalmology* (1987) **94**:1148–54.

87. Hilton GF, Tornambe PE. The Retinal Detachment Study Group. Pneumatic retinopexy. An analysis of intraoperative and postoperative complications, *Retina* (1991) **11**:285–94.

88. Eckardt C. *Staphylococcus epidermidis* endophthalmitis after pneumatic retinopexy, *Am J Ophthalmol* (1987) **103**:720–1.

89. Tornambe PE, Hilton GF. Retinal Detachment Study Group. Pneumatic retinopexy: a multicenter randomized controlled clinical trial comparing pneumatic retinopexy with scleral buckling, *Ophthalmology* (1989) **96**:772–84.

90. Cohen SM, Flynn HW Jr, Murray TG et al. Endophthalmitis after pars plana vitrectomy, *Ophthalmology* (1995) **102**:705–12.

91. Ho PC, Tolentino FI. Bacterial endophthalmitis after closed vitrectomy, *Arch Ophthalmol* (1984) **102**:207–10.

92. Marmer RH. Radial keratotomy complications, *Ann Ophthalmol* (1987) **19**:409–11.

93. McLeod SD, Flowers CW, Lopez PF et al. Endophthalmitis and orbital cellulitis after radial keratotomy, *Ophthalmology* (1995) **102**:1902–7.

94. Manka RL, Gast TJ. Endophthalmitis following Ruiz procedure. Case report, *Arch Ophthalmol* (1990) **108**:21.

95. Barak MH, Shapiro MB. Bacterial endophthalmitis following postkeratoplasty relaxing incisions, *Refract Corneal Surg* (1990) **6**:271–2.

96. O'Day DM, Feman SS, Elliott JH. Visual impairment following radial keratotomy: a cluster of cases, *Ophthalmology* (1986) **93**:319–26.

97. Rosecan LR. Endophthalmitis and cystoid macular edema after astigmatic keratotomy, *Ophthalmic Surg* (1994) **25**:481–2.

98. Aiello LP, Javitt JC, Canner JK. National outcomes of penetrating keratoplasty. Risks of endophthalmitis and retinal detachment, *Arch Ophthalmol* (1993) **111**:509–13.

99. Kattan HM, Flynn HW Jr, Pflugfelder SC et al. Nosocomial endophthalmitis survey. Current incidence of infection after intraocular surgery, *Ophthalmology* (1991) **98**:227–38.

100. Kloess PM, Stulting RD, Waring GO III et al. Bacterial and fungal endophthalmitis after penetrating keratoplasty, *Am J Ophthalmol* (1993) **115**:309–16. [Erratum appears in *Am J Ophthalmol* (1993) **115**:548.]

101. Merchant A, Zacks CM, Wilhelmus K et al. Candidal endophthalmitis after keratoplasty, *Cornea* (2001) **20**:226–9.

102. Cameron JA, Badr IA, Risco JM et al. Endophthalmitis cluster from contaminated donor corneas following penetrating keratoplasty, *Can J Ophthalmol* (1998) **33**:8–13.

103. Cameron JA, Antonios SR, Cotter JB et al. Endophthalmitis from contaminated donor corneas following penetrating keratoplasty, *Arch Ophthalmol* (1991) **109**:54–9.

104. Insler MS, Urso LF. *Candida albicans* endophthalmitis after penetrating keratoplasty, *Am J Ophthalmol* (1987) **104**:57–60.

105. Matoba A, Moore MB, Merten JL et al. Donor-to-host transmission of streptococcal infection by corneas stored in McCarey-Kaufman medium, *Cornea* (1984) **3**:105–8.

106. Lindquist TD, Weber K, Spika J et al. Gentamicin-resistant streptococcal endophthalmitis after keratoplasty, *Cornea* (1990) **9**:88–9.

107. Antonios SR, Cameron JA, Badr IA et al. Contamination of donor cornea. Post-penetrating keratoplasty endophthalmitis, *Cornea* (1991) **10**:217–20.

108. Speaker MG, Milch FA, Shah MK et al. Role of external bacterial flora in the pathogenesis of acute postoperative endophthalmitis, *Ophthalmology* (1991) **98**:639–50.

109. Lam DS, Kwok AK, Chew S. Post-keratoplasty endophthalmitis caused by *Proteus mirabilis*, *Eye* (1998) **12**:139–40.

110. Insler MS, Kook MS, Mani H et al. *Citrobacter diversus* endophthalmitis following penetrating keratoplasty, *Am J Ophthalmol* (1988) **106**:632–3.

111. Nouri M, Terada H, Alfonso EC et al. Endophthalmitis after keratoprosthesis: incidence, bacterial causes, and risk factors, *Arch Ophthalmol* (2001) **119**:484–9.

112. Scott IU, Flynn HW Jr, Feuer W. Endophthalmitis after secondary intraocular lens implantation. A case-report study, *Ophthalmology* (1995) **102**: 1925–31.

113. Tuft SJ, Ramakrishnan M, Seal DV et al. Role of *Staphylococcus aureus* in chronic allergic conjunctivitis, *Ophthalmology* (1992) **99**:180–4.

114. Recchia FM, Baumal CR, Sivalingam A et al. Endophthalmitis after pediatric strabismus surgery, *Arch Ophthalmol* (2000) **118**:939–44.

115. Sullivan LJ, Snibson G, Joseph C et al. *Scedosporium prolificans* sclerokeratitis, *Aust NZ J Ophthalmol* (1994) **22**:207–9.

8

Management and treatment of endophthalmitis

Clinical descriptions and pictures of exogenous and endogenous endophthalmitis are given in Chapters 6, 7, 9 and 10.

How to perform the anterior chamber tap

The anterior chamber tap is similar to a paracentesis and is done after the eye surface has been cultured.

1. A topical anesthetic agent should be placed onto the cornea and into the conjunctival cul de sac.
2. The eye surface should be sterilized with 5% povidone-iodine *after* surface cultures have been taken; 10% povidone-iodine can be diluted with balanced salt solution to make a 5% dilution.
3. The eye is stabilized with a cotton-tipped applicator or forceps.
4. The sample is taken with a 27- or 30-gauge needle attached to a tuberculin syringe.
5. The needle should be placed into the anterior chamber from the limbus and kept over the iris to avoid lens trauma (Figure 8.1).
6. A sample of approximately 0.2 ml should be taken (if possible).
7. The disturbance of any hypopyon should be avoided to retain a view of the posterior pole (if possible) for visualization of the needle tip when injecting antibiotics or performing a vitrectomy.
8. A vitreous tap is obtained (see below); then the appropriate antibiotics are injected.

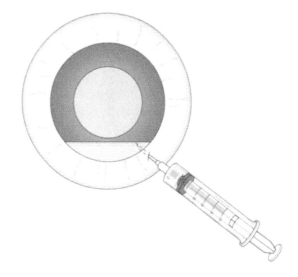

Figure 8.1

Performance of an anterior chamber tap for diagnostic purposes. This diagram depicts an eye with acute postoperative endophthalmitis. There is a layered hypopyon inferiorly. Prior to performing a diagnostic tap, the eye is cleansed with a dilute solution of povidone-iodine (5%). A paracentesis is performed with a 25- or 30-gauge needle on a tuberculin syringe. Care must be taken to avoid disturbing the hypopyon and the needle should be kept over the iris at all times to avoid touching the lens. A small amount of the aqueous (0.1–0.2 ml) should be aspirated into the sterile syringe. This can be used for Gram stain, culture, or polymerase chain reaction (Chapter 3).

How to perform the vitreous tap

1. The eye should remain anesthetized following the anterior chamber tap and will be slightly soft following the procedure.
2. The sample should be obtained with a 25-gauge needle attached to a tuberculin syringe.

3. The eye is stabilized with a cotton-tipped applicator or forceps.
4. The needle should be positioned perpendicular to the eye wall (Figure 8.2).
5. The eye is entered 3.5–4.0 mm from the limbus, depending on lens status. This distance can be approximated using the width of the hub of a sterile tuberculin syringe which can be placed on the sclera to make a mark.
6. The needle should be visualized in the pupil before aspiration of the sample begins.
7. The largest amount of vitreous that easily enters the syringe (0.2 ml) without undue pressure should be aspirated. The needle is withdrawn.
8. A vitreous sample sometimes cannot be retrieved through a 25-gauge needle; a small sclerotomy with a Ziegler knife may be required to allow a 23-gauge needle access. If this second attempt fails, a vitrector may be needed. The vitrector is placed into a sclerotomy site and the sample is aspirated into a 3–5-ml syringe attached to the aspiration port of the vitrector (Figures 8.3 and 8.4). An assistant provides gentle aspiration while the surgeon visualizes the cutter in the pupil (see section on Vitrectomy on page 166).

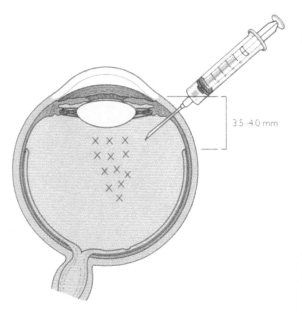

3.5–4.0 mm

Figure 8.2

Performance of a vitreous tap for diagnostic purposes with a needle and syringe. This diagram depicts an eye with endophthalmitis from which the vitreous sample is needed. The samples are obtained with a 25- or 23-gauge needle attached to a tuberculin (TB) syringe. The eye is entered 3.5–4.0 mm from the limbus. This distance can be measured with the barrel of a TB syringe. The inner diameter of the barrel measures approximately 4.0 mm. The barrel can be laid on the sclera to give the distance from the limbus. The needle should be placed perpendicular to the sclera and the tip of the needle should be visualized in the pupil if possible, before obtaining any sample. The sample is aspirated slowly and in a controled manner. It is important to obtain a sufficient volume for investigational studies (at least 0.1–0.2 ml). If a sufficient sample cannot be obtained with this instrument, it may be necessary to use a Ziegler knife (to make a larger sclerotomy) and a vitrectomy instrument (to get a sufficient amount of vitreous). We prefer to use a separate syringe for injection of antibiotics, so the original needle used to obtain the sample should be withdrawn and a new needle with a TB syringe and antimicrobials attached should be inserted at the appropriate distance from the limbus. The needle should be visualized in the pupil, if possible, and the bevel of the needle should be pointed toward the cornea. It is important to inject slowly to avoid a jet stream of drug shooting toward the retina.

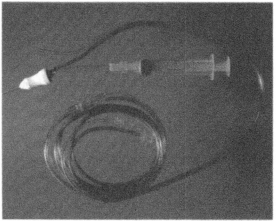

Figure 8.3

Performance of a vitreous tap for diagnostic purposes with a vitrector. This diagram shows a photograph of a vitrectomy instrument from which the aspiration tubing has been removed. It has been replaced with a short piece of sterile tubing attached to a 6 ml syringe. As the vitrectomy instrument cuts the vitreous, the sample is aspirated gently into the syringe. If a large sample is desired, the volume in the vitreous cavity can be replaced with sterile air. It is important not to dilute the sample with sterile saline. After the sample is obtained, the original aspiration tubing is replaced on the hub of the vitrector, which can be used to complete the vitrectomy if needed. We prefer to use a separate syringe.

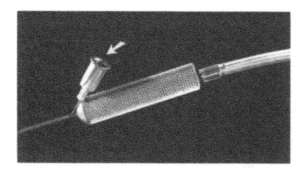

Figure 8.4

Performance of a vitreous tap for diagnostic purposes with a Microvit vitrector. A 25-gauge vitrector, which was developed for vitreous sampling, is shown (available from Becton-Dickson). There is a convenient aspiration port to which a syringe may be attached (arrow). This Microvit allows safe cutting and aspiration of vitreous through a small gauge incision. This instrument can be used in the operating room or outpatient setting. It is important to replace the aspirated volume in the vitreous cavity with sterile air through a separate infusion site (using a 25-gauge butterfly needle attached to a syringe with a filter). This prevents dilution of the sample and maintains the globe.

Box 8.1 Intravitreal drug preparation for the USA*

A. Gentamicin 100 μg in 0.1 ml NaCl for injection USP
1. One vial is filled with gentamicin 80 mg/2 ml
2. Withdraw 0.25 ml in syringe 1 (10 mg)
3. Empty contents of syringe 1 into a second 10-ml syringe and add 9.75 ml of 0.9% NaCl for injection (preservative-free) to make up 10 ml solution (1 mg/1 ml)
4. Withdraw 0.1 ml from syringe 2 into TB syringe. This will contain 100 μg/0.1 ml of gentamicin.

B. Amikacin 200 μg in 0.1 ml NaCl for injection USP
1. One vial is filled with amikacin 100 mg/2 ml
2. Withdraw 0.4 ml into TB syringe 1 which will contain 20 mg of amikacin
3. Empty contents of syringe 1 into a second 10-ml syringe and add 9.6 ml of 0.9% NaCl for injection (preservative-free) to make up 10 ml solution (2 mg/ml)
4. Withdraw 0.1 ml from syringe 2 into TB syringe. This will contain 200 μg/0.1 ml of amikacin.

C. Vancomycin 1 mg in 0.1 ml NaCl for injection USP
1. One vial of vancomycin powder, 500 mg, is diluted with 10 ml 0.9% NaCl for injection USP (preservative-free) (50 mg/ml)
2. Withdraw 1 ml into syringe 1 (50 mg/ml)
3. Empty contents of syringe 1 into a second syringe and add 4 ml of 0.9% NaCl for injection (preservative-free) to make up 5 ml solution (10 mg/ml)
4. Withdraw 0.1 ml from syringe 2 into TB syringe. This will contain 1 mg of vancomycin.

D. Clindamycin 450 μg in 0.1 ml NaCl for injection USP
1. Clindamycin is available in vials containing 150 mg/ml
2. Withdraw 0.3 ml into syringe 1
3. Empty contents of syringe 1 into a second 10-ml syringe and add 9.7 ml of 0.9% NaCl for injection (preservative-free) to make up 10 ml solution (4.5 mg/ml)
4. Withdraw 0.1 ml from syringe 2 into TB syringe which will contain 450 μg of clindamycin.

E. Ceftazidime 1 mg in 0.1 ml NaCl for injection USP
1. One vial of ceftazidime powder, 500 mg, is diluted with 10 ml 0.9% NaCl for injection USP (preservative-free) (50 mg/ml)
2. Withdraw 1 ml into syringe 1 (50 mg/ml)
3. Empty contents of syringe 1 into a second syringe and add 4 ml of 0.9% NaCl for injection (preservative-free) to make up 5 ml solution (10 mg/ml)
4. Withdraw 0.1 ml from syringe 2 into TB syringe which will contain 1 mg of ceftazidime.

F. Dexamethasone 400 μg
Withdraw 0.1 ml in a TB syringe from a vial of dexamethasone containing 4 mg/1 ml and inject intravitreally.

G. Amphotericin B 5 μg in 0.1 ml sterile water
1. One vial of amphotericin B containing 50 mg is diluted with 10 ml sterile water for injection USP (preservative-free) (5 mg/ml)
2. Withdraw 0.1 ml (500 μg) in a TB syringe
3. Add contents of TB syringe to a syringe containing 9.9 ml of sterile water for injection USP (50 μg/ml)
4. Withdraw 0.1 ml in a TB syringe which will contain 5 μg of amphotericin B and inject intravitreally.

*Not for use in the UK; see Chapter 6.

9. Reattachment of a syringe with antibiotics to the original vitreous biopsy needle should not be attempted because of the difficulty in stabilizing an unsecured needle in the eye and the risk of trauma to the retina. A safer method is to simply withdraw the biopsy needle and re-enter the eye with the new needle attached to the antibiotic syringe to deliver intravitreal therapy.

10. Injection of intravitreal antimicrobial treatment immediately follows the vitreous tap with the bevel of the needle toward the anterior segment. The medication is injected slowly to prevent a jet stream of drug squirting toward the retina.

Guidelines for intravitreal injection of antimicrobial therapy (Box 8.1)[1,2]

- The drugs injected should be given in the smallest volume possible, usually 0.1 ml, and each given in a separate syringe.
- Dexamethasone and vancomycin cannot be placed in the same syringe because they will precipitate. This also applies to vancomycin and other antibiotics.
- Aminoglycosides and dexamethasone may be used in the same syringe, but it is not good practice to mix antibiotics or drugs in one syringe as compatibility is unknown.
- The eye should remain anesthetized following the anterior chamber and vitreous tap(s) but remain slightly soft after the tap(s). If the patient is anxious or uncooperative, peribulbar anesthesia with 2% lidocaine without epinephrine should be considered prior to tapping. It is not advisable to attempt a retrobulbar injection once the eye is softened by the withdrawal of aqueous and vitreous. General anesthesia is preferred for children and patients with open ocular wounds.

Adjunctive topical therapy

Topical antimicrobial treatment should begin immediately after the injection of the intravitreal drugs and should be continued at least hourly for several days. The topical use of medication is a simple, noninvasive method of delivering a drug to the anterior segment; however, penetration of the vitreous is poor with most agents. Although commonly used, subconjunctival therapy is probably not mandatory unless there is a wound infection or an infected filtering bleb.

Loading doses of topical ophthalmic drops and application every 15–30 minutes provide prolonged therapeutic levels in the cornea and aqueous fluid.[3] Bacterial keratitis is treated with alternating 15-minute applications of topical fortified gentamicin solution (9–15 mg/ml) and cefazolin (100 mg/ml), although the benefits of this regimen in endophthalmitis have not been supported with sufficient data.

Ointments usually provide more prolonged levels, but not necessarily higher levels, than aqueous solutions. Table 8.1 lists antibiotics that penetrate well into the anterior chamber; these drugs can be used easily at frequent intervals and may be especially useful in the treatment of endophthalmitis caused by corneal ulceration or infected filtering blebs.[2]

Antibiotic selection

Early diagnosis and appropriate treatment with intraocular antibiotics are important factors in the successful management of endophthalmitis. Emerging resistance of organisms to standard antibiotic therapy has forced clinicians to continually evaluate the best intraocular antibiotics for the treatment of endophthalmitis. Although drug combinations are necessary to cover the full range of bacteria causing endophthalmitis, antimicrobial synergy is probably less important in endophthalmitis treatment because of the high intravitreal concentrations of individual antibiotics achieved by intravitreal injection. Acute postoperative endophthalmitis is treated by a combination of broad-spectrum antibiotics (vancomycin or clindamycin with amikacin or ceftazidime) which are administered intravitreally, subconjunctivally, and topically. One-quarter of the nontoxic intravitreal dose in nonvitrectomized eyes is safe in vitrectomized eyes.[4] This reduction in dose in vitrectomized eyes is recommended because antibiotic toxicity has been evaluated most often in nonvitrectomized eyes, in which the vitreous prevents rapid diffusion of antibiotics toward the retina. The vitreous reduces the concentration of antibiotic that reaches the retina,

Table 8.1 Ocular anti-infective drugs

Drug	Systemic dose (adult)	Topical (%)	Subconjunctival dose (mg)	Aqueous concentration after subconjunctival injection (µg/ml)	Intravitreal dose (mg)	Vitreous half-life (h)	Infusion solution concentration (µg/ml)
PENICILLINS							
Ampicillin	150–200 mg/kg/d IV		100		5	6	
Azlocillin	Up to 350 mg/kg/d IV		100	12			
Carbenicillin	400–600 mg/kg/d IV	10	100		0.5–2.0	10–20	
Dicloxacillin*	0.125–0.5 g q6h PO/IM						
Methicillin	1–2 g q4h IV/IM	10	100		2.0	3–5	20
Nafcillin*	1–2 g q4h IV/IM						
Oxacillin	1–2 g q4h IV/IM	6.6	100		0.5		10
Penicillin G	2–4 MU q4–6h IV	0.1	50,000 to 1 MU (300–600 mg)		0.2–0.3	3	80
Piperacillin	200–500 mg/kg/d IV/IM	5–10			1.5		
Ticarcillin	250–300 mg/k/d IV/IM	5–10	100–150		3.0		
CEPHALOSPORINS							
Cefamandole	0.5 g q6h–2 g q4h IM/IV		12.5		2.0		
Cefazolin	0.25 g q8h–2 g q4h IM/IV	5–10	50–100		0.5–2.0	7	
Cefotaxime	1 g q8h–2 g q4h IM/IV	5–10	100	5	0.4	16	
Cefsulodin	1.0–1.5 g q6h IV		100				
Ceftazidime	1–2 g q8–12h IV/IM		125	8	2.0	16	150
Ceftriaxone	1–2 g q12–24 h IM/IV		100		2.0	12	
Cefuroxime	1–2 g q8–12 h IV/IM		125	20	2.0	16	
Cephalothin	0.5 g q6–2 g q4h IM/IV	5	50–125		2.0	7	
AMINOGLYCOSIDES							
Amikacin	15 mg/kg/d Divided q8–12 h IM/IV	0.5–1.5	25	4	0.4	24	10
Gentamicin	3–5 mg/kg/d divided q8h IM/IV	0.3–1.5	10–40	4	0.2	12–35	8
Netilmicin	4.0–6.5 mg/kg/d divided q8h IM/IV				0.25	24	
Tobramycin	3–5 mg/kg/d divided q8h IM/IV	0.3–1.5	20–40		0.2	16	10
Neomycin*		0.3–3.3					
MISCELLANEOUS							
Aztreonam	1 g q8h–2 g q6h IV				0.1	7.5	
Bacitracin*		10,000 U/ml	10,000 U				
Ciprofloxacin	250–750 mg q 12 h PO	0.3	–	–	0.1	12	
Clindamycin	150–450 mg, q6h PO 150–900 mg q8h IV/IM	1–5	150		1.0	7–8	9
Chloramphenicol	0.25–0.75 g q6h PO 50/mg/kg/d IM/IV		50–100		2.0	10	10
Cotrimoxazole*	2.5–5.0 mg/kg q6h IV	TMP 16 SMZ 80			1.6 (TMP)		
Fusidic acid*	500 mg t.i.d. PO/IV		Not recommended				
Imipenem	0.5–1.0 g q6h IV/IM				0.5		16
Metronidazole*	7.5 mg/kg q6h IV						
Teicoplanin	200 mg IV/IM	5	67	18	0.75		8
Vancomycin	1 g q12h IV		25		1.0	30	20
ANTIFUNGALS							
Amphotericin B	0.25 mg/kg, increase 0.5 mg/kg/d IV	0.1–5.0	0.750		0.005–0.010	18	
Clotrimazole*	60–100 mg/kg/d PO	1	5–10				
Econazole*	30 mg/kg/d IV; 200 mg t.i.d. PO	1					
Fluconazole	50–400 mg/d PO/IV				0.1		
Flucytosine	50–150 mg/kg/d PO	1			0.1		
Itraconazole	50–400 mg/d PO				0.01		
Ketoconazole	200–1200 mg/d PO	1			0.54		
Miconazole	600 mg q12h IV	1	5–10	3–4	0.025–0.05		
Natamycin		5					
Oxiconazole					0.1		
Terconazole		5			10		
Voriconazole†	200–400 mg q12h PO; 3–6 mg/kg q12h IV						

*This drug has been evaluated in animals and is not currently used for therapy for endophthalmitis.
†Refer to Chapter 11 for therapeutic advice.

while allowing the antibiotic to be cleared through the anterior chamber. The recommended doses of common antibiotics are shown in Table 8.1.

Adjunctive systemic therapy

Because of the first report of the Endophthalmitis Vitrectomy Study (EVS),[5] some surgeons may defer administration of systemic antibiotics in postoperative endophthalmitis. However, we recommend it for 3–5 days until the vitreous abscess is controled in postoperative cases and particularly in traumatic and endogenous endophthalmitis. This recommendation is especially important if systemic steroids are to be used as described in the EVS. It must be stressed that the EVS recommendations do not apply to endogenous, traumatic, or bleb-associated cases of endophthalmitis, or to acute purulent postoperative endophthalmitis. Also, systemic antibiotics similar to those given intravitreally (Chapter 5) are useful adjuncts in these cases to maintain effective bactericidal levels within the eye. Oral doses of fluoroquinolones have been effective (see Chapter 11).[6]

Vitrectomy for endophthalmitis

When vision in endophthalmitis diminishes to light perception[5] or the vitreous haze precludes a view of the disc or a large vessel, pars plana vitrectomy is indicated.[7] If cultures have not been taken, they may be obtained in the operating room before vitrectomy.

It is important to culture the external eye and proceed with wound closure before performing anterior chamber and vitreous taps and/or vitrectomy. The eye can be inflated with sterile air prior to tapping. Alternatively, sterile saline may be used, although this may minimally dilute the sample. Either way, returning the intraocular pressure (IOP) to near-normal greatly decreases the chances of producing choroidal detachments. We prefer infusion of air through the infusion line to maintain IOP if the tip of the infusion cannula can be seen. Following the anterior chamber tap, the eye pressure should be normalized before making sclerotomies for vitrectomy.

- The safest way to perform a vitrectomy in the absence of a posterior view is to insert an anterior chamber maintainer or a bent 23-gauge needle to infuse sterile balanced saline solution or air. An infusion light pipe is used for visualization.
- To obtain diagnostic vitreous samples, use the 23-gauge pneumovitrector[8] or the 25-gauge vitreous microinstrumentation (Figure 8.4).[9] Both instruments allow vitreous biopsy without significant traction on the peripheral retina. A complete vitrectomy can be performed immediately after the sample is obtained, or may be delayed.
- The anterior infusion (using either air or saline) can be turned on promptly after the vitreous sample is obtained. In this way, the IOP may be maintained without sample dilution. The alternative is to infuse air through the infusion light pipe or infusion cannula.
- The vitrector aspiration port is attached to a sterile syringe and manual aspiration is applied as the surgeon performs the vitreous biopsy (see Figure 8.3).
- In a pseudophakic eye with a posterior chamber intraocular lens (IOL), the vitrector can be placed just behind the IOL, allowing safe vitreous cutting.
- In a traumatized eye with a cataract, care must be taken to avoid the retina if the view is impaired.
- A lighted infusion cannula (Figure 8.5), which can be inserted through a superior sclerotomy and seen through the pupil, is a useful instrument that provides adequate illumination for visualization of the vitrector during the vitreous biopsy.
- Following vitreous biopsy, the vitrectomy can be continued using the same lighted infusion cannula to provide both light and infusion during the early vitrectomy.
- A separate infusion cannula should be placed early in the procedure, but the surgeon should wait to commence infusion until the tip of the cannula can be seen in the vitreous cavity. The core vitrectomy can then be completed with the separate infusion on.
- In summary, obtaining a vitreous sample, removing anterior vitreous debris, and instilling antibiotics may be accomplished with the two-port vitrectomy employing the lighted infusion cannula and the vitrector. A conven-

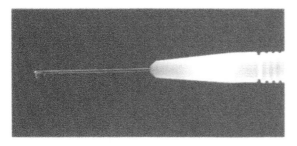

Figure 8.5

Use of lighted infusion cannula in initial vitrectomy for endophthalmitis. This photograph shows the infusion light pipe that is a very useful instrument for obtaining a vitreous sample or carrying out a limited vitrectomy in an eye with endophthalmitis that has a compromised view into the vitreous cavity due to vitreous opacities. Often it is impossible to visualize the posterior infusion cannula. It is, however, possible to place the posterior fusion cannula but refrain from turning it on. The two superior sclerotomies are created as usual. The vitrector is placed in one sclerotomy and the infusion light pipe into the second one. This provides both infusion and light, allowing the anterior vitreous cavity to be debrided. Frequently, the tip of the infusion cannula can then be visualized and posterior infusion safely commenced to allow completion of the vitrectomy.

tional three-port vitrectomy may be required to remove inflammatory debris in the posterior vitreous cavity. Manipulations very close to the retina should be avoided. The safest course may be to refrain from performing a complete vitrectomy at the first operation unless this can be accomplished quickly without compromising the retina.

- A poststerilization vitrectomy can be timed to remove vitreous debris and to prevent further enzymatic degradation of the retina. Epiretinal membranes commonly develop after endophthalmitis because of incomplete posterior hyaloid removal and require judicious surgical removal.[10]
- In chronic bacterial postoperative endophthalmitis, if antibiotic treatment is unsuccessful, a pars plana vitrectomy including removal of the IOL and the posterior capsule should be performed.[11]
- In postoperative mycotic endophthalmitis, antimycotics (amphotericin B or fluconazole) are administered intravitreally. If the inflammation is severe, a pars plana vitrectomy should be performed with possible removal of the posterior capsule and the IOL.

- In endogenous mycotic endophthalmitis, antimycotics (amphotericin B or fluconazole) are administered systemically and intravitreally. If the inflammation is severe in these eyes, a pars plana vitrectomy should be performed and antimycotics given intravitreally. These patients are often gravely ill, and the surgical goal may be debridement and intravitreal drug therapy.
- Endogenous bacterial endophthalmitis is also frequently seen in critically ill patients. Their clinical course is often rapidly progressive, and despite local and systemic treatment, the eyes may be lost. Management is particularly difficult if the patient is too ill to tolerate surgery. In these cases, a pneumovitrectomy at the bedside may allow some vitreous debridement and obtain a satisfactory sample for culture and histopathologic examination.[8] Immediate systemic and intravitreal broad-spectrum antibiotic therapy should be given as necessary.
- In traumatic injuries with intraocular foreign bodies, endophthalmitis prevention is the surgical goal. Acute posttraumatic endophthalmitis is treated by intravitreal antibiotic administration (vancomycin and amikacin or ceftazidime) in combination with pars plana vitrectomy and removal of the foreign body. Treatment is supplemented by systemic, subconjunctival, and topical antibiotic administration. Intravitreal steroids decrease tissue damage and inflammation, although their use is not universal.[12]

Preoperative hypotony

Surgery in eyes with either wound dehiscence or bleb infections can be complicated by preoperative hypotony. Wound and suture dehiscences must be initially addressed. In bleb infections, surgical excision of the infected leaking bleb and a full-thickness scleral graft may be considered to repair the scleral defect and close the eye.[13]

Retreatment

The need for reinjection of antibiotics or a poststerilization vitrectomy for debris is decided on a case-by-case basis. If the eye does not recover after initial treatment, vision decreases, or the cultures show unusual organisms not covered by the initial broad-spectrum antibiotics, a case can be made for reinjection of another appropriate antibiotic, or for immediate vitrectomy and antibiotic instillation either in the infusion fluid or at the end of the case (up to one-fourth of the dose recommended for the nonvitrectomized eye).[4,14–38]

Infusion fluid additives

Whenever a vitrectomy is performed for endophthalmitis, we recommend adding antibiotics and steroids to the infusion fluid. The doses are provided in Table 8.2.[7]

Table 8.2[7] Maximum nontoxic doses of antibiotics and dexamethasone in infusion fluid

Agent	Nontoxic dose (µg/ml)
Single:	
Amikacin	10
Amphotericin B methyl ester	75*
Ceftazidime	40
Chloramphenicol	10
Clindamycin	9
Dexamethasone	64
Gentamicin	8
Imipenem	16
Lincomycin	10
Methicillin	20
Netilmicin	4
Oxacillin	10
Penicillin	80
Teicoplanin	8
Tobramycin	10
Vancomycin	30
Combination of drugs:	
Clindamycin/gentamicin	9
	8
Gentamicin/oxacillin	8
	10
Methicillin/gentamicin	20
	8
Penicillin/gentamicin	80
	8

*Recommended dose is 10 µg/ml.

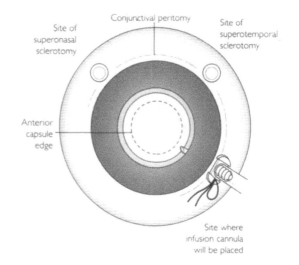

Figure 8.6

Diagram depicting removal of a posterior chamber intraocular lens in an eye with *Propionibacterium acnes* endophthalmitis: a conjunctival peritomy is created from the horizontal meridian nasally to below the level where the infusion cannula will be placed in order to accommodate the large cataract-like incision needed to remove the IOL and allow a subsequent vitrectomy.

Endophthalmitis in silicone-filled eyes

In silicone oil-filled eyes with suspected endophthalmitis, anterior chamber and vitreous taps for culture should be performed initially, then an intravitreal injection of antibiotic dose (up to one-fourth of the dose recommended for the nonvitrectomized eye)[4] and dexamethasone (1 mg) should be given. If there is purulent exudate in the vitreous cavity, removal of the silicone using infusion fluid with antibiotics and steroids (8 µg of gentamicin, 9 µg clindamycin, 20 µg vancomycin, and 64 µg of dexamethasone) should be considered. Silicone oil can be reinjected immediately or following resolution of the inflammation. Aggressive management of endophthalmitis in an eye requiring silicone oil tamponade may salvage useful vision.[39] Systemic oral antibiotics may be used as adjunctive therapy.

Surgical complications include:

- Iatrogenic retinal holes
- Postoperative epiretinal membrane formation

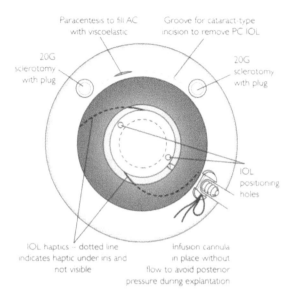

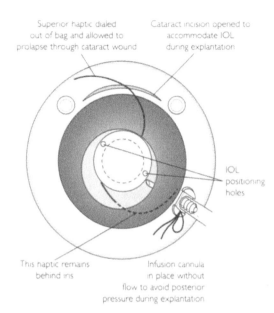

Figure 8.7

Diagram depicting removal of a PC-IOL in an eye with *Propionibacterium acnes* endophthalmitis. This diagram depicts the sequence of events in removing the PC-IOL. The infusion cannula is placed but the infusion is not commenced. If the superior sclerotomies are created at this time, they should be plugged. A groove for a cataract-type incision is created, a paracentesis is created, and the anterior chamber is filled with viscoelastic. A Sinsky hook is used to dial the IOL in the bag to allow one haptic to be prolapsed into the anterior chamber.

Figure 8.8

Diagram depicting removal of a PC-IOL in an eye with *Propionibacterium acnes* endophthalmitis. The next step is to open the cataract wound and infuse enough viscoelastic to maintain a formed anterior chamber. The IOL haptic in the anterior chamber is allowed to prolapse out of the eye through the wound.

- Postoperative retinal detachment
- Postoperative proliferative vitreoretinopathy if there is a retinal detachment
- Postoperative cataract formation
- Postoperative hypotony and phthisis bulbi.

Surgical removal of IOL and entire capsule in *Propionibacterium acnes* endophthalmitis

- The conjunctiva should be opened nasally from the horizontal meridian to 12:00 and extended temporally to below the level where the infusion cannula sclerotomy will be created (Figure 8.6).

- The plan is to make a large cataract incision superiorly to remove the IOL.
- The posterior infusion is placed inferotemporally as usual; the tip of the cannula is visualized but infusion is not begun at this time to avoid posterior pressure during IOL removal (Figure 8.7).
- Two superior sclerotomies are created and plugged.
- A groove for a cataract-type incision is made with the crescent blade superiorly, creating a wound of sufficient length to allow removal of the IOL (Figure 8.8).
- A paracentesis into the anterior chamber is created with a Sharp blade (via the cataract groove) and the anterior chamber is filled with viscoelastic.
- A Sinsky hook is inserted through the paracentesis to snag the IOL haptics and dial them into the anterior chamber. In fact, snagging only one haptic is probably sufficient to allow it to

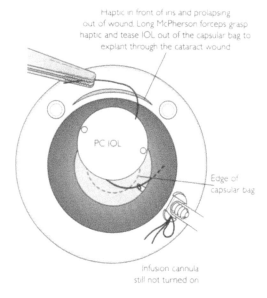

Haptic in front of iris and prolapsing out of wound. Long McPherson forceps grasp haptic and tease IOL out of the capsular bag to explant through the cataract wound

PC IOL

Edge of capsular bag

Infusion cannula still not turned on

Figure 8.9

Diagram depicting removal of a PC-IOL in an eye with *Propionibacterium acnes* endophthalmitis. Using a long McPherson forceps, the haptic is grasped, and the IOL is dialed out of the capsular bag and gently extracted from the eye. Note that the posterior infusion is still not turned on.

be grasped with a long McPherson forceps; the IOL can be dialed into the anterior chamber. The eye remains a closed chamber at this point and IOP is controled to avoid bleeding and choroidal detachment.

- The full length of the cataract wound is opened.
- Using a rocking motion, the IOL is teased out of the capsule with long McPherson forceps and dialed into the anterior chamber and extracted from the eye (Figure 8.9).
- The cataract wound is closed with 9-0 nylon to provide tensile strength for the subsequent vitrectomy (Figure 8.10). Replacement of the IOL with an anterior chamber lens or sewn-in posterior chamber lens is not recommended at this stage.
- Some surgeons recommend injection of alpha-chymotrypsin behind the iris to chemo-dissect the zonules. Unfortunately, this agent is no longer readily available.
- The posterior infusion is turned on under direct visualization.

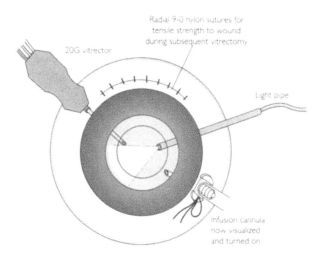

20G vitrector

Radial 9-0 nylon sutures for tensile strength to wound during subsequent vitrectomy

Light pipe

Infusion cannula now visualized and turned on

Figure 8.10

Diagram depicting removal of a PC-IOL in an eye with *Propionibacterium acnes* endophthalmitis. The cataract wound is closed with radial 9-0 nylon sutures to provide sufficient tensile strength during the subsequent vitrectomy. Following closure of this wound, the posterior infusion is turned on and a complete vitrectomy is performed. We prefer to use low-dose antibiotics and steroids in the infusion fluid during the vitrectomy.

- Anterior and posterior vitrectomy are performed to remove adherent vitreous (see Figure 8.10).
- An attempt should be made to use vitreous forceps to grasp the lens capsule while the assistant performs scleral depression (Figure 8.11). If the capsule detaches easily, it can be extracted through the sclerotomy site with vitreous forceps. If the capsule is adherent, use of the vitrector and scleral depression should be considered to remove the capsule and zonules from the ciliary body one clock hour at a time under direct visualization.
- If the vitrectomy has not been completed, it can be finished at this time with scleral depression.
- The peripheral retina must be examined carefully and peripheral tears treated with laser or cryopexy. Scleral buckling is optional, depending on the location and extent of any tears.

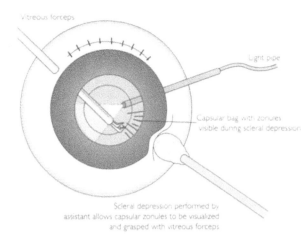

Figure 8.11

Diagram depicting removal of posterior capsule in an eye with *Propionibacterium acnes* endophthalmitis. After a complete vitrectomy is performed, the assistant uses scleral depression to allow the surgeon to visualize the capsular zonules. The zonules are grasped with vitreous forceps and the attachments are gently teased from the ciliary body. If they cannot be easily separated, vitreous scissors may be needed to cut them. The capsule is then separated from the ciliary body and removed from the eye with a vitrector or through the sclerotomy in small pieces.

- Intravitreal antibiotics can be injected prior to closing the infusion site. Use up to one-quarter of the dose of intravitreal antibiotics recommended for a nonvitrectomized eye[4,40] and dexamethasone (1 mg).

Steroids

Basic to the treatment of endophthalmitis is the use of appropriate antibiotics that will eradicate the offending organisms. However, it is also well established that the extent and duration of the host inflammatory response can exacerbate the primary damage caused by the offending organism.[40] Furthermore, some bacteria release toxins that impart secondary damage to the host. For instance, Gram-positive bacteria (especially streptococci) release teichoic acids from ruptured cell walls, while Gram-negative bacteria release endotoxins all of which exacerbate host damage.[41,42] These pathologic processes

Box 8.2 Actions of steroids

- Inhibit macrophage and neutrophil migration/activation
- Vascular stabilization
  - Inhibit leakage of proteins and fluids into the area of inflammation
  - Reduce capillary permeability
- Stabilize lysosomal membranes
- Block inflammatory mediators
  - Histamine
  - Slow-reacting substance of anaphylaxis
  - Bradykinin
  - Inhibit phospholipase A2 – decrease prostaglandins
  - Inhibit platelet-aggregating factors produced by the vascular endothelium
  - Interleukin-1
  - Tumor necrosis factor

ultimately culminate in fibrin membrane proliferation (see inflammation section), subsequent retinal necrosis/detachment, and vascular pathology leading to catastrophic vision loss.

Corticosteroids have long been investigated as an adjunct to reduce such secondary damage caused by the host's inflammatory response. In theory, corticosteroids diminish the effect of inflammation-induced damage to the host by the methods listed in Box 8.2 (and reviewed in Chapter 2).

The ability of intravitreally injected corticosteroids to modulate the host inflammatory response in the setting of endophthalmitis has been investigated extensively using several animal models and different offending organisms.[18,43] Case reports dating back to the 1970s have proposed beneficial effects of intravitreal dexamethasone when used in addition to intravitreal antibiotics.[44,45]

Corticosteroids

Dexamethasone is a synthetic adrenocortical steroid with molecular weight of 392.47. It is designated chemically as 9-fluoro-11b,17,21-trihydroxy-16a-methylpregna-1,4-diene-3,20-dione. The empirical formula is $C_{22}H_{29}FO_5$. The chemical structure of a corticosteroid is shown in Figure 8.12. In general, dexamethasone

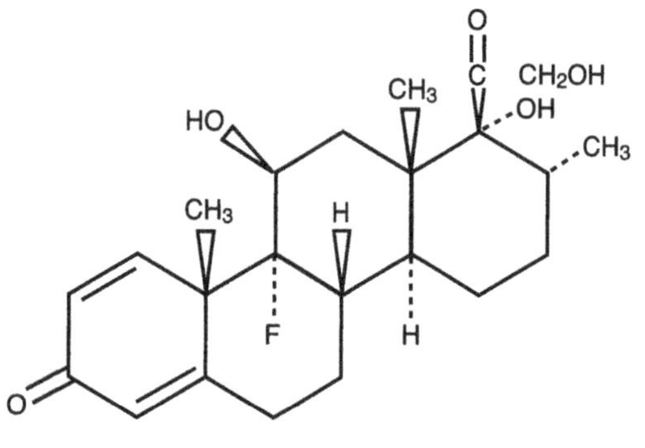

Figure 8.12

Chemical structure diagram of a corticosteroid.

suppresses inflammation and the normal immune response and is used to treat inflammatory disorders.

There are many potential side effects of systemic steroid use as listed in Box 8.3. Systemic steroids must be used with caution. Schulman et al reported a 33-year-old man treated with systemic corticosteroids for an unspecified infectious chorioretinitis before a definitive diagnosis of cryptococcal retinitis and meningitis was made.[46] The patient deteriorated rapidly and subsequently died. Other such case reports exist in the literature.

Intraocularly, we routinely use 16 µg of dexamethasone in vitrectomy infusion fluid in diabetic patients without any observable side effects. Down-regulation of the immune response to combat infection, intrinsic toxicity, retinal detachment, IOP elevation, and cataract formation are the main ocular complications to be monitored when using intravitreal dexamethasone.

Evaluating intravitreal dexamethasone

In deciding whether intravitreal steroid supplementation, with 400 µg dexamethasone, should be used in endophthalmitis patients, several questions have to be addressed:

- Does steroid therapy decrease inflammatory damage?

Box 8.3 Side effects of systemic steroids

Ophthalmic: Elevated intraocular pressure, posterior subcapsular cataracts, retinal detachment, retinal toxicity, decreased wound healing

Cardiovascular: Myocardial rupture following recent myocardial infarction; congestive heart failure

Musculoskeletal: Myopathy leading to atrophy; osteoporosis leading to vertebral compression fractures and aseptic necrosis of femoral and humeral heads; pathologic fracture of long bones; tendon rupture

Metabolic: Sodium and fluid retention leading to congestive heart failure in susceptible patients; potassium loss leading to hypokalemic alkalosis; hypertension

Gastrointestinal: Peptic ulcer; perforation of the small and large bowel; esophagitis; pancreatitis

Neurologic: Increased intracranial pressure leading to papilledema; psychic disturbances; convulsions

Endocrine: Cushingoid state; hirsutism; growth suppression; secondary down-regulation of the steroid responsiveness (especially in times of stress); manifestations of latent diabetes mellitus; altered insulin or oral hypoglycemic need

Dermatologic: Thin fragile skin; petechiae and ecchymoses; erythema; allergic reactions; impaired wound healing

Other: Thromboembolism; increased appetite; weight gain

- Does steroid therapy improve final visual acuity?
- Does steroid therapy improve electrophysiologic function?
- Does steroid treatment blunt immune response?
- Does steroid therapy induce a toxic effect?
- What are the therapeutic and toxic dosages of steroid?
- Are there any drug interactions?

Modulating inflammatory response

Various animal models and organisms have been used to study endophthalmitis. Using different endpoints, most studies have shown either beneficial or at least neutral effects of concomitant intravitreal dexamethasone use. Generally, the amount of inflammation has been shown to decrease with intravitreal dexamethasone, which may decrease collateral damage. However, clinical correlation through either direct visual acuity measurement or indirect electrophysiology measurements has been less clear.

Park et al showed that rabbits treated with intravitreal vancomycin (1000 μg) and concomitant dexamethasone (400 μg) demonstrated decreased levels of intraocular inflammation and histologic preservation of retinal structures when examined 2 weeks after inoculation with pneumococcus.[47] In this study, 30 albino rabbits were injected intravitreally with *Streptococcus pneumoniae* and randomized to treatment with intravitreal vancomycin, combination intravitreal vancomycin/dexamethasone, or no treatment. Interestingly, untreated and vancomycin-treated eyes demonstrated the same degree of change on clinical and histologic examination, with marked anterior and posterior segment inflammation with total retinal necrosis.

Liu et al showed that the addition of dexamethasone to intravitreal vancomycin in a rabbit model with *Bacillus cereus* endophthalmitis reduced histologic evidence of inflammation at 14 days postinjection.[48] Cataracts developed in a significant percentage of eyes not treated with dexamethasone, implying a more severe grade of intraocular inflammation. *B. cereus* is a potentially devastating cause of endophthalmitis that requires prompt treatment. This bacterium releases endotoxins and extracellular virulence factors that elicit secondary inflammatory damage.[49,50]

Studying yet another organism, Smith et al compared the efficacy of intravitreal dexamethasone in a rabbit endophthalmitis model infected with methicillin-resistant *Staphylococcus epidermidis*.[51] The rabbits were treated with vancomycin alone, dexamethasone alone, or a combination of vancomycin and dexamethasone. The degree of inflammation via vitreal aspiration and histologic study was evaluated. Although clinical examination showed no significant difference, histologic evaluation showed a decrease in inflammation at 24 hours. As expected, dexamethasone alone was worse than no treatment at all.

In a study employing both electrophysiologic and histologic parameters, Kim et al evaluated the efficacy of intravitreal dexamethasone (400 μg) in combination with ciprofloxacin (300 μg) in rabbits inoculated with *Pseudomonas aeruginosa*.[52] The therapy was evaluated at 6, 12, 18, and 24 hours post-inoculation by electrophysiology and histology. The authors determined that the addition of dexamethasone did not have a beneficial or detrimental effect using either criterion. In contrast, Graham and Peyman noted an improvement in inflammation after intravitreal injection of a combination of dexamethasone (360 μg) and gentamicin sulfate (500 μg) 5 hours after induction of endophthalmitis in rabbits by inoculation with *Pseudomonas*.[18] The difference may relate to timing – with a greater beneficial effect if steroids are used within 6 hours of inoculation.

Evaluating a relatively new drug, Yildirim et al studied the effect of intravitreal levofloxacin/dexamethasone on albino rabbits infected with an intravitreal inoculum of *S. epidermidis*.[53] Five days after drug injection, the treated groups had significantly lower clinical scores than the control group; the culture results of the treatment groups were sterile. The histopathologic scores of the treatment groups were also lower than the control group (p = 0.007).

Jett et al observed that electroretinogram (ERG) outcome was dependent on the cytotoxicity of the *Enterococcus faecalis* strain tested. In this study, cytolytic toxin-producing *E. faecalis* endophthalmitis caused ERG B-wave amplitude decline regardless of treatment with intravitreal antibiotics or dexamethasone.[54] However, noncytolytic strains of the same organism allowed preservation of ERG B-waves when treated with the same regimen. Aguilar et al noted increased inflammatory scores, corneal opacity, and the number of eyes developing retinal necrosis when intraocular corticosteroids were injected in an endophthalmitis model eye (inoculated with *S. aureus*) after vitrectomy and intraocular antibiotics.[55]

The intravitreal use of corticosteroids in the treatment of fungal endophthalmitis is generally considered to be contraindicated because it may enhance fungal virulence. However, Coats and Peyman demonstrated that corticosteroids in combination with antifungal drugs did not impair antifungal effects or enhance fungal proliferation.[12] In this study, 20 rabbits were observed after exogenous induction of endophthalmitis with *Candida albicans*. Eight eyes received intravitreal amphotericin B alone; eight eyes received amphotericin B plus dexamethasone. Four eyes served as controls. On the fourth day, vitreous of the eyes in the two drug-treated groups was significantly clearer compared with that of eyes in the control group. By the seventh day, the eyes treated with amphotericin B plus dexamethasone had significantly clearer vitreous in comparison with the eyes that received only amphotericin B (p = 0.0017). Culture results were negative in both treatment groups; clinical grading was confirmed by histopathologic examination. The authors suggested that use of corticosteroids in exogenous fungal endophthalmitis may be beneficial when fungal proliferation has been controled or when administered with the appropriate antifungal agent.

Majji et al corroborated these findings in a retrospective study that determined that steroids may promote faster clearance of inflammation in fungal endophthalmitis.[56] In this retrospective analysis of 20 human patients with culture-proven exogenous fungal endophthalmitis following cataract surgery or trauma, all eyes were managed with pars plana vitrectomy with intravitreal amphotericin B and oral ketoconazole. Intravitreal dexamethasone was the lone variable. The authors found that intravitreal dexamethasone was not statistically associated with any difference in anatomic and visual outcome. However, use of intravitreal steroids was associated with:

- A higher number of patients with favorable visual outcome (not statistically significant)
- An increased rate of clearance of inflammation (40 ± 15.5 vs 55 ± 8.6 days).

Visual acuity

Animal studies are limited in that visual acuities cannot be measured and must be inferred from indirect testing methods such as the ERG, clinical inflammation scoring systems, and histologic studies. In a human study, Das et al performed a prospective study of intravitreal dexamethasone injection in exogenous bacterial endophthalmitis (postoperative and posttraumatic) involving 63 eyes.[57] All patients underwent vitrectomy with intraocular antibiotics consisting of amikacin (400 μg) and vancomycin (1 mg). The endpoints were inflammation score and final visual acuity. This study showed that the inflammation score was reduced significantly at weeks 1, 4, and 12 in the group treated with intravitreal dexamethasone. Furthermore, the group not treated with

dexamethasone showed a significant increase in inflammation score at week 1 before declining at further time points. However, the final visual acuity was comparable in both groups at 12 weeks.

Das et al also evaluated the use of intravitreal dexamethasone with *Bacillus* endophthalmitis in a retrospective fashion.[58] Thirty-one culture-proven *Bacillus* endophthalmitis cases underwent surgery/intravitreal antibiotics with or without intravitreal dexamethasone. No clinical difference was shown as regards the final visual outcome. The degree of inflammation was not measured in this study.

In another study, Auclin et al evaluated 52 patients with postoperative endophthalmitis who were treated with intravitreal injection of antibiotics (vancomycin-amikacin) and steroids (dexamethasone), systemic antibiotics (pefloxacin-piperacillin), and systemic steroids in bolus.[59] Visual acuity was measurable in 45 eyes (86.5%) with visual acuity of 20/100 noted in 33 eyes (63.4%) and 20/40 in 23 eyes (44.2%).

Shah et al reported on a retrospective review of 57 patients with postoperative endophthalmitis at the Wills Eye Hospital and Barnes Retina Institute.[60] The authors reported that intravitreal injection of dexamethasone (400 μg/0.1 ml) actually reduced the likelihood of obtaining a three-line improvement in visual acuity (Snellen best-corrected visual acuity) by a factor of 3.5 with a range of 1.2–14. In this study, all patients were given intravitreal amikacin (400 μg/0.1 ml) and vancomycin (1 mg/ 0.1 ml) without systemic antibiotics. Vitrectomy or vitreous tap was performed at the discretion of the treating physician, as was injection of intravitreal dexamethasone. The authors postulated that the use of steroids either blunted the immune response or had a toxic effect on the retina. In response, Harris pointed to a possible selection bias because the patients who did not receive intravitreal dexamethasone had better presenting visual acuity (better than 5/200).[61] However, the authors responded that the difference is in fact only 4/31 (12%) with better than 5/200 as opposed to 5/26 in the group with worse than 5/200 (20%), which does not represent a clinical significance.

Drug interaction

In an interesting observation, Park et al noted that concomitant administration of dexamethasone with vancomycin enhanced the antibiotic effect by decreasing its rate of elimination.[62] In an animal study, these authors found that the vitreous concentration of vancomycin was 140 ± 51 µg/ml in eyes treated with intravitreal dexamethasone compared with 78 ± 41 µg/ml in eyes treated only with intravitreal vancomycin (p<0.001). The authors speculated that although intravitreal dexamethasone may primarily enhance the excretion of vancomycin through the canal of Schlemm, it also stabilizes the inner and outer retinal barrier that has been made porous by the inflammation. The net effect favors retention of vancomycin in the eye.

On the other hand, Smith et al demonstrated that the intravitreal vancomycin concentration was significantly lower in both uninfected and infected rabbit eyes injected with vancomycin (1 mg) and dexamethasone (400 µg) (p<0.002).[63] Intravitreal vancomycin concentrations were analyzed using model-independent parameters with the area under the concentration-time curves derived by trapezoidal approximation.

Toxicity

Yoshizumi et al evaluated retinal toxicity of the intravitreal drugs used frequently in the treatment of endophthalmitis.[64] Rabbit eyes were injected with vancomycin 0.3 mg, ceftazidime 0.7 mg, and dexamethasone sodium phosphate 0.13 mg at three consecutive 48-hour intervals. The contralateral eyes were injected with three times these concentrations at the same time intervals. These drug concentrations approximated the levels recommended in human eyes. The authors found that the lower concentrations did not yield any evidence of retinal toxicity and that the higher concentration resulted only in mild ERG changes.

Kwak and D'Amico reported that the primary toxicity of intravitreally injected dexamethasone occurs in the Mueller cells.[65] After injecting 440 µg of dexamethasone into a rabbit eye, only a transient increase in staining of the Mueller cells was noted, with normalization in 2 days. Higher doses resulted in an increasing spectrum of disorganization in Mueller and other retinal cells. The authors speculated that dexamethasone caused primary interference of Mueller cell function, possibly through alterations in retinal glutamate or glucose metabolism. Das et al alluded to the same finding, reporting that intrav-

itreal dexamethasone higher than 800 µg may cause histologic changes in the retina by causing vacuolation between the outer plexiform and outer nuclear layers.[57] The authors also noted that the primary site of toxic reaction occurred in the Mueller cells.

The toxicity of dexamethasone administered intravitreally was also evaluated by Graham and Peyman.[18] In this study, 400 µg of intravitreal dexamethasone was found to be nontoxic to intraocular structures. Residual concentrations were found to be present for at least 4 days. In another study, Nabih et al also did not observe any toxicity in rabbits after injections of up to 4.8 mg/0.2 ml of intravitreal dexamethasone.[66] Although the minimum therapeutic concentration has not been identified, it is believed that even a minute concentration may be enough to reduce the inflammatory response.[18,67]

Timing

Yoshizumi et al demonstrated a beneficial effect of dexamethasone in rabbit eyes with induced *S. aureus* endophthalmitis.[68] Electroretinographic function was measured in relation to the timing of intravitreal vancomycin and dexamethasone. The mean inflammatory scores were significantly improved in eyes treated with intravitreal vancomycin and dexamethasone at 36 hours and 48 hours after inoculation as compared with those treated with vancomycin alone. Vitreal cultures were negative in eyes treated at 24 hours and 36 hours after inoculation. It is worth noting that even the positive cultures in eyes given vancomycin and dexamethasone were fewer than in eyes given vancomycin alone. Histopathologic examination showed increasing levels of tissue inflammation with each passing time interval.

Based on these results, Yoshizumi et al reported that the early treatment (at 24 hours) with vancomycin with or without dexamethasone resulted in complete sterilization and preservation of retinal function.[68] The optimal timing of intravitreal dexamethasone was found to occur 36 hours after inoculation. The authors noted that the extension of a treatment window to 36 hours is consistent with previous findings by Jett et al[54] and Peyman et al[69] who also found that treatment begun *within 36 hours of infection* resulted in the best final visual acuity.

Table 8.3 Combination of antibiotics with dexamethasone

Pathogen	Host	Symptoms or diagnostic test used	Response	Antibiotic used with dexamethasone
Staphylococcus aureus[55]	Rabbits	Inflammation	Worsened inflammation	Vancomycin
S. aureus[68]	Rabbits	Histology, ERG	Best given at 36 hours	Vancomycin, ceftazidime
S. aureus[70]	Rabbits	Histology, inflammation	No improvement	Cefazolin
Methicillin-resistant Staphylococcus epidermidis[63]	Rabbits	Vancomycin concentration measured	Decreased vancomycin concentration in presence of intravitreal dexamethasone	Vancomycin
Methicillin-resistant S. epidermidis[61]	Rabbits	Histology, inflammation	Less inflammation	Vancomycin
S. epidermidis[43]	Rabbits	Histology, clinical examination	Less inflammation	Gentamicin
Streptococcus pneumoniae[62]	Rabbits	Vancomycin concentration	Increased vancomycin concentration	Vancomycin
Strep. pneumoniae[47]	Rabbits	Histology	Less inflammation	Vancomycin
Enterococcus faecalis[54]	Rabbits	ERG	No improvement	None
Pseudomonas aeruginosa[52]	Rabbits	ERG, histology	No improvement	Ciprofloxacin
Pseudomonas aeruginosa[18]	Rabbits	Inflammation	Less inflammation	Gentamicin
Bacillus sp.[58]	Clinical	Visual acuity	No improvement	Gentamicin and cefazolin in the earlier period and combination of gentamicin/amikacin and later vancomycin
Bacillus cereus[48]	Rabbits	Histology	Less inflammation	Vancomycin
Fungus[56]	Clinical	Inflammation, visual acuity, inflammation clearance	No improvement except in clearance	Intravitreal amphotericin B and oral ketoconazole
Fungus[12]	Rabbit	Histology, inflammation	Improved	Intravitreal amphotericin B

Various studies have been undertaken to answer these questions, mostly in animal models (Table 8.3).[12,18,42,43,47,48,51,52,54–56,58,62,63,68,70] Among the most significant limitations of the available data are the different endpoints (inflammation scoring, histology, electrophysiology, visual acuity) and varying models of endophthalmitis and host. Today, the use of steroids for endophthalmitis is a generally accepted pattern of practice.

Table 8.4 Variables in treating endophthalmitis

Type of bacteria – Gram-positive or Gram-negative	Virulence of the organism
Size of the inoculum	Inflammatory response
Timing of treatment	Route of treatment
Vitrectomy	

Conclusions

The variables that may influence the effect of intravitreal corticosteroids on endophthalmitis are listed in Table 8.4.

Given the variability of the results, it seems that endophthalmitis caused by different organisms may show different susceptibility. For instance, Jett et al pointed out that endophthalmitis caused by toxin-producing strains of *E. faecalis* did not show improvement with intraocular dexamethasone although endophthalmitis caused by the noncytolytic strains showed improvement.[54] This finding that corticosteroids would not ameliorate both kinds of strains seems counterintuitive; perhaps the reason will be discovered. At this point, it seems prudent to make well thought-out clinical decisions based on the individual patient.

Intravitreal dexamethasone appears to decrease inflammation in endophthalmitis. Most studies favor or at least remain neutral on whether intravitreal steroids should be used to treat endophthalmitis. The theoretical benefit of reduced inflammation has yet to be translated into a human trial demonstrating improved vision; however, various investigators have elucidated toxicity, drug interactions, and a time window to maximize benefits that provide ample guidelines for intravitreal use of dexamethasone in endophthalmitis. Intravitreal dexamethasone as an adjunct to the treatment of endophthalmitis appears to be generally accepted. We inject 400 µg/0.1 ml of intravitreal dexamethasone at the same time as the antibiotics or antifungals. Appropriate cultures are taken and serve as a treatment guideline.

Endophthalmitis Vitrectomy Study

The EVS was a randomized prospective study involving 24 centers and 420 patients between 1990 and 1994.[5] This study looked specifically at patients presenting with clinical signs and symptoms of bacterial endophthalmitis within 6 weeks of either cataract surgery or secondary IOL implantation. It was a focused and limited attempt to determine the role of pars plana vitrectomy, systemic antibiotics, and systemic steroids in the management of endophthalmitis following cataract surgery or secondary lens implantation. As such, its study population was limited and its application to other causes of endophthalmitis must not be extrapolated. Therefore, its universal application to all cases of endophthalmitis, as it is apt to be done, must be viewed with caution. In this section, the EVS will be discussed in detail followed by review of some of the issues raised regarding its findings.

The EVS evaluated bacterial endophthalmitis patients presenting within 6 weeks of either cataract surgery or secondary IOL implantation.

Table 8.5 Patient randomization scheme in the Endophthalmitis Vitrectomy Study

Vitreous tap + intravitreal antibiotic	Systemic antibiotic (ceftazidime and amikacin) *or* No systemic antibiotics
Vitrectomy + intravitreal antibiotic	Systemic antibiotics (ceftazidime and amikacin) *or* No systemic antibiotics

These patients were required to have visual acuity between 20/50 to light perception and a cornea with sufficient clarity for vitrectomy. Patients were randomized immediately to one of four treatment groups (Table 8.5).

All eyes underwent paracentesis to secure a 0.1-ml aqueous sample. The vitreous tap groups had a vitreous sample of 0.1–0.3 ml collected either by a pars plana vitreous needle aspiration or with a vitrectomy suction cutter through a single sclerotomy. Eyes in the vitrectomy groups underwent three-port pars plana vitrectomy, removing at least 50% of the vitreous gel in eyes with no posterior hyaloid detachment. Intravitreal injections of amikacin (0.4 mg) and vancomycin (1 mg) in 0.1 ml of normal saline were given to all eyes.

The intravenous antibiotic patient groups were started on systemic ceftazidime and amikacin for 5–10 days. Patients allergic to ceftazidime were given oral ciprofloxacin. Additionally, topical steroids were begun postoperatively while oral prednisone (30 mg twice a day) was administered for 5–10 days.

Endpoint assessments consisted of best-corrected visual acuity and media clarity evaluated both clinically and photographically and performed at the 3- and 9-month follow-up visits, except for those patients who required an additional surgical procedure. In such patients, a 12-month follow-up outcome evaluation was performed.

EVS findings

The visual outcomes for patients in the EVS are shown in Table 8.6. For patients presenting with light perception vision, an immediate vitrectomy led to:

Table 8.6 Visual outcome of patients in the Endophthalmitis Vitrectomy Study

Visual acuity	Percentage of patients achieving this level of visual acuity
20/40 or better	50%
20/100 or better	75%
5/200	11%

Table 8.7 Causative organisms in eyes in the EVS that achieved visual acuity of 20/100 or better

Organism	Visual acuity of 20/100 or better
Coagulase-negative staphylococci (CNS)	84%
Staphylococcus aureus	50%
Streptococci	30%
Enterococci (E. faecalis)	14%
Gram-negative organisms	56%

- Three-fold greater chance of achieving 20/40 or better vision
- Two-fold greater chance of achieving 20/100 vision
- Fifty percent decrease in the risk of achieving severe visual loss
- More rapid clearing of the media at 3 months but no difference at 9 months.

Intravenous antibiotics did not influence the final visual outcome or media clarity. Visual outcome was also highly correlated with the identity of infecting species and Gram stain results as noted in Table 8.7.

Eyes infected with bacteria that produced a positive Gram stain showed worse visual outcome compared with an equivocal or negative Gram stain. The investigators speculated that a positive Gram stain might signify infection with a larger inoculum, more rapid bacterial multiplication, or a longer duration of infection. These factors might result in increased production of inflammatory products and toxins, leading to a worse outcome.

Patients with diabetes

Because of their immunocompromised state, patients with diabetes are at increased risk for developing postoperative endophthalmitis. In the EVS, 13.8% (58) of the patients were diabetic.[71] Fifty-seven percent of patients with diabetes who underwent vitrectomy (in contrast to 40% with tap/biopsy) achieved a visual acuity of 20/40, which was similar to results for patients without diabetes. The EVS investigators concluded that either initial vitrectomy or tap/biopsy would be warranted in diabetic patients presenting with initial vision better than light perception.

Diabetic eyes had a higher confirmed growth at culture (84.5%) than nondiabetic eyes (66.8%). The greatest difference in growth occurred with Gram-positive coagulase-negative staphylococci (CNS), which were present in 58.6% of cultures from diabetic eyes compared with 45% of cultures from nondiabetic patients. Organisms cultured from diabetic eyes also showed a slight tendency to be more virulent. Both groups had a similar rate of infection with Gram-negative bacteria, with diabetics showing a higher rate of infection with streptococci and S. aureus.[71]

The eyes of patients with diabetes were more likely to have an additional procedure after the initial intervention than the eyes of patients without diabetes during the course of follow-up (diabetic eyes 43.17% versus eyes of nondiabetics 34%, p = 0.18).[71] The difference was most marked in procedures performed in the first week after initial assessment: 20.7% of diabetic eyes required additional procedures compared with 8.8% of nondiabetic eyes. The incidence of hypopyon was equal in both groups, with the height of the hypopyon 50% higher in the diabetic group. Final visual outcome at all levels tested was poorer in the diabetic eyes than in the nondiabetic group. The investigators found that 20/40 vision was achieved in 39% of diabetic eyes compared with 55% nondiabetic eyes.[71]

Financial impact

A subgroup of patients from four clinical centers representing 31% of the EVS population was retrospectively analyzed to determine the relationship between economic impact and the quality of outcomes.[72] The results demonstrated that for all efficacy or outcome measures evaluated in eyes presenting with light perception vision only, vitrectomy was both more charge-effective and more clinically efficacious than tap biopsy. In contrast, for the subgroup of patients presenting with hand motion or better vision, both procedures demonstrated similar clinical efficacy, but tap biopsy was more charge-effective.

Patients undergoing vitrectomy had a mean adjusted hospital charge of $6600 compared with $5600 for a tap biopsy procedure. Factors besides vitrectomy independently associated with higher adjusted hospital charges were a baseline vision of only light perception, female gender, and a history of diabetes mellitus. A lower adjusted hospital charge was associated with the presenting symptom of a red eye.[72]

The investigators determined that the annual cost savings in the United States would range between $8.6 million and $38.5 million if the EVS results were used as the guidelines for the treatment of endophthalmitis following cataract extraction or secondary IOL implantation.[72]

Analysis of the EVS

Patient selection

In the EVS, only 69% of the patient population had positive cultures and stains, and in 8% of these, the only positive culture was from the vitrectomy cassette, which was sometimes stored up to 12 hours, and not from the undiluted vitreous or aqueous samples.[73] Therefore, one might question whether the EVS patients who had negative cultures should be considered as postoperative bacterial endophthalmitis, which could have significant statistical implications for the data. Furthermore, the EVS de-emphasized the importance of pain as a symptom by indicating that one-quarter of the patients did not have pain. It would have been valuable to analyze, in fact, how many patients with positive cultures had pain versus those with negative cultures.

Media clarity

As published in the EVS, there was a difference of only 10% in media clarity between vitrectomized and nonvitrectomized eyes 3 months after surgery.[5] There was no significant difference between these two groups as far as clarity of media is concerned at the final analysis after treatment. Our animal study showed that the results of vitrectomy and intravitreal injection of antibiotics were comparable as far as the recovery of the eye from the infection was concerned; the only difference was in the clarity of the media.[74] This finding is important because the final visual acuity may be related to the clarity of the media.[75] According to the criteria of the EVS, one-quarter of the patients would require vitrectomy.

Unfortunately, in the EVS, no intravitreal steroids were used. We have demonstrated since 1974 that steroids significantly reduce postoperative inflammation.[18] Lack of intravitreal steroids will cause increased postoperative inflammation and cloudiness of the media, influencing the final visual acuity or need for additional surgery to clear the media. Therefore, if intravitreal steroids had been used by the EVS, the insignificant differences (overall, 7% at 5/200 or less visual acuity level) between the vitrectomized or nonvitrectomized groups might have been even smaller.

Furthermore, it is surprising that the EVS recommended exclusion of systemic administration of antibiotics but recommended systemic administration of steroids. This recommendation defies the conventional wisdom in medicine of administering steroids with appropriate antibiotic coverage in the presence of a localized infection in the body. Perhaps intravitreal injection of steroids should also have been evaluated, as this approach appears to be efficacious in treating endophthalmitis. Unfortunately, the subconjunctival antibiotic treatment of endophthalmitis used by the EVS has been shown to be ineffective.[76]

Objective visual acuity

The use of a visual acuity level of light perception as an indication for vitrectomy is a subjective one. Often, a patient can be uncooperative or may not be able to communicate adequately, especially when the eye is painful and swollen. Instead, the absence of red reflex or lack of visibility of disc and large vessels (not second-order retinal vessels as was recorded by the EVS) may be better objective criteria.[77] Such a criterion would depend solely on the objective assessment of the ophthalmologist and would promote delivery of more uniform care.

Intravitreal antibiotics

The conclusion of the EVS is that no single antibiotic, such as amikacin, ceftazidime, or ciprofloxacin, should be used because none of them covers all the Gram-positive and Gram-negative bacteria. This conclusion is probably incorrect as far as intravitreal injection is concerned. The sensitivity studies performed in the hospital laboratories usually are limited to the concentration of antibiotics achieved in the blood after systemic administration. After a single intravitreal injection of 400 µg amikacin, the concentration of amikacin per milliliter in the vitreous cavity (5 ml) can be assayed at 80 µg/ml. Sensitivity testing at these concentrations is never performed in routine microbiologic evaluation. However, most bacteria are sensitive to these high concentrations even though they may not show sensitivity at the usually tested concentrations of 8–10 µg/ml.

When we initiated intravitreal injection of antibiotics, we were using up to 400 µg of gentamicin alone.[30,78] As a result, even Gram-positive organisms that ordinarily were not sensitive to low or moderate gentamicin levels were eradicated and there was no need for additional intravitreal antibiotics. In addition, aminoglycosides have a dose-dependent effect on bacteria. Because of the concern of retinal toxicity from intravitreal gentamicin, we reduced the dosage to 200 µg, resulting in intravitreal concentrations that are significantly higher than those achieved by systemically administered medication.[79] In general, however, we believe that a combination of 50% of a nontoxic dose of a broad-spectrum antibiotic such as an aminoglycoside (amikacin 200 µg)[22] and other antibiotics such as vancomycin (500 µg)[80] or clindamycin (500 µg)[81] is desirable to increase the spectrum of antimicrobial efficacy, and to be effective against most expected Gram-positive and Gram-negative bacteria, including *Pseudomonas aeruginosa*.[80,81] It is interesting to note that the combination dose of 400 µg amikacin plus 1 mg vancomycin used in the EVS had not yet been evaluated and published for toxicity in animals. Unfortunately, no fluorescein angiography was performed in the EVS to evaluate this potential problem. Interestingly, there was one case of macular infarct in the EVS report.

Therapeutic options

The emphasis placed by the EVS on vitrectomy as the initial treatment method for patients presenting with light perception visual acuity may not be applicable to the practice of a general ophthalmologist. Endophthalmitis is often diagnosed by a general ophthalmologist and a considerable time delay may occur while referring the patient to a retinal specialist for therapy. It may be more prudent to recommend that an intravitreal injection of antibiotics and steroids be given by the general ophthalmologist after aspirating vitreous for culture.[82] The patient may then be referred for a vitrectomy while the antibiotic and steroid treatments are at work during the inevitable time delay between diagnosis and surgery. If the facilities are available, vitrectomy can be performed immediately; however, it may be delayed up to 24–48 hours without compromising proper patient care during referral, while allowing time for proper systemic evaluation of the patient and possibly obtaining preliminary positive culture results preoperatively. A number of these vitrectomies may not be needed and intravitreal antibiotics and steroids might clear up the media within 24–48 hours. This occurs more frequently in patients in whom no bacterial growth from biopsy samples is obtained; therefore, immediate vitrectomy might result in an additional unnecessary procedure in these patients.

The EVS emphasized that there is a potential for cost savings because there is no need for systemic administration of antibiotics in endophthalmitis. However, it represents an ethical dilemma as to whether one should offer different treatment to the patient than one would want for oneself. We might ask the question 'How would we as ophthalmologists want to be treated if we had endophthalmitis?' Probably we would want a short course of systemic medication, in addition to the intravitreal antibiotics. Systemic administration of the same antibiotic as given intravitreally not only provides prolonged anterior chamber and vitreous levels but also protects the patients against possible bacterial spread or new infection. Therefore, the conclusion that financial savings are possible (or might be dictated to us by a 'clever' HMO) might not be ethical and may lead to a moral dilemma for the physicians. In addition, the availability of effective oral doses of the third- and fourth-generation fluoroquinolones makes hospitalization unnecessary.

Other flaws in the EVS study included:

- Patient recruitment was initially 1200 patients but one-third declined to take part. Of the remainder, one-half could not be included because they did not meet the requirements of the trial protocol, so that only one-third of the patients initially recruited took part in the study. This problem biased the study toward the inclusion of less severe, less acute cases from whom there was a high isolation rate of CNS.
- Only 10% of cultures yielded highly virulent bacteria so that the role of intravenous antibiotics for treatment of acute purulent endophthalmitis could not be conclusive. It is thus the opinion of these authors that systemic antibiotics should be used as adjunctive therapy to intravitreal antibiotics for management of acute purulent endophthalmitis.

References

1. Peyman GA, Meffert SA, Conway MD et al, eds. *Vitreoretinal Surgical Techniques* (Martin Dunitz: London, 2001) 494.
2. Peyman GA, Schulman JA. *Intravitreal Surgery: Principles and Practice,* 2nd edn (Appleton & Lange: Norwalk, CT, 1994) 867–8.
3. Glasser DB, Gardner S, Ellis JG et al. Loading doses and extended dosing intervals in topical gentamicin therapy, *Am J Ophthalmol* (1985) **99**:329–32.
4. Hegazy HM, Kivilcim M, Peyman GA et al. Evaluation of toxicity of intravitreal ceftazidime, vancomycin, and ganciclovir in a silicone-oil filled eye, *Retina* (1999) **19**:553–7.
5. Endophthalmitis Vitrectomy Study Group, Results of the Endophthalmitis Vitrectomy Study: A randomized trial of immediate vitrectomy and of intravenous antibiotics for the treatment of postoperative bacterial endophthalmitis, *Arch Ophthalmol* (1995) **113**:1479–96.
6. Fiscella RG, Nguyen TK, Cwik MJ et al. Aqueous and vitreous penetration of levofloxacin after oral administration, *Ophthalmology* (1999) **106**: 2286–90.
7. Peyman GA, Schulman JA. *Intravitreal Surgery: Principles and Practice,* 2nd edn (Appleton & Lange: Norwalk, CT, 1994) 901–5.
8. Peyman GA. A miniaturized vitrectomy system for vitreous and retinal biopsy, *Can J Ophthalmol* (1990) **25**:285–6.
9. de Juan E Jr, Hickingbotham D. Refinements in microinstrumentation for vitreous surgery, *Am J Ophthalmol* (1990) **109**:218–20.
10. Doft BH, Kelsey SF, Wisniewski SR. Additional procedures after the initial vitrectomy or tap-biopsy in the Endophthalmitis Vitrectomy Study, *Ophthalmology* (1998) **105**:707–16.
11. Peyman GA, Bassili SS. A practical guideline for management of endophthalmitis, *Ophthalmic Surg* (1995) **26**:294–303.
12. Coats ML, Peyman GA. Intravitreal corticosteroids in the treatment of exogenous fungal endophthalmitis, *Retina* (1992) **12**:46–51.
13. Kosmin AS, Wishart PK. A full-thickness scleral graft for the surgical management of a late filtration bleb leak, *Ophthalmic Surg Lasers* (1997) **28**: 461–8.
14. Peyman GA, May DR, Ericson ES et al. Intraocular injection of gentamicin: toxic effects and clearance, *Arch Ophthalmol* (1974) **92**:42–7.
15. May DR, Ericson ES, Peyman GA et al. Intraocular injection of gentamicin: single injection therapy of experimental bacterial endophthalmitis, *Arch Ophthalmol* (1974) **91**:487–9.
16. Axelrod AJ, Peyman GA, Apple DJ. Toxicity of intravitreal injection of amphotericin B, *Am J Ophthalmol* (1973) **76**:578–83.
17. Axelrod AJ, Peyman GA. Intravitreal amphotericin B treatment of experimental fungal endophthalmitis, *Am J Ophthalmol* (1973) **76**:584–8.
18. Graham RO, Peyman GA. Intravitreal injection of dexamethasone: treatment of experimentally induced endophthalmitis, *Arch Ophthalmol* (1974) **92**:149–54.
19. Graham RO, Peyman GA, Fishman G. Intravitreal injection of cephaloridine in the treatment of endophthalmitis, *Arch Ophthalmol* (1975) **93**: 56–61.
20. Koziol J, Peyman G. Intraocular chloramphenicol and bacterial endophthalmitis, *Can J Ophthalmol* (1974) **9**:316–21.
21. Peyman GA, Nelsen P, Bennett TO. Intravitreal injection of kanamycin in experimentally induced endophthalmitis, *Can J Ophthalmol* (1974) **9**:322–7.
22. Nelsen P, Peyman GA, Bennett TO. BB-K8: a new aminoglycoside for intravitreal injection in bacterial endophthalmitis, *Am J Ophthalmol* (1974) **78**: 82–9.
23. Bennett TO, Peyman GA. Use of tobramycin in eradicating experimental bacterial endophthalmitis, *Albrecht von Graefes Arch Klin Exp Ophthalmol* (1974) **191**:93–107.
24. Schenk AG, Peyman GA. Lincomycin by direct intravitreal injection in the treatment of experimental bacterial endophthalmitis, *Albrecht von Graefes Arch Klin Exp Ophthalmol* (1974) **190**:281–91.

25. Bennett TO, Peyman GA. Toxicity of intravitreal aminoglycosides in primates, *Can J Ophthalmol* (1974) **9**:475–8.

26. Schenk AG, Peyman GA, Paque JT. The intravitreal use of carbenicillin (Geopen) for treatment of *Pseudomonas* endophthalmitis, *Acta Ophthalmol* (1974) **52**:707–17.

27. Paque JT, Peyman GA. Intravitreal clindamycin phosphate in the treatment of vitreous infection, *Ophthalmic Surg* (1974) **5**:34–9.

28. Daily MJ, Peyman GA, Fishman G. Intravitreal injection of methicillin for treatment of endophthalmitis, *Am J Ophthalmol* (1973) **76**:343–50.

29. Peyman GA, Herbst R. Bacterial endophthalmitis: treatment with intraocular injection of gentamicin and dexamethasone, *Arch Ophthalmol* (1974) **91**: 416–18.

30. Peyman GA, Vastine DW, Crouch ER et al. Clinical use of intravitreal antibiotics to treat bacterial endophthalmitis, *Trans Acad Ophthalmol Otolaryngol* (1974) **78**:0P862–75.

31. Vlchek JK, Peyman GA. Cephaloridine-induced retinopathy by intravitreal injection: an ultrastructural study, *Ann Ophthalmol* (1975) **7**:903–14.

32. Peyman GA. Antibiotic administration in the treatment of bacterial endophthalmitis: II. Intravitreal injections, *Surv Ophthalmol* (1977) **21**:332, 339–46.

33. Stainer GA, Peyman GA, Meisels H et al. Toxicity of selected antibiotics in vitreous replacement fluid, *Ann Ophthalmol* (1977) **9**:615–18.

34. Vastine DW, Peyman GA, Guth SB. Visual prognosis in bacterial endophthalmitis treated with intravitreal antibiotics, *Ophthalmic Surg* (1979) **10**:76–83.

35. Peyman GA. Aminoglycoside toxicity, *Arch Ophthalmol* (1992) **110**:446.

36. Kasbeer RT, Peyman GA. Intravitreal oxacillin in experimental staphylococcal endophthalmitis, *Albrecht von Graefes Arch Klin Exp Ophthalmol* (1975) **196**:279–87.

37. Peyman GA, Vastine DW, Diamond JG. Vitrectomy in exogenous *Candida* endophthalmitis, *Albrecht von Graefes Arch Klin Exp Ophthalmol* (1975) **197**:55–9.

38. Peyman GA, Raichand M, Bennett TO. Management of endophthalmitis with pars plana vitrectomy, *Br J Ophthalmol* (1980) **64**:472–5.

39. Zimmer-Galler IE, Santos A, Haller JA et al. Management of endophthalmitis in a silicone oil-filled eye, *Retina* (1997) **17**:507–9.

40. Gardner S. Treatment of bacterial endophthalmitis: Part I, *Ocular Therapy Report* (1991) **2**:1–16.

41. Schulman J, Peyman GA. Intravitreal corticosteroids as an adjunct in the treatment of bacterial and fungal endophthalmitis: a review, *Retina* (1992) **12**:336–40

42. Tauber MG, Sande MA. Pathogenesis of bacterial meningitis: contributions by experimental models in rabbits, *Infection* (1984) **12**(Suppl):S3–S10.

43. Maxwell DP Jr, Brent BD, Diamond JG et al. Effect of intravitreal dexamethasone on ocular histopathology in a rabbit model of endophthalmitis, *Ophthalmology* (1991) **98**:1370–5.

44. Peyman GA, Rose M, Sanders D. Intravitreal antibiotic injection and vitrectomy in acute bacterial endophthalmitis, *Can J Ophthalmol* (1976) **11**: 188–90.

45. Peyman GA, Vastine DW, Meisels HI. The experimental and clinical use of intravitreal antibiotics to treat bacterial and fungal endophthalmitis, *Doc Ophthalmol* (1975) **39**:183–201.

46. Schulman JA, Leveque C, Coats M et al. Fatal disseminated cryptococcosis following intraocular involvement, *Br J Ophthalmol* (1988) **72**:171–5.

47. Park SS, Samiy N, Ruoff K et al. Effect of intravitreal dexamethasone in treatment of pneumococcal endophthalmitis in rabbits, *Arch Ophthalmol* (1995) **113**:1324–9.

48. Liu SM, Way T, Rodrigues M et al. Effects of intravitreal corticosteroids in the treatment of *Bacillus cereus* endophthalmitis, *Arch Ophthalmol* (2000) **118**:803–6.

49. Turnbull PC, Kramer JM. Non-gastrointestinal *Bacillus cereus* infections: an analysis of exotoxins production by strains isolated over a two-year period, *J Clin Pathol* (1983) **36**:1091–6.

50. Beecher DJ, Pulido JS, Barney NP et al. Extracellular virulence factors in *Bacillus cereus* endophthalmitis: methods and implications of involvement of hemolysin BL, *Infect Immun* (1995) **63**:632–9.

51. Smith MA, Sorenson JA, D'Aversa G et al. Treatment of experimental methicillin-resistant *Staphylococcus epidermidis* endophthalmitis with intravitreal vancomycin and intravitreal dexamethasone, *J Infect Dis* (1997) **175**:4 62–6.

52. Kim IT, Chung KH, Koo BS. Efficacy of ciprofloxacin and dexamethasone in experimental *Pseudomonas* endophthalmitis, *Korean J Ophthalmol* (1996) **10**:8–17.

53. Yildirim O, Oz O, Aslan G et al. The efficacy of intravitreal levofloxacin and intravitreal dexamethasone in experimental *Staphylococcus epidermidis* endophthalmitis, *Ophthalmic Res* (2002) **34**:349–56.

54. Jett BD, Jensen HG, Atkuri RV et al. Evaluation of therapeutic measures for treating endophthalmitis caused by isogenic toxin-producing and toxin-nonproducing *Enterococcus faecalis* strains, *Invest Ophthalmol Vis Sci* (1995) **36**:9–15.

55. Aguilar HE, Meredith TA, Drews CD et al. Treatment of experimental *S. aureus* endophthalmitis with vancomycin, cefazolin and corticosteroids, *Invest Ophthalmol Vis Sci* (1990) **31** (Suppl):140.

56. Majji AB, Jalali S, Das T et al. Role of intravitreal dexamethasone in exogenous fungal endophthalmitis, *Eye* (1999) **13** (Pt 5):660–5.

57. Das T, Jalali S, Gothwal VK et al. Intravitreal dexamethasone in exogenous bacterial endophthalmitis: results of a prospective randomized study, *Br J Ophthalmol* (1999) **88**:1050–5.

58. Das T, Choudhury K, Sharma S et al. Clinical profile and outcome in *Bacillus* endophthalmitis, *Ophthalmology* (2001) **108**:1819–25.

59. Auclin F, Pollet E, Roman S et al. Fifty-two cases of postoperative endophthalmitis treated with one protocol: anatomical and functional results, *J Fr Ophtalmol* (2001) **24**:687–91.

60. Shah GK, Stein JD, Sharma S et al. Visual outcomes following the use of intravitreal steroids in the treatment of postoperative endophthalmitis, *Ophthalmology* (2000) **107**:486–9.

61. Harris MJ. Visual outcome after intravitreal steroid use for postoperative endophthalmitis, *Ophthalmology* (2001) **108**:240–1.

62. Park SS, Vallar RV, Hong CH et al. Intravitreal dexamethasone effect on intravitreal vancomycin elimination in endophthalmitis, *Arch Ophthalmol* (1999) **117**:1058–62.

63. Smith MA, Sorenson JA, Smith C et al. Effects of intravitreal dexamethasone on concentration of intravitreal vancomycin in experimental methicillin-resistant *Staphylococcus epidermidis* endophthalmitis, *Antimicrob Agents Chemother* (1991) **35**:1298–302.

64. Yoshizumi MO, Bhavsar AR, Dessouki A et al. Safety of repeated intravitreous injections of antibiotics and dexamethasone, *Retina* (1999) **19**:437–41.

65. Kwak HW, D'Amico DJ. Evaluation of the retinal toxicity and pharmacokinetics of dexamethasone after intravitreal injection, *Arch Ophthalmol* (1992) **110**: 259–66.

66. Nabih M, Peyman GA, Tawakol ME et al. Toxicity of high-dose intravitreal dexamethasone, *Int Ophthalmol* (1991) **15**: 233–5.

67. Short C, Keates RH, Donovan EF et al. Ocular penetration studies: 1. Topical administration of dexamethasone, *Arch Ophthalmol* (1966) **75**: 689–92.

68. Yoshizumi MO, Lee GC, Equi RA et al. Timing of dexamethasone treatment in experimental *Staphylococcus aureus* endophthalmitis, *Retina* (1998) **18**:130–5.

69. Peyman GA, Vastine DW, Raichand M. Symposium: post-operative endophthalmitis. Experimental aspects and their clinical application, *Ophthalmology* (1978) **85**:374–85.

70. Meredith TA, Aguilar HE, Drews C et al. Intraocular dexamethasone produces a harmful effect on treatment of experimental *Staphylococcus aureus* endophthalmitis, *Trans Am Ophthalmol Soc* (1996) **94**:241–57.

71. Doft BH, Wisniewski SR, Kelsey SF et al. The Endophthalmitis Vitrectomy Study Group. Diabetes and postoperative endophthalmitis in the Endophthalmitis Vitrectomy Study, *Arch Ophthalmol* (2001) **119**:650–6.

72. Wisniewski SR, Hammer ME, Grizzard WS et al. An investigation of the hospital charges related to the treatment of endophthalmitis in the Endophthalmitis Vitrectomy Study, *Ophthalmology* (1997) **104**:739–45.

73. Barza M, Pavan PR, Doft BH et al. Evaluation of microbiological diagnostic techniques in postoperative endophthalmitis in the Endophthalmitis Vitrectomy Study, *Arch Ophthalmol* (1997) **115**: 1142–50.

74. McGetrick JJ, Peyman GA. Vitrectomy in experimental endophthalmitis. Part II: Bacterial endophthalmitis, *Ophthalmic Surg* (1979) **10**:87–92.

75. Peyman GA, Paque JT, Meisels HI et al. Postoperative endophthalmitis: a comparison of methods for treatment and prophylaxis with gentamicin, *Ophthalmic Surg* (1975) **6**:45–55.

76. Peyman GA, Schulman JA. *Intravitreal Surgery: Principles and Practice*, 1st edn (Appleton-Century-Crofts: Norwalk, CT, 1986) 435.

77. Peyman GA, Vastine DW, Meisels HI. The experimental and clinical use of intravitreal antibiotics to treat bacterial and fungal endophthalmitis, *Doc Ophthalmol* (1975) **39**:183–201.

78. Zachary IG, Forster RK. Experimental intravitreal gentamicin, *Am J Ophthalmol* (1976) **82**:604–11.

79. Homer P, Peyman GA, Koziol J et al. Intravitreal injection of vancomycin in experimental staphylococcal endophthalmitis, *Acta Ophthalmol* (1975) **53**:311–20.

80. Benz MS, Scott IU, Flynn HW Jr et al. Endophthalmitis isolates and antibiotic sensitivities: a 6-year review of culture-proven cases, *Am J Ophthalmol* (2004) **137**:38–42.

81. Eifrig CW, Scott IU, Flynn HW Jr et al. Endophthalmitis caused by *Pseudomonas aeruginosa*, *Ophthalmology* (2003) **110**:1714–17.

82. Peyman GA, Schulman JA. *Intravitreal Surgery: Principles and Practice*, 2nd edn (Appleton & Lange: Norwalk, CT, 1994) 897.

9

Endogenous endophthalmitis

Endogenous or metastatic endophthalmitis, a severe vision-threatening intraocular infection, occurs through hematogenous dissemination from a concurrent infection in the host or an external source such as a catheter or an intravenous needle. Endogenous bacterial infection is relatively rare, accounting for 2–8% of all cases.[1] The incidence rate of endogenous fungal endophthalmitis has been estimated in the past to range from 9% to 45% of patients with disseminated fungal infection or fungemia.[2-6] However, recent studies have reported an incidence of 2% or 2.8%.[7,8]

In an 18-year review between 1982 and 2000 at the Cleveland Clinic, a tertiary care center, the average occurrence for their unit was 1.8 cases per year.[9] Ninety per cent of patients were diagnosed with medical conditions including diabetes, hypertension, gastrointestinal disorders, cardiac disorders, malignancy, and immunosuppression or prolonged surgical complications. Acute ocular symptoms, rather than systemic symptoms, were the most common reasons for presenting to the physician. This situation has now changed with early aggressive systemic antifungal chemotherapy for either growth of fungi from blood cultures or local sites of fungal infection thought on clinical criteria to be disseminated.[8]

Because of the rapid advance of medical technology, a longer lifespan of patients with chronic diseases, and a rising prevalence of long-term intravenous access, the disease may become more common in clinical practice – albeit less common in those with organ transplants and immunosuppression, as the result of early ophthalmologic screening of all susceptible patients.[7]

Endogenous endophthalmitis is most commonly caused by fungi. Fungal organisms account for more than 50% of all cases of endogenous endophthalmitis. *Candida albicans* is by far the most frequent cause (75–80% of fungal cases) followed by *Aspergillus* spp. A review of the literature

Table 9.1 Endophthalmitis in candidemia

Series	No. of cases with candidemia	No. of cases with classic retinal lesions	Incidence of retinal lesions (%)
Klein et al, 1979[10]	21	11	53
Henderson et al, 1981[11]	9	7	78
Parke et al, 1982[4]	27	10	37
Harvey and Myers, 1987[12]	43	2	5
Brooks, 1989[5]	32	9	28
Binder et al, 2003[9]	10	6	60
Total	142	45	Mean = 32%

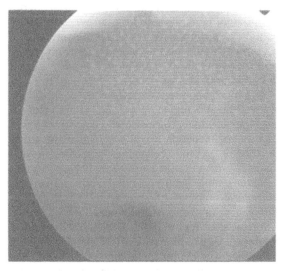

Figure 9.1

Vitreous condensation in endogenous endophthalmitis of an immunosuppressed patient.

reveals that endophthalmitis occurs in 5–78% of patients with candidemia (Table 9.1);[4,5,9–12] however, this probably reflects the catchment population of the reporting hospital, particularly if it has an organ transplant unit with highly immunosuppressed patients (Figure 9.1).

Aspergillosis is the second most common cause of fungal endophthalmitis, especially in intravenous drug users. Less frequent are *Candida* spp. other than *C. albicans*, *Torulopsis glabrata*, *Cryptococcus neoformans*, *Sporothrix schenckii*, *Scedosporium apiospermum* (*Pseudallescheria boydii*), *Blastomyces dermatitidis*, *Coccidiodes immitis*, and *Mucor*. The incidence of endogenous fungal endophthalmitis has increased significantly in recent years. From 1980 to 1989, the incidence of bloodstream infection from *Candida* spp. reported by the Centers for Disease Control and Prevention increased fivefold for large teaching hospitals and tertiary care centers and has continued today.

Bacterial infections

Individuals who develop endogenous bacterial endophthalmitis tend to have conditions either associated with immunosuppression or predisposing to infection. These causes include diabetes, leukemia, lymphoma, asplenia, hypogammaglobulinemia, bone marrow transplant, acquired immunodeficiency syndrome (AIDS), systemic lupus erythematosus, chronic alcoholism, generalized debility and aging, steroid use, and prematurity.

The most important host sources of infectious agents include endocarditis, the gastrointestinal tract, genitourinary tract, skin and wound infection, pulmonary infections, meningitis, and septic arthritis (Box 9.1). Other predisposing factors include invasive procedures, such as hemodialysis, bladder catheterization, gastrointestinal endoscopy, total parenteral nutrition, chemotherapy, dental procedures, and intravenous drug abuse.

Bacterial endophthalmitis is bilateral in approximately 14–25% of cases. In bilateral infection, simultaneous ocular involvement is the rule; however, one eye is characteristically more severely affected than the other. Delayed involvement of the second eye can occur even in patients already being treated with systemic antibiotics.

Box 9.1 Sources of bacterial infection

- Endocarditis
- Gastrointestinal tract
- Genitourinary tract
- Pulmonary infection
- Meningitis
- Septic arthritis
- Hemodialysis
- Septicemia
- Dental procedure
- Chemotherapy

The right eye is involved twice as often as the left, probably because of this eye's proximity and more direct blood flow from the right carotid artery. There is no gender predisposition.

Fungal infections

Candida spp. are the most frequent cause of endogenous fungal endophthalmitis. A review of the literature (Table 9.2)[4,5,9,10–12] shows that *C. albicans* is by far the most common pathogen. Other fungi less frequently implicated include *Aspergillus*, *Cryptococcus*, *Scedosporium apiospermum* (*Pseudallescheria*), *Sporothrix*, *Blastomyces*, *Histoplasma*, *Coccidioides*, *Fusarium*, and *Penicillium* spp., as listed in Table 9.3.[13–70]

Risk factors

Multiple risk factors predispose to the development of endogenous fungal endophthalmitis. In a review of 76 cases of candidal endophthalmitis, Edwards et al found the following associations[67]:

- 84% had intravenous antibiotics. Antibiotic use allowed *Candida* superinfection in the gastrointestinal tract and elsewhere. Investigators also noted that certain antibiotics enhanced candidal growth *in vitro*.
- 63% of affected individuals had undergone major surgery. Surgery in areas such as the gastrointestinal tract enables hematogenous seeding both pre- and postoperatively when tissues such as the intestinal mucosa experience circulation compromise, predisposing to

Table 9.2 Types of *Candida* infection

Reference	No. of cases with endophthalmitis	Frequency per species (%)				
		C. albicans	C. tropicalis	C. glabrata	C. parapsilosis	Other species
Klein et al, 1979[10]	11	81	0	19	0	0
Henderson et al, 1981[11]	7	100	0	0	0	0
Parke et al, 1982[4]	11	91	9	0	0	0
Harvey and Myers, 1987[12]	2	50	50	0	0	0
Brooks, 1989[5]	9	67	0	0	1	2
Binder et al, 2003[9]	10	10	0	0	0	0

Table 9.3 Endogenous fungal infection in endophthalmitis

Reference	Type of fungus (no. of infected patients)	Source	Age of patient (years)	Place
Arroyo et al, 2004[13]	Candida albicans (1, bilateral)	Candidemia due to infected subclavicular venous thrombosis. Bilateral vitrectomy and membrane peeling for macular traction retinal detachments. Retinal granuloma excised from one eye. Vision improved	43	Boston, MA, USA
Schelenz and Goldstein, 2003[14]	Aspergillus fumigatus (2)	Polycystic kidney disease	47, 56	London, UK
Binder et al, 2003[9]	Candida albicans (10) Aspergillus fumigatus (3) Pseudallescheria boydii (1)	Cancer, diabetes, and immunosuppression in a tertiary care center	30–85	Cleveland, OH, USA
Dorey et al, 2002[15]	Rhodotorula glutinis	IV drug abuse, HIV, hepatitis C	26	Ottawa, Canada
Feman et al, 2002[7]	Candida albicans (2)	Disseminated fungal infection, cirrhosis	46/NG	St Louis, MO, USA
Castiglioni et al, 2002[16]	Pseudallescheria boydii (1)	Organ transplant recipient with review of the literature with 23 cases of disseminated infection without endophthalmitis	58	Pittsburgh, PA, USA
Nishio et al, 2002[17]	Fusarium solani (1)	Lymphoblastic leukemia	56	Shiga, Japan
Tsai-Chia-Chen et al, 2002[18]	Candida albicans (1)	Postpartum	33	Taiwan, China
Kou et al, 2001[19]	Candida spp. (1)	?	55	Chang Gung, China
Bhansali et al, 2001[20]	Mucor (1)	Diabetes (type 2)	NG	Chandigarh, India
Rao and Hidayat, 2001[21]	Candida spp. (13) Aspergillus spp. (12)	Clinical and histopathologic study. Candida in patients with gastrointestinal tract surgery, diabetes mellitus, or IV feeding lines. Aspergillus in patients with organ transplant or cardiac surgery	NG	Los Angeles, CA, USA
Gonzales et al, 2000[22]	Histoplasma capsulatum (1, bilateral)	AIDS with skin histoplasmosis	30	Miami, FL, USA
Ohnishi et al, 1999[23]	Candida sp. (1, bilateral)	Liver dysfunction, IV hyperalimentation	53	Wakayama, Japan
Li et al, 1998[24]	Blastomyces dermatitidis (1)	Pulmonary TB, painful eye, decreasing vision	29	Chicago, IL, USA

continued

Table 9.3 Endogenous fungal infection in endophthalmitis – *continued*

Reference	Type of fungus (no. of infected patients)	Source	Age of patient (years)	Place
Weishaar et al, 1998[25]	Aspergillus (10)	Retrospective review of 12 eyes from 10 patients: 7 intravenous drug abusers, 3 chronic respiratory disease on corticosteroids	31–91	Miami, FL, USA
Seal et al, 1998[26]	*Candida albicans* (1, bilateral)	Postpartum following contaminated blood transfusion. Misdiagnosis as Behçet's disease. Given steroids with resulting blindness	35	Amman, Jordan
Sheu et al, 1998[27]	*Cryptococcus neoformans* (1)	SLE on corticosteroids and cytotoxic drugs	45	Kaohsiung, Taiwan
Okhravi et al, 1997[28]	*Paecilomyces lilacinus* (1)	Endogenous endophthalmitis with secondary pupillary block glaucoma and corneal invasion requiring a PK. No known trauma	34	London, UK
Hutnik et al, 1997[29]	*Aspergillus fumigatus* (1)	Pneumonia 1 week previously given antibiotics. Autopsy-proven orbital aspergillosis. Death due to invasion of internal carotid artery wall	75	London, Canada
Scherer and Lee, 1997[8]	*Candida albicans* (3)	Systemic fungus infection in 107 patients, 3 with chorioretinitis consistent with the early diagnosis of endophthalmitis without vitreous seeding. Leukemia, rheumatoid arthritis, gastrointestinal tract surgery	34, 56, 65	Ann Arbor, MI, USA
Essman et al, 1997[30]	*Candida* spp. (17) *Aspergillus* spp. (3)	Treatment outcome in a 10-year study. Culture-proven in 20 eyes of 18 patients. Recommend vitrectomy for vitreous infiltrates with intravitreal amphotericin and systemic therapy (fluconazole for *Candida*)	21–88	Miami, FL, USA
Glasgow et al, 1996[31]	*Fusarium* sp. (1, bilateral)	AIDS, CMV retinitis. Intravitreal and IV amphotericin B; pars plana vitrectomy; IV fluconazole but enucleation needed prior to death	51	Los Angeles, CA, USA
Hunt and Glasgow, 1996[32]	Aspergillus (7) and review of all reported cases of endogenous *Aspergillus* endophthalmitis up to 1995	Orthotopic liver transplantations, only diagnosed in one patient before death from systemic infection	35–63	Los Angeles, CA, USA
Jampol et al, 1996[33]	*Candida albicans* (6)	Crohn's disease, other surgery and use of steroids. Choroidal neovascularization following choroidoretinitis with late visual loss	18–79	Chicago, IL, USA
Zarbin et al, 1996[34]	Presumed Candida (2)	Diabetes (2)	75, 71	New Jersey/San Francisco, USA
Henderson and Irfan, 1996[35]	*Candida albicans* (1, bilateral)	Bilateral endophthalmitis with chorioretinitis following toxic megacolon due to *Salmonella* gastroenteritis	61	Hull, UK
Matsuo et al, 1995[36]	*Aspergillus flavus* (1)	Severe periodontitis	64	Okayama City, Japan
Graham et al, 1995[37]	Aspergillus (1)	Lung transplantation and immunosuppression	29	Seattle, WA, USA
Custis et al, 1995[38]	*Cryptococcus laurentii* (1), and review of 22 cases (7 unilateral, 12 bilateral, 3 not known)	Chronic uveitis and retinal detachment repair with diagnosis by vitreous biopsy (oral fluconazole for 5 months). Only 6 of 22 reviewed cases were diagnosed antemortem without enucleation	61	Baltimore, MD, USA

continued

Table 9.3 Endogenous fungal infection in endophthalmitis – *continued*

Reference	Type of fungus (no. of infected patients)	Source	Age of patient (years)	Place
Yohai et al, 1994[39]	*Rhizopus arrhizus* (6) *Rhizopus* sp. *Mucor ramosissimus*	Rhino-orbital-cerebral mucormycosis in 6 cases with diabetes mellitus. No AIDS cases. Reviewed 208 cases since 1970. Early diagnosis needed to treat and cure infection	56–75	Ohio, USA
Donahue et al, 1994[42]	*Candida albicans* (10) *Torulopsis glabrata* (1)	Chorioretinitis in 9% of 118 patients with candidemia	NG	Pittsburgh, PA, USA
Pavan and Curtis, 1993[40]	*Bipolaris hawaiiensis* (1)	AIDS. Intravitreal and IV amphotericin B; pars plana vitrectomy; oral fluconazole	26	Tampa, FL, USA
Nakazawa et al, 1992[41]	Mixed hyaline fungi (6)	Systemic fungus infection in tumor patients in which 6/84 developed endophthalmitis	NG	Juntendo, Japan
Crump et al, 1992[42]	*Cryptococcus neoformans* (1) + review of 26 cases over the last 23 years	Elderly patient with ECCE/IOL 5 years previously	84	Ann Arbor, MI, USA
Greenwald et al, 1992[43]	*Candida albicans* (1)	Diabetes mellitus, urinary tract infection with *Candida albicans* and lithotripsy	58	Charlottes-ville, VA, USA
McGuire et al, 1991[44]	*Pseudallescheria boydii* (7)	Review of 17 cases of oculomycosis: 7 had endogenous endophthalmitis (2 anterior segment, 5 posterior) and 12 had exogenous infection (Chapter 6)	15–49	Dayton, OH, USA
Pfeifer et al, 1991[45]	*Pseudallescheria boydii* (2)	Pulmonary fibrosis; cardiac transplant	45, 52	St Louis, MO, USA
Denning et al, 1991[46]	*Cryptococcus neoformans* (1) with review of 20 cases, 5 with AIDS	AIDS. Bilateral retinal lesions with hemorrhages 2 weeks after meningitis occurred. Responded well to itraconazole for 3 months	31	San Jose, CA, USA
Safnek et al, 1990[47]	*Blastomyces dermatitidis* (1)	Severe acute and chronic granulomatous and nongranulomatous endophthalmitis with no evidence of systemic disease. Not responsive to therapy; enucleated	71	Winnipeg, Canada
Clinch et al, 1989[48]	*Candida albicans* (1)	Disseminated candidemia	1	Philadelphia, PA, USA
Khurana et al, 1989[49]	Aspergillus (1)	Fungi in anterior and posterior segments and crystalline lens. Acute renal failure, septicemia, and thrombophlebitis. 25 cases of intralens infection reported and reviewed worldwide	45	Rohtuk, India
Brooks, 1989[5]	*Candida albicans* (6) *Candida parapsilosis* (2) *Candida glabrata* (1)	Hospitalized patients with candidemia over 2 years; 8/63 patients had chorioretinitis. Patients had alcohol abuse, diabetes, cancer. Screen all patients with candidemia for early retinal signs	56 (mean)	Orlando, FL, USA
Kurosawa et al, 1988[50]	*Sporothrix schenckii* (1)	AIDS with disseminated cutaneous sporotrichosis. IV, intravitreal, and intracameral amphotericin B; potassium iodide with treatment failure needing enucleation	30	Chicago, IL, USA
Silva et al, 1988[51]	Paracoccidioidomycosis (1)	Complication of anterior uveitis, and involvement of lids and conjunctiva	33	Sao Paulo, Brazil
Hiss et al, 1988[52]	*Cryptococcus neoformans* (1)	Polyarteritis nodosa and long-term steroids. Solitary, 'fluffy' vitreoretinal mass	63	Philadelphia, PA, USA
Weiss et al, 1988[53]	Aspergillus (1)	Simultaneous *Aspergillus* endophthalmitis and CMV retinitis after kidney transplantation	34	Boston, MA, USA

continued

Table 9.3 Endogenous fungal infection in endophthalmitis – *continued*

Reference	Type of fungus (no. of infected patients)	Source	Age of patient (years)	Place
Harvey et al, 1987[12]	Candida albicans (1) Candida tropicalis (1)	8–fold increase in hospital-acquired fungemia with *C. albicans* 58%, *C. tropicalis* 25%, and *C. parapsilosis* 15% contributing to a 75% mortality rate	20–59	Youngstown, OH, USA
Henderly et al, 1987[54]	Cryptococcus neoformans (1)	Hydrocephalus, meningitis, and bilateral chorioretinitis and endophthalmitis. Cultured from vitreous and CSF. Vitrectomy, intravitreal and systemic amphotericin needed	?	USA
Lance et al, 1988[55]	Aspergillus flavus (1)	IV drug abuser	35	Pittsburgh, PA, USA
Swan et al, 1985[56]	Penicillium sp. (1)	IV drug abuse. *Penicillium* sp. isolated from vitreous aspirate. Sterilization of vitreous with amphotericin and flucytosine but loss of light perception	30	Rootstown, OH, USA
Furia et al, 1984[57]	Candida albicans (bilateral)	Heroin addict	27	France
Baley et al, 1984[58]	Torulopsis glabrata (1)	Necrotizing enterocolitis	?	Cleveland, OH, USA
Wilmarth et al, 1983[59]	Aspergillus fumigatus (1)	IV drug abuse with *A. fumigatus* cultured from drug storage vial and vitreous biopsy	27	Sacramento, CA, USA
Parke et al, 1982[4]	Candida albicans (9) Candida tropicalis (1)	Endogenous endophthalmitis among patients with candidemia	NG	Houston, TX, USA
Henderson et al, 1981[11]	Candida albicans (7)	Associated with parenteral hyperalimentation in hospital with contamination of IV lines. 13/131 developed chorioretinitis due to *Candida* spp. of whom 7 had candidemia	NG	Downey, USA
Weis et al, 1981[60]	Cryptococcus neoformans (1)	Endophthalmitis without other CNS involvement. Chronic active hepatitis on prednisone	NG	Lafayette, USA
Shields et al, 1980[61]	Cryptococcus neoformans (1, bilateral)	Obstructive hydrocephalus. Initial diagnosis of toxoplasmosis retinochoroiditis	40	Philadelphia, PA, USA
Palmer, 1980[62]	Candida (1)	Infant with endophthalmitis	1	USA
Peyman et al, 1980[63]	Candida spp. (4)	IV heroin injections ×4	NG	Chicago, IL, USA
Aguilar et al, 1979[64]	Candida albicans (2)	IV drug abuse	25, 21	Stanford, USA
Snip and Michels, 1976[65]	Candida albicans (1)	IV drug abuse	27	Baltimore, MD, USA
Naidoff and Green, 1975[66]	Aspergillus spp. (2) with review of 15 cases; 3 had undergone renal transplantation	*Aspergillus* in vitreous cavity or retina (10), choroid (6), anterior segment (2) and in all areas (2) occurring after kidney transplantation	26, 29	Philadelphia, PA, USA
Edwards et al, 1974[67]	34 cases of Candida endophthalmitis & review of 42 cases in literature	Hematogenous *Candida* endophthalmitis. Recommended screening of patients with candidemia	9 months to 91	Los Angeles, CA, USA
Griffin et al, 1973[68]	Candida albicans (6) plus 15 cases of Candida albicans endophthalmitis diagnosed postmortem	Complications from general surgery with IV therapy. Presented with chorioretinitis lesions and hemorrhage, vitreous haze, and anterior uveitis. Of 15 post-mortem cases, only 2 were diagnosed ante-mortem	NG	Los Angeles, CA, USA
Wålinder and Kock, 1971[69]	Aspergillus sp. (1) Candida sp. (1)	?	50+	Denmark

continued

Table 9.3 Endogenous fungal infection in endophthalmitis – *continued*

Reference	Type of fungus (no. of infected patients)	Source	Age of patient (years)	Place
Tarkkanen et al, 1967[70]	*Candida albicans* (1)	?	5	Finland

CMV, cytomegalovirus; CSF, cerebrospinal fluid; ECCE, extracapsular cataract extraction; GI, gastrointestinal; IOL, intraocular lens; IV, intravenous; NG, not given; PK, penetrating keratoplasty; SLE, systemic lupus erythematosus; TB, tuberculosis.

infiltration by *Candida* spp. Additionally, the patient is more likely to undergo prolonged intravenous antibiotic administration postoperatively.

- 46% of patients had intravenous catheters.
- 88% of patients received some form of intravenous infusion. The intravenous catheters predispose the patient to infection with *Candida* spp. followed by hematogenous seeding.
- 54% of patients were either treated with steroids before the development of endophthalmitis or steroids were initiated when the ocular disease was diagnosed.
- 8% received therapy with other immunosuppressive agents before the onset of endophthalmitis. The immune system is a natural defense system against candidal infection; immunosuppressive therapy predisposes the individual (Chapter 2).

Additionally, several patients in this series had diseases associated with impaired host defenses such as diabetes, malignancy, liver disease (cirrhosis or hepatitis), and alcoholism.

Tanaka et al retrospectively analyzed predisposing factors for the development of endogenous fungal endophthalmitis in 79 eyes of 46 patients over a 12-year period between 1986 and 1998.[71] The authors found that a similar rate (87%) of patients received intravenous hyperalimentation before the development of endogenous fungal endophthalmitis. Disease onset was 11 days from the initiation of intravenous hyperalimentation. The authors found additional correlations:

- β-D-glucan ≥20 pg (90%) – a test for deep mycoses
- Fever of unknown origin (76%)

- Male gender (74%)
- Presence of cancer (72%)
- Neutrophils ≤500/ml (67%) – a test for deep mycoses
- Cand-tec ≥ × 4 (57%) – a test for deep mycoses.

Intravenous drug abuse is associated with the development of *Candida* endophthalmitis. The source of the fungus is either drug paraphernalia or contaminated illegal drugs. Interestingly, pure heroin inhibits the growth of *C. albicans*. The endophthalmitis is characteristically associated with only a transient or no fungal septicemia (candidemia). The patients tend to be young and, if confirmation of systemic infection is needed, the organisms can often be cultured from cutaneous lesions.

Several reports document the occurrence of endogenous fungal endophthalmitis in neonates. Palmer noted that premature and newborn infants were at high risk for developing endogenous *Candida* endophthalmitis.[62] Several factors that place these neonates at increased risk were identified:

- Newborn leukocytes are less lethal to *C. albicans*
- Deficient host immune system found in newborns
- Inadequate anatomic barriers (skin, mucosa, gastrointestinal mucosa) to resist fungal invasion from surface colonization
- Intravenous hyperalimentation, indwelling catheters, broad-spectrum antibiotic use, and previous surgery, especially abdominal procedures.

Identification and screening of infants at high risk for developing *Candida* endophthalmitis is recommended. Regular assessment should result in prompt diagnosis and treatment of this infection, leading to good ocular outcomes in these patients.

Factors that alter natural tissue barriers and replace the normal bacterial flora with fungal organisms promote tissue invasion. Factors that promote the growth of Candida spp. on mucosal surfaces include:

- Corticosteroid use in diabetic individuals which increases glucose levels, a nutrient important for the growth of Candida spp.
- Ileus accompanying gastrointestinal disease and surgery which promotes fungal overgrowth
- Use of broad-spectrum antibiotics which promote growth of Candida spp. by killing normal bacterial microflora.

Other risk factors include the use of radiation and chemotherapy in the treatment of malignancies, parental hyperalimentation, indwelling bladder catheters, and debilitation.

Edwards et al demonstrated that endogenous Candida endophthalmitis was associated with evidence of other organ involvement in 79% of autopsies performed on patients with candidemia.[67] However, in a prospective study, Parke et al found that endophthalmitis developed in 37% of patients with C. albicans fungemia.[4] In another prospective study, Brooks found that 28% of patients with Candida sepsis developed candidal endogenous endophthalmitis.[5]

These studies included patients with a variety of ocular lesions not necessarily indicating vitreous cavity involvement, but associated with candidiasis. In contrast, in another prospective multicenter study, Donahue et al found that of 118 patients with candidemia, Candida chorioretinitis developed in 9% of patients; however, no patients progressed to Candida endophthalmitis.[2] This study employed a tighter definition of endophthalmitis as either Candida chorioretinitis with extension of the inflammatory process into the vitreous or vitreous abscesses presenting as intravitreal fluff balls.

In all cases of chorioretinitis, treatment with systemic amphotericin B resulted in resolution of the lesions without vitreous involvement. Risk factors for the development of Candida chorioretinitis in this series included multiple positive blood cultures, immunosuppression, fungemia

with C. albicans versus other species, and visual symptoms. The investigators concluded that frequent ocular examination of patients demonstrating candidemia with these risk factors should result in prompt diagnosis of candidal chorioretinitis. Treatment of candidal chorioretinitis with systemic amphotericin B should keep the infection confined to the posterior uvea, preventing extension of the infection into the vitreous cavity. A full list of fungi that cause chorioretinitis is given in Table 9.4.[72-87]

Scherer and Lee found a much lower rate of endophthalmitis (2.8%) in patients with nosocomial systemic fungal infections.[8] The investigators attributed this low incidence to a recent change in treatment protocol. Previously, ophthalmic consultation was obtained so that a diagnosis of fungal endophthalmitis could be used as an indicator of deep, systemic fungal disease, which would justify treatment with systemic antifungal agents. Physicians were reluctant to start patients on amphotericin B with only positive blood cultures or a presumptive diagnosis of deep tissue fungal infection because some patients were reported to recover spontaneously and because use of this antifungal agent was associated with serious hematologic and renal toxicity. With greater physician experience, systemic antifungal therapy is being initiated in the presence of a single positive blood culture. More than 90% of patients in this series were receiving systemic antifungal agents at the time of ocular examination. Screening of susceptible patients at an early stage is also taking place and is well justified.

Pathophysiology

In contrast to exogenous infection where the organisms are introduced directly into the vitreous, pathogens in endogenous endophthalmitis become lodged in the small vessels of the retina or choroid. Retinitis, choroiditis, retinochoroiditis, chorioretinitis, endophthalmitis, and panophthalmitis then result from infectious seeding. Secondary extension into the retina and vitreous may follow with further propagation of the organism. The blood–ocular barrier is broken down by the inflammation elicited by the embolus. The organisms then spread to contiguous perivascular tissue, stimulating a further inflammatory

Table 9.4 Fungal causes of chorioretinitis, excluding cases caused by *Candida albicans*

Reference	Type of fungus (no. of infected patients)	Source	Age of patient (years)	Place
Spencer et al, 2003[72]	*Histoplasma capsulatum* (1)	Bilateral chronic histoplasmosis syndrome. Development of nested PCR for DNA diagnosis in an enucleated eye	?	San Francisco, CA, USA
Kiratli et al, 2001[73]	*Scedosporium apiospermum* (1)	Painless loss of vision with lymphadenopathy, misdiagnosed as tuberculous lymphadenitis, in an immunocompetent woman. Responded well to oral itraconazole 200 mg b.i.d. for 1 year	24	Ankara, Turkey
Gonzales et al, 2000[22]	*Histoplasma capsulatum* (1, bilateral)	AIDS. Endogenous endophthalmitis with subretinal exudation, choroidal granulomas, intraretinal hemorrhage, exudative bilateral retinal detachment. Vitrectomy (culture positive), intravitreal amphotericin, CF and 20/300	25	Miami, FL, USA
Anteby et al, 1997[74]	*Aspergillus fumigatus* (1)	Necrotizing chorioretinitis as a presenting symptom of disseminated aspergillosis after lung transplantation. Aggressive endophthalmitis after 24 hours followed by rapid death. Vitreous tap culture was positive	27	Jerusalem, Israel
Yau et al, 1996[75]	*Histoplasma capsulatum* (1)	Unilateral optic neuritis, AIDS and disseminated histoplasmosis	35	Washington, DC, USA
Morinelli et al, 1993[76]	*Candida* spp. (1, bilateral) *Cryptococcus neoformans* (7, 4 bilateral) *Aspergillus fumigatus* (1) *Histoplasma capsulatum* (1, bilateral) *Toxoplasma gondii* (1) *Pneumocystis carinii* (5), *Mycobacterium tuberculosis* (1) and *M. avium-intra-cellulare* (1)	470 autopsy eyes examined of 235 patients who died with AIDS. 18 cases of choroiditis of whom 15 died due to dissemination with the same organism. 5/18 had co-infection with CMV in the retina of one eye	28–49	Los Angeles, CA, USA
Specht et al, 1991[77]	Histoplasmosis (1)	Retinitis with AIDS, disseminated histoplasmosis and CMV pneumonitis	29	Washington, DC, USA
Dantas et al, 1990[78]	*Paracoccidioides brasiliensis* (1)	Fatal infection with meningoencephalitis	39	Rio de Janeiro, Brazil
Golden et al, 1986[79]	*Coccidioides immitis* (1) and review of literature for 15 cases	Disseminated infection with ocular involvement in a Mexican infant	7 weeks	Tucson, AZ, USA
Macher et al, 1985[80]	*Histoplasma capsulatum* (1, bilateral))	Disseminated infection in AIDS. Post-mortem specimen	31	Washington, DC, USA
Scholz et al, 1984[81]	*Histoplasma capsulatum* (1)	Chronic alcoholism, heroin abuse, renal failure and transplantation with immunosuppression. Post-mortem specimen	39	Baltimore, MD, USA
Schwarz et al, 1977[82]	*Histoplasma capsulatum* (1) and review of literature for 5 cases	Post-mortem specimen. Histoplasma cells in vessels of the choroid. Other cases had yeast-laden macrophages in choroidal vessels with or without a granulomatous response	3	Cincinnati, OH, USA
Chapman-Smith, 1977[83]	*Cryptococcus neoformans* (1)	Worked in a tower inhabited by pigeons Necrotizing choroidoretinitis. No primary or disseminated infection.	27	Melbourne, Australia

continued

Table 9.4 Fungal causes of chorioretinitis, excluding cases caused by *Candida albicans* – continued

Reference	Type of fungus (no. of infected patients)	Source	Age of patient (years)	Place
Font and Jakobiec, 1976[84]	*Sporotrichum schenkii* (1)	*S. schenkii* detected by immunofluorescence. Granulomatous inflammation with foreign body giant cells	42	Washington, DC, USA
Craig and Suie, 1974[85]	*Histoplasma capsulatum* (1)	Postmortem specimen. Fatal disseminated infection. Histoplasma cells cultured from choroid and retina. Identified by light and electron microscopy within cytoplasm of macrophages in the choroid	22	Columbus, OH, USA
Klintworth et al, 1973[86]	*Histoplasma capsulatum* (1)	Post-mortem specimen. Granulomatous choroiditis with fatal disseminated infection	14	Durham, NC, USA
Cameron and Harrison, 1970[87]	*Cryptococcus neoformans* (2)	Chorioretinitis (1), papilledema (1)	64, 29	Brisbane, Australia

CF, counting fingers; CMV, cytomegalovirus; PCR, polymerase chain reaction.

response. The vascular nature of endogenous endophthalmitis renders it more susceptible to systemic antibiotics. In contrast, exogenous endophthalmitis presents a difficult target for systemic antibiotics alone because the organisms are directly introduced into the vitreous cavity. Therapy usually requires intravitreal antibiotics, sometimes combined with vitrectomy.

The unimpeded infection spreads into the adjacent fluid compartment and may present as a focus of diffuse infection. In diffuse posterior endophthalmitis and panophthalmitis, large metastatic bacterial emboli may lodge in the central retinal artery, causing ischemic retinal necrosis with irreversible tissue damage and limiting the eye's functional response to treatment. The emboli break up and lodge in smaller retinal vessels with a resultant severe inflammatory tissue reaction leading to further irreversible tissue damage. Ocular damage occurs from the pathogen or from inflammatory mediators.

Clinical manifestations

A high degree of suspicion is required to make an early diagnosis of endogenous endophthalmitis so as to maximize the visual outcome. In addition to the ocular findings, it is essential to assess the clinical manifestations of the debilitating conditions such as endocarditis which cause the initial infection and allow it to propagate. Therefore, routine vital signs and physical examination may be warranted in the office and in conjunction with the patient's primary physician.

Patients commonly complain of eye pain, blurring of vision, ocular discharge, and photophobia. A comprehensive ophthalmic examination including visual acuity, intraocular pressure, pupillary reaction, slit-lamp examination for inflammation, and dilated fundus examination is performed. Early in the disease, Roth's spots (round, white retinal spots surrounded by hemorrhage) and retinal periphlebitis may be seen on fundus examination. Later in the disease, obvious signs such as chemosis, proptosis, and hypopyon may be manifest. Ultrasonography is performed when a clinical examination is inadequate or to supplement clinical findings. Clinicians must be more aware of the need to examine the eyes of extremely ill and sedated patients, such as those in intensive care units.

Fungal endophthalmitis may present acutely or as an indolent course over days to weeks. A history of penetrating injury with a plant substance or soil-contaminated foreign body might be elicited (Chapter 6). Individuals with candidal infections may present with high fever, followed several days later by ocular symptoms. Pyrexia of unknown origin may be associated with an occult retinochoroidal fungal infiltrate.

Bacterial endophthalmitis

Historically, *Neisseria meningitidis* was the most common bacterial organism associated with infectious endophthalmitis until the 1940s. With the introduction of antibiotics such as penicillin and the sulfonamides, and prompt diagnosis and treatment of associated endophthalmitis, *N. meningitidis* is isolated less frequently today. Nonetheless, it still occurs and bilateral endophthalmitis can be the presenting sign of a meningococcal septicemia without meningitis.[88-91]

Gram-positive organisms are most common among bacterial etiologies of endogenous endophthalmitis, especially the streptococcal species. *Staphylococcus aureus* is the most commonly isolated organism and is implicated with skin infections or chronic systemic disease, such as diabetes mellitus or renal failure. Streptococcal species include *Strep. pneumoniae* and *Strep. viridans*, and Lancefield group A beta-hemolytic streptococci (BHS) are also common. Other streptococcal species such as group B in newborns with meningitis or group G BHS in elderly patients with wound infections or malignancies have also been isolated. *Bacillus cereus* has been implicated in intravenous drug abuse and intravenous injections. *Streptococcus bovis* and *Clostridium* spp. have been implicated in association with bowel carcinomas.

Greenwald et al found *B. cereus* to be the most common bacterium associated with endogenous bacterial endophthalmitis.[92] However, others have cited *Streptococcus* spp. including *Strep. pneumoniae*, *Klebsiella pneumoniae*, and formerly opportunistic organisms of low pathogenicity infecting immunocompromised hosts as the more prevalent bacterial pathogens in this disorder. The isolates obtained depend on the population being studied, such as transplantation and leukemic units.

Okada et al identified organisms in 27 of 28 (96.4%) cases of endogenous bacterial endophthalmitis with two eyes demonstrating two different organisms.[1] The highest yields for positive cultures were obtained from the vitreous (73.9%) and blood (72%). An aqueous Gram stain that correlated with aqueous cultures was present in 6 of 10 eyes (60%) while the vitreous Gram stain and culture results were similar in only 8 of 17 patients. Gram-positive bacteria were isolated in 20 eyes (71%). Streptococci were isolated in 32% of patients, with *Strep. pneumoniae*, *Strep. viridans*, and group B streptococcus isolated in three, two, and two eyes, respectively. Group G BHS and *Streptococcus milleri* were isolated from individual eyes. *S. aureus*, the second most commonly isolated organism, was found in 7 patients (25%). *Clostridium septicum*, *B. cereus*, and *P. acnes* were also isolated from individual eyes.

Listeria monocytogenes is a rare cause of endophthalmitis.[93] It is a soil and environmental Gram-positive rod bacterium found to colonize the genital tract of farm animals where it is a cause of abortion. This species is also found in unpasteurized cheese and milk and inadequately cooked meat pâté. Lohmann et al described a 73-year-old male with acute iridocyclitis and secondary glaucoma whose severity increased over several days to acute endophthalmitis.[93] Early identification was made with polymerase chain reaction (PCR) from an anterior chamber tap specimen (Chapter 3). Early specific antibiotic therapy allowed a rapid recovery in vision. The authors also reviewed 15 cases described in the literature in which there was profound visual loss as the result of a delay in diagnosis.

Gram-negative bacteria are other bacterial etiologies. *Escherichia coli* is the most common among the Gram-negative bacteria. *H. influenzae*, *N. meningitidis*, *K. pneumoniae*, *Serratia* spp., and *Ps. aeruginosa* can also cause endogenous endophthalmitis. Gram-negative bacteria were isolated from 32% of patients. *E. coli* was isolated from five eyes (18%). *K. pneumoniae*, *Serr. marcescens*, *Ps. aeruginosa*, and *N. meningitidis* were also isolated from individual eyes.

In Asia, Wong et al incriminated Gram-negative bacteria in 70% of eyes with endogenous endophthalmitis.[94] The most common organism isolated was *K. pneumoniae* in 60% of cases. This organism is frequently incriminated in liver abscesses; hepatobiliary infection was the most common source of septicemia in this series. The investigators noted a suspected higher incidence of cholangiohepatitis with the secondary development of liver abscesses in the Far East compared

Table 9.5 Bacteria implicated in endogenous endophthalmitis

Gram-positive bacteria	Staphylococcus aureus, Streptococcus pneumoniae, Streptococcus viridans, Streptococcus milleri and groups A, C, and G betahemolytic streptococci, Listeria monocytogenes, Bacillus cereus, Actinomyces spp.
Gram-negative bacteria	Haemophilus influenzae, Neisseria meningitidis,[88–91] Klebsiella pneumoniae,[96] Serratia spp., Brucella spp., Pseudomonas aeruginosa, Escherichia coli[87]
Acid-fast (weak – 5%)	Nocardia asteroides[95]
Acid-fast (strong – 20%) and alcohol-fast	Mycobacteria

with the Caucasian population and this probably accounts for the higher incidence of Gram-negative endophthalmitis in this series. In addition, cirrhosis and hepatitis B infection are much more common in the Chinese population.

A literature review by the same investigators revealed differences in the location of identified sources of organisms in Caucasian patients. Endocarditis, urinary tract infection, and meningitis were the source of bacteremia in 18%, 18%, and 15% of Caucasian patients, respectively. The dichotomy in spectrum of causative organisms and source of infection based on geographical location translates into different approaches to the management of endogenous endophthalmitis based on geographical location.

Nocardia asteroides, *Actinomyces* spp., and *Mycobacterium tuberculosis* (Chapter 10) are acid-fast bacteria that may cause endogenous endophthalmitis (Table 9.5).[88–91,95–97]

Classification of bacterial endogenous endophthalmitis

Greenwald et al classified metastatic bacterial endophthalmitis into five distinct categories based on location (anterior and posterior) and extent of ocular involvement (diffuse or focal).[92] This categorization was based on a review of the literature and an analysis of five cases. The categories were anterior focal, anterior diffuse, posterior focal, posterior diffuse, and panophthalmitis. This clinical diagnostic categorization still applies.

Anterior focal

Eyes with anterior focal endophthalmitis were characterized by inflammation localized to one or more discrete areas in the iris, ciliary body, or anterior chamber. Characteristically, these eyes presented with normal to mildly edematous lids, mild-to-moderate conjunctivitis, and mild-to-moderate corneal haze. The lesions described are usually relatively small and associated with surrounding anterior chamber reaction, sometimes in the presence of a hypopyon. The prognosis for these eyes when early diagnosis and treatment is initiated is very good. When the infection involves the anterior segment, even if severe, the prognosis is better because the barrier effect of the lens and iris hampers the spread of microorganisms in the posterior segment.

Anterior diffuse

In contrast, eyes with anterior diffuse metastatic bacterial endophthalmitis present with diffuse inflammation of the anterior chamber associated with mild-to-moderate conjunctival edema. In some instances, a hypopyon may be present and obscure iris details with the inflammatory response. The posterior segment remains uninvolved. If visualization of the posterior segment is impossible, ultrasound usually shows no echoes in the vitreous cavity. In contrast to other types of endophthalmitis, aqueous cultures are usually positive but vitreous cultures only turn positive late in the course of the disease, when the infection has progressed to the posterior segment. Factors which appear to confine the infection to the anterior chamber include the forward flow of aqueous and the presence of the lens and posterior capsule. The prognosis following treatment for these eyes is excellent.

Posterior focal

Posterior focal endophthalmitis presents with variable signs of anterior segment inflammation in the presence of mild-to-moderate vitreous inflammation. One or more discrete focal retinal lesion is involved. The prognosis is good for this form of metastatic bacterial endophthalmitis.

Posterior diffuse

In contrast, the prognosis in posterior diffuse metastatic endophthalmitis is poor. The vitreous presents with diffuse inflammation and frequently appears opaque. When the retina can be visualized, embolic lesions with severe retinal necrosis caused by inflammation and sometimes ischemia may be present. Sometimes, the whole retina is destroyed. Vitreous abscess formation may develop.

Panophthalmitis

Panophthalmitis represents the most extensive ocular involvement in endogenous endophthalmitis, with extension of inflammation to extraocular tissues. The prognosis is very poor. Severe inflammatory involvement of the anterior and posterior segments is present, frequently accompanied by corneal opacification and proptosis. Lid chemosis and edema along with inflammation of orbital structures are observed. Panophthalmitis can be a life-threatening condition, especially if the bacterium is highly virulent.

Fungal endophthalmitis

Fungal endophthalmitis may present as an indolent course over days to weeks or it may be reasonably acute. A history of a penetrating injury with a plant substance or soil-contaminated foreign body may be elicited (Chapter 6). Individuals with candidal infections may present with high fever, followed several days later by ocular symptoms. Pyrexia of unknown origin may be associated with an occult retinochoroidal fungal infiltrate in which case an investigation should always be made for endocarditis. Fungal genera that can cause endophthalmitis are listed in Box 9.2.

Box 9.2 Fungal species as a cause of endogenous endophthalmitis

- Candida
- Aspergillus
- Fusarium
- Pseudallescheria
- Cryptococcus
- Paecilomyces
- Sporothrix
- Coccidioides
- Histoplasmosis
- Blastomyces
- Bipolaris
- Mucor

Candidiasis

The first case of endogenous candidal endophthalmitis was described in 1947. Some patients may be too ill or sedated to recognize the symptoms, which include floaters, localized scotoma, subtle changes in vision, photophobia, ciliary injection, or ocular pain. Most patients present with macular lesions or significant vitreous involvement. Early lesions start as an inner choroidal focal inflammatory reaction surrounding a small locus of *Candida* cells. A small minority of cases begin with a localized retinitis. The characteristic lesion is described as a creamy-white, round or oval, one-eighth to one-quarter disc diameter in size, circumscribed chorioretinal lesion with overlying vitreous inflammation of varying intensity.

As the infectious focus breaks into the vitreous, it enlarges in a globular fashion with budding extensions. Vitreous extension is accompanied by focal perivascular inflammatory deposits and increasing vitreous haze, with strand-like clusters of inflammatory cells and a diffuse cellular infiltration. Lesions are commonly multifocal and located in both eyes (Figure 9.2). A small focal intraretinal hemorrhage can be seen and may appear as a Roth's spot if it surrounds an infectious focus. Focal retinal necrosis and scarring combined with membrane formation and contraction are the major causes of permanent vision loss.

Candidal infection can take days to weeks to produce the level of damage that bacterial organisms cause in hours. Anterior segment inflammation lags behind posterior segment inflammation

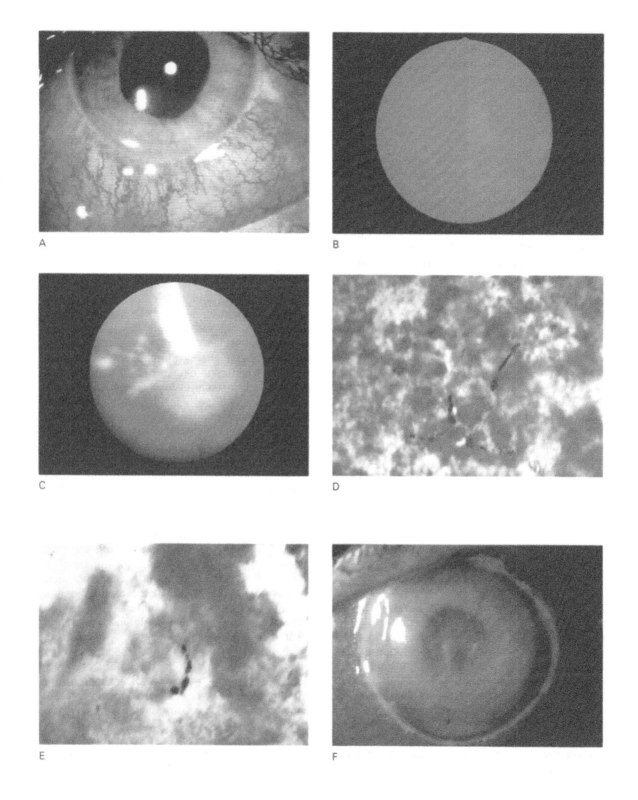

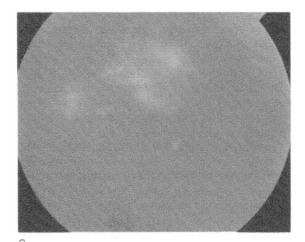

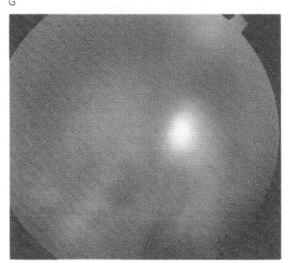

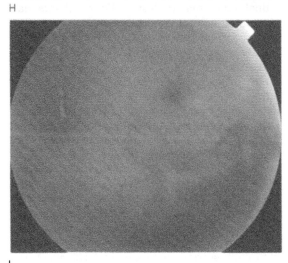

Figure 9.2

(A) Severe bilateral *Candida albicans* endophthalmitis following a contaminated blood transfusion after childbirth. (B) Retinal appearance of patient in (A) with chorioretinitis and vitritis. (C) Further retinal appearance of *Candida albicans* endophthalmitis. (D) Gram stain from vitreous of the patient in (A), showing pseudomycelium. (E) Further Gram stain from vitreous. (F) Anterior chamber inflammation with hypopyon in a patient with an indwelling catheter and endogenous *Candida* endophthalmitis. (G) Blurred vision with hazy vitreous with an infiltration around the macular area. Young male who had undergone kidney transplantation 5 years previously. Chronic immunosuppression with *Candida* gastrointestinal tract infection. Treated with intravitreal amphotericin and intravenous Ambisome. The vitreous biopsy was negative by Gram stain and culture. (H) Same patient as in (G) 4 months after the first attack with recurrent infection in the same eye. Retinal detachment was observed and surgery was performed with a circling band, pars plana vitrectomy, and silicone oil injection. The vitreous samples taken during the surgery were still negative. (I) Retinal vasculitis and phlebitis due to endogenous endophthalmitis in an immunosuppressed patient. Increased permeability and tortuosity in vessels with white-yellow cellular infiltrates and small hemorrhagic spots in an early stage.

but mirrors the intensity of the vitreous reaction and progresses to iridocyclitis with synechiae, hypopyon, pupillary block (Figure 9.3), and even a ciliary body abscess.

Histologically, the chorioretinal lesions of early candidal endophthalmitis show an intense localized inflammatory reaction arising in the choroid, composed of suppurative and granulomatous elements surrounding a small nidus of *Candida* cells. From the inner choroid, the inflammatory reaction breaks through Bruch's membrane into the retina to produce a localized microabscess. In the absence of effective treatment, the infectious nidus enlarges to rupture through the internal limiting membrane and 'spills' into the vitreous. The characteristic budding yeast and pseudo-hyphae of *Candida* cells are seen more frequently in the vitreous than the choroid where the organism originated, because the host immune defenses are better able to confine the infectious process. Perivasculitis, papillitis, and localized serous retinal detachment sometimes accompany the spreading infection. In the late stage, there is tractional retinal detachment associated with proliferative vitreoretinopathy and a cyclitic membrane.

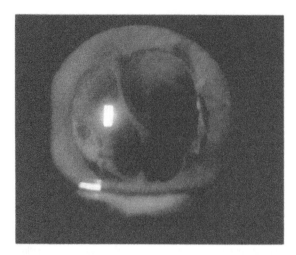

Figure 9.3

Posterior synechia and fixed pupillary area with regressed pupillary membrane formation after endophthalmitis.

In summary, the clinical diagnosis of *Candida* endophthalmitis can be defined as:

- Chorioretinitis with focal, deep, white infiltrative lesions but with no evidence of direct vitreal involvement except for diffuse vitreal haze, or
- Endophthalmitis with extension of the surrounding inflammation into the vitreous or with a vitreous abscess manifesting as 'fluff balls', or
- There may be a combination of both; therefore, all types of *Candida* endophthalmitis have been included in Table 9.3. Table 9.4 includes only those fungi that usually cause a granulomatous chorioretinitis without an accompanying endophthalmitis involving the vitreous.

Neonatal candidemia and end-organ damage, including endophthalmitis, has been the subject of a recent meta-analysis.[98]

Aspergillosis

Aspergillus was named by Micheli in 1792 for its resemblance to the aspergillum, a globe used to sprinkle holy water. This ubiquitous fungus is the second most common source of endogenous fungal endophthalmitis after *Candida* spp. Only five of the more than 900 varieties of *Aspergillus* cause endogenous endophthalmitis. These include *A. flavus, A. fumigatus, A. candidus, A. niger,* and *A. terreus. A. fumigatus* is the most frequently encountered pathogenic species in humans.

Initially, typical signs and symptoms of endophthalmitis occur. Endogenous aspergillosis endophthalmitis may be the presenting feature of disseminated aspergillosis. The chorioretinitis may manifest as depigmented discrete lesions, Roth's spots, or elevated pale yellow, fluffy lesions. Choroidal and retinal vascular occlusions have been reported. The disease progresses to involve all chambers of the eye and may eventually lead to serous or exudative retinal detachment, choroidal or vitreous abscess formation, and intravitreal granulomata.

In a retrospective analysis of 12 eyes in 10 patients diagnosed with culture-proven endogenous *Aspergillus* endophthalmitis, Weishaar et al found that there was a characteristic acute onset of intraocular inflammation and a chorioretinal lesion located frequently in the macula.[25] Despite resolution of the intraocular infection with vitrectomy and intravitreal amphotericin B, the visual outcome was generally poor, especially with macular lesions. All patients presented with a 1- or 2-day history of pain, and marked loss of visual acuity; vitritis was present in all 12 eyes. Nine of 12 eyes presented with a macula-involving chorioretinal inflammatory lesion. Four patients had associated pulmonary diseases and were receiving concurrent steroid therapy; six patients had a history of intravenous drug use. Blood cultures and echocardiograms were negative. Management consisted of vitrectomy in 10/12 eyes and intravitreal amphotericin B in 11/12 eyes. One patient was treated with oral antifungals while six patients completed systemic amphotericin B therapy. In three eyes without central macular involvement, final visual acuities were 20/25 to 20/200. In eight eyes with initial macular involvement, final visual acuities were 20/400 in three eyes and 1/200 or less in another three eyes. Two eyes were enucleated for chronic pain and recurrent retinal detachment.[25]

In a histopathologic study examining enucleated eyes secondary to candidal (13 eyes) and aspergillosis (12 eyes) endophthalmitis, Rao and Hidayat found that the vitreous was the primary focus of infection for *Candida* spp., whereas *Aspergillus* spp. preferred the subretinal pigment epithelium area.[21] Therefore, vitreous biopsy may not yield positive results in *Aspergillus* endophthalmitis. Retinal and choroidal vessel wall invasion was seen in aspergillosis but not with candidiasis. *Candida* endophthalmitis was noted in patients with a history of gastrointestinal surgery, hyperalimentation, or diabetes mellitus, whereas aspergillosis was present in patients who had undergone organ transplantation or cardiac surgery. Both infectious agents induced suppurative nongranulomatous inflammation. This intraocular infection is usually associated with a high rate of mortality caused by cerebral and cardiac complications.[21]

In another series analyzing endogenous fungal endophthalmitis over a 10-year period, Essman et al found 16 of 20 cases due to *Candida* spp. with the remaining four cases caused by *Aspergillus* spp.[30] Eyes with *Candida* endophthalmitis presented in an indolent fashion with a mean duration from onset of symptoms to initial treatment of 61 days compared with 5 days for *Aspergillus* endophthalmitis. A final visual acuity of 20/400 or better was achieved in 75%, 80%, and 0% of eyes infected with *C. albicans, C. tropicalis,* and *Aspergillus* spp., respectively. Four eyes with *C. albicans* endophthalmitis had a final visual acuity of less than 20/400 as a result of retinal detachment. Direct infection of the macula was the cause of the poor final visual acuity in two patients infected with *Aspergillus* spp., while the third patient had a persistent retinal detachment. Only two patients in this series had positive nonocular cultures. The diagnosis of endogenous fungal endophthalmitis occurred in an outpatient setting for all the patients; the presence of a disseminated focus of infection was found in only two patients.[30]

The authors compared this group of patients with a series of endogenous bacterial endophthalmitis cases from another large institution.[30] Final visual results were poorer in individuals with bacterial endogenous endophthalmitis; only 22% had a vision of 20/400 or better compared with 72% of patients in this series. Symptoms developed more rapidly in cases of bacterial endophthalmitis; 86% of patients developed symptoms within 1 week of presentation or less.

Cryptococcosis

Cryptococcus neoformans is a non-mycelial, yeast-like capsulate fungus with worldwide distribution. The organism is found in bird droppings, contaminated soil, and vegetation. *C. neoformans* is a budding, spore-forming yeast that produces smooth, yellow-tan colonies on culture. Systemic disease is most often acquired through inhalation of aerosolized organisms but direct entry through the digestive tract or skin can occur. Dissemination occurs most frequently to the central nervous system. In 1995, there were fewer than 30 cases of confirmed ocular cryptococcosis in the literature.[38]

The incidence of cryptococcosis and meningitis caused by *C. neoformans* in patients with AIDS has accounted for its increased incidence with a rate of 2–9%.[76] Patients may also be immunocompetent.

Systemic features include meningitis, pneumonia, mucocutaneous lesions, multiple skin lesions, pyelonephritis, endocarditis, hepatitis, and prostatitis. Ocular involvement includes sequelae from the systemic involvement as well as the primary infection. For instance, meningitis can cause papilledema, optic atrophy, or extraocular muscle paresis. In one series of 80 patients, Kestelyn et al found papilledema in 32.5%, abducens nerve palsy in 9%, and optic atrophy in 2.5% of cases.[99] The primary infection can cause choroiditis, retinitis, uveitis, inflammatory iris mass, keratitis, conjunctival granuloma, phthisis bulbi, periorbital necrotizing fasciitis, and orbital infection. Exogenous endophthalmitis also occurs following penetrating keratoplasty (Chapter 6).

Diagnosis is made presumptively in a patient with characteristic clinical findings. In clinically suspicious patients with a negative serum, sputum, cerebrospinal fluid, and blood examination, vitreous biopsy or vitrectomy may be positive on a fungal stain (Chapter 3). Therapy depends on the etiology and requires a combination of systemic antifungal agents, intravitreous amphotericin B and pars plana vitrectomy. If cryptococcal organisms are seen on the india ink stain at the time of diagnostic vitreous tap or vitrectomy, intravitreal amphotericin B should be administered immediately and systemic therapy should be started. Early vitrectomy is recommended if severe vitritis fails to clear or worsens with antifungal therapy (Chapter 7).

Pseudallescheriasis

Pseudallescheria boydii is a ubiquitous organism found worldwide in soil, stagnant water, and vegetation. This is an opportunistic mycelial fungus with low virulence that can imitate aspergillosis both clinically and histologically; thus it is also referred to as the 'great imitator.' The definitive diagnosis is made on fungal culture, which can differentiate it from *A. fumigatus*, the most dominant form of Aspergillus in humans. The former appears velvety white and becomes dark gray whereas the latter appears as green colonies (Chapter 3).

   P. boydii is the sexual state of the organism and causes invasive infections including sinusitis, otitis, pulmonary infection, prosthetic and native valve endocarditis, prostatitis, meningitis, brain abscess, arthritis, osteomyelitis, and disseminated disease. Traumatic implantation causes Madura foot (maduromycosis) and involves both the soft tissue and bone. As with aspergillosis, dissemination is more likely in immunocompromised hosts. *Scedosporium apiospermum* is the asexual phase which is cultured in the laboratory and is the preferred name.

   In a series of 17 cases of human ocular infection with *P. boydii* reported by McGuire et al, 5 cases were endogenous and 12 were exogenous (cataract surgery, 1; keratitis, 7; penetrating trauma, 2; conjunctival and eyelid mycetoma, 1).[44] Eye pain was the most common symptom followed by decreased or blurred vision, photophobia, and tearing. Visual acuity ranged from 20/200 to no light perception. Other signs of endophthalmitis were also present. Five of the six patients died of disseminated pseudallescheriasis, their underlying disease, or multisystemic disease. Three of the patients who died had undergone vitrectomy and aggressive systemic therapy with amphotericin B.

Fusarium

Fusarium is an aggressive mycelial fungus that causes endophthalmitis that is particularly difficult to treat; it occurs in immunocompromised patients.[100] *Fusarium* endophthalmitis usually requires extensive surgery and intravitreal and systemic amphotericin but does not always respond.[26]

Viral infections

Vitritis, chorioretinitis, and associated optic neuritis caused by West Nile and other viruses are considered in Chapter 10, 'Differential diagnoses'.

Laboratory examination

The most important laboratory studies are Gram stain and culture of the aqueous and vitreous fluids collected before the institution of antibiotic therapy (Chapter 3). The use of blood culture bottles for the inoculation of ocular specimens is a good idea and increases the yield or chances of a positive culture. Cultures of other sites, including the intravenous catheter tip if present, should be obtained. Immunologic tests for specific bacterial antigens can be performed in patients who have already received antibiotics, but the usefulness of these tests has been challenged. Molecular biology with PCR of anterior chamber (aqueous humor) and vitreous samples is producing positive results when traditional tests of stain and culture are negative[101–103] and is particularly useful (Chapter 3). Small samples of aqueous and vitreous (20–50 µl aliquots) in sterile tubes should be kept frozen at –20°C specifically for PCR tests.

   In patients with endogenous endophthalmitis, a systemic work-up must also be undertaken in conjunction with an infectious disease physician or microbiologist to ascertain the source of infection. These tests include:

- Complete blood count with differential.
- Erythrocyte sedimentation rate to evaluate for rheumatic disease, chronic infections, or malignancy.
- Blood urea nitrogen and creatinine to evaluate for renal failure.
- Human immunodeficiency virus (HIV) infection should be considered in otherwise healthy persons with endophthalmitis.
- Routine radiographs may reveal a primary pulmonary infection.
- Echocardiography is warranted to assess the possibility of endocarditis.
- CT scan/MRI of orbit may help rule out other differential diagnoses.
- Blood culture – evaluating for source of infection.

- Urine culture – evaluating for source of infection.
- Cerebrospinal fluid, throat culture, stool culture to evaluate for source of infection.
- Culture of foreign objects (indwelling intravascular catheter tip, penetrating object, etc.).

Treatment

The outcome of endogenous endophthalmitis is generally disappointing compared with that of exogenous endophthalmitis especially for infection due to *Aspergillus* sp. Three factors that result in a poor prognosis are:

- Virulent organisms
- Host immunosuppression
- Diagnostic delay.

Even with aggressive treatment, vision is limited to counting fingers in about 40% of patients. Given its vascular spread, endogenous endophthalmitis is more responsive to intravenous antibiotics than is exogenous endophthalmitis which occurs from intraocular injection of pathogens. Systemic medications also treat the source of the organism, thereby reducing the likelihood of invasion to the other eye. Furthermore, the nature of the clinical presentation, as well as the presumed (or confirmed) source of infection, can be used to guide antibiotic choice. **The most important therapeutic principle in endophthalmitis is early diagnosis and treatment with correct identification of the pathogenic organism.**

In cases of endogenous bacterial endophthalmitis, empiric broad-spectrum antibiotic therapy with vancomycin (Vancocin) and an aminoglycoside or a third-generation cephalosporin should be considered unless the diagnosis is late. If there is endophthalmitis present, vitrectomy should be performed (Chapter 8) with instillation of intravitreal antibiotics and corticosteroids.[91,104,105] Third-generation cephalosporins penetrate ocular tissues well and are effective against Gram-negative organisms but are less effective than first-generation cephalosporins against Gram-positive bacteria. Clindamycin can be used in intravenous drug abusers until *Bacillus* infection can be excluded. Second- or third-generation cephalosporins and aminoglycosides are considered the drugs of choice from documented sources for gastrointestinal or genitourinary infections. Vancomycin might also be given to patients known to abuse drugs, covering the possibility of infection with *Bacillus* spp. In addition, quinolone therapy (levofloxacin, ciprofloxacin, moxifloxacin) should be used for known infection due to Gram-negative bacteria.

In a 10-year study of treatment outcomes, Essman et al reported that 13 of 17 eyes (76%) with *Candida* endophthalmitis and none of 3 eyes (0%) with *Aspergillus* endophthalmitis, achieved visual acuity of 20/400 or better.[30] Scherer and Lee reported that in 107 patients with systemic fungal infection who were receiving antifungal antibiotics and who were screened ophthalmologically, only 3 eyes (2.8%) had chorioretinal features consistent with early endogenous endophthalmitis; none had vitreous involvement.[8] Based on these findings, the authors noted that early systemic treatment of deep tissue fungal infection appears to dramatically decrease the incidence of endogenous fungal endophthalmitis.

Animal models of endogenous *Candida* endophthalmitis suggest that early treatment with either imidazoles or amphotericin B is more successful than delaying treatment for a week despite similar numbers of yeasts at each time period. Correct identification of the organism by blood or ocular fluid cultures and determination of *in vitro* susceptibility to various antifungal agents will help to identify the most effective antifungal drugs for successful treatment. If the patient's history, stains, or culture results suggest a fungal infection, amphotericin B (Amphotec), fluconazole (Diflucan), or itraconazole (Sporanox) should be included in the regimen.

Smiddy suggested that systemic treatment with oral fluconazole may be effective for simple choroiditis or minimal endophthalmitis (i.e. vitritis).[106] An alternative imidazole is itraconazole (Chapter 11). For persistent or progressive vitritis, he recommends vitrectomy to clear the organism. Instead of intravitreal amphotericin B in conjunction with vitrectomy, the author asserted that an extended course of oral fluconazole following vitrectomy without intravitreal amphotericin B resolved the infection in a vast majority of patients. According to Smiddy, if the macula is spared and preretinal membranes can be effectively removed, visual acuity results can be exceedingly good. The management of endogenous endophthalmitis is also considered by Samiy and D'Amico.[107]

Intravitreal injections have revolutionized the treatment of exogenous endophthalmitis, but their usefulness in endogenous cases is controversial (Chapter 8).[108] Furthermore, in an attempt to reduce inflammation-mediated damage, corticosteroids such as dexamethasone have been administered intravitreally with some controversy.[104,105] Topical steroids have been used empirically in patients with anterior (focal or diffuse) disease to prevent complications such as glaucoma and formation of synechiae. Similarly, surgical intervention such as vitrectomy is widely accepted in postsurgical and posttraumatic endophthalmitis; however, its benefits in endogenous endophthalmitis have been the subject of debate. Surgical intervention is generally recommended for patients infected with especially virulent organisms such as Strep. pyogenes (BHS group A), Strep. pneumoniae, S. aureus, or Ps. aeruginosa, in those with visual acuity of 20/400 or less and in cases of pupillary glaucoma from extensive posterior synechiae or severe vitreous involvement. Vitrectomy and intravitreal antibiotics may also prevent ocular atrophy or the need for enucleation when the hypopyon level is high and there is evidence of vitreous opacities and retinal detachment on the B-scan examination.

However, a recent review of all cases of culture-proven endogenous endophthalmitis from Miami between 1996 and 2002,[108] in which 11 eyes (52%) were treated with vitrectomy and intravitreal antibiotics, has found continuing high morbidity and poor visual acuity outcome, with no improvement for recovery from Aspergillus infection; similar findings have been reported recently from London (UK).[91] Most cases, however, are medical emergencies requiring immediate diagnosis and vitrectomy with intravitreal antibiotics and corticosteroids which should be performed without any delay, if necessary in the outpatient (Chapter 8) or clinic setting, without waiting four hours or more for operating theatre space. Aggressive early management can be expected to improve the visual outcome.

References

1. Okada AA, Johnson RP, Liles WC et al. Endogenous bacterial endophthalmitis. Report of a ten-year retrospective study, Ophthalmology (1994) 101:832–8.

2. Donahue SP, Greven CM, Zuravleff JJ et al. Intraocular candidiasis in patients with candidemia. Clinical implications derived from a prospective multicenter study, Ophthalmology (1994) 101: 1302–9.

3. McDonnel PJ, McDonnel JM, Brown RH et al. Ocular involvement in patients with fungal infections, Ophthalmology (1985) 92:706–9.

4. Parke DW II, Jones DB, Gentry LO. Endogenous endophthalmitis among patients with candidemia, Ophthalmology (1982) 89:789–96.

5. Brooks RG. Prospective study of Candida endophthalmitis in hospitalized patients with candidemia, Arch Intern Med (1989) 149: 2226–8.

6. Bross J, Talbot GH, Maislin G et al. Risk factors for nosocomial candidemia: a case-control study in adults without leukemia, Am J Med (1989) 87: 614–20.

7. Feman SS, Nichols JC, Chung SM et al. Endophthalmitis in patients with disseminated fungal disease, Trans Am Ophthalmol Soc (2002) 100:67–71.

8. Scherer WJ, Lee K. Implications of early systemic therapy on the incidence of endogenous fungal endophthalmitis, Ophthalmology (1997) 104: 1593–8.

9. Binder MI, Chua J, Kaiser PK et al. Endogenous endophthalmitis: an 18–year review of culture-positive cases at a tertiary care center, Medicine (Baltimore) (2003) 82:97–105.

10. Klein JJ, Watanakunakorn C. Hospital-acquired fungemia: its natural course and clinical significance, Am J Med (1979) 67:51–8.

11. Henderson DK, Edwards JE Jr, Montgomerie JZ. Hematogenous Candida endophthalmitis in patients receiving parenteral hyperalimentation fluids, J Infect Dis (1981) 143:655–61.

12. Harvey RL, Myers JP. Nosocomial fungemia in a large community teaching hospital, Arch Intern Med (1987) 147:2117–20.

13. Arroyo JG, Bula DV, Grant CA et al. Bilateral Candida albicans endophthalmitis associated with an infected deep vein thrombus, Jpn J Ophthalmol (2004) 48:30–3.

14. Schelenz S, Goldsmith DJ. Aspergillus endophthalmitis: an unusual complication of disseminated infection in renal transplant patients, J Infect (2003) 47:336–43.

15. Dorey MW, Brownstein S, Kertes PJ et al. Rhodotorula glutinis endophthalmitis, Can J Ophthalmol (2002) 37:416–18.

16. Castiglioni B, Sutton D, Rinaldi MG et al. Pseudallescheria boydii (Anamorph Scedosporium apiospermum). Infection in solid organ transplant recipients in a tertiary medical center and review of the literature, Medicine (Baltimore) (2002) 81:333–48.

17. Nishio H, Sakakibara-Kawamura K, Suzuki T et al. An autopsy case of Ph1-positive acute lymphoblastic leukemia with disseminated infection of *Fusarium solani*, *Kansenshogaku Zasshi* (2002) **76**:67–71.

18. Tsai CC, Chen SJ, Chung YM et al. Postpartum endogenous *Candida* endophthalmitis, *J Formos Med Assoc* (2002) **101**:432–6.

19. Kou HK, Lin JW, Chang KC. Clinicopathological report of *Candida* granuloma from an endogenous candidal endophthalmitis, *Chang Gung Med J* (2001) **24**:460–3.

20. Bhansali A, Sharma A, Kashyap A et al. Mucor endophthalmitis, *Acta Ophthalmol Scand* (2001) **79**:88–90.

21. Rao NA, Hidayat AA. Endogenous mycotic endophthalmitis: variations in clinical and histopathologic changes in candidiasis compared with aspergillosis, *Am J Ophthalmol* (2001) **132**:244–51.

22. Gonzales CA, Scott IU, Chaudhry NA et al. Endogenous endophthalmitis caused by *Histoplasma capsulatum* var. *capsulatum*. A case report and literature review, *Ophthalmology* (2000) **107**: 725–9.

23. Ohnishi Y, Tawara A, Murata T et al. Postmortem findings two weeks after oral treatment for metastatic *Candida* endophthalmitis with fluconazole, *Ophthalmologica* (1999) **213**:341–4.

24. Li S, Perlman JI, Edward DP et al. Unilateral *Blastomyces dermatitidis* endophthalmitis and orbital cellulitis: a case report and literature review, *Ophthalmology* (1998) **105**:1466–70.

25. Weishaar PD, Flynn HW Jr, Murray TG et al. Endogenous *Aspergillus* endophthalmitis. Clinical features and treatment outcomes, *Ophthalmology* (1998) **105**:57–65.

26. Seal DV, Bron AJ, Hay J. *Ocular Infection: Investigation and Treatment in Practice* (Martin Dunitz: London, 1998).

27. Sheu SJ, Chen YC, Kuo NW et al. Endogenous cryptococcal endophthalmitis, *Ophthalmology* (1998) **105**:377–81.

28. Okhravi N, Dart JKG, Towler HM et al. *Paecilomyces lilacinus* endophthalmitis with secondary keratitis: a case report and literature review, *Arch Ophthalmol* (1997) **115**:1320–4.

29. Hutnik CM, Nicolle DA, Munoz DG. Orbital aspergillosis. A fatal masquerader, *J Neuroophthalmol* (1997) **17**:257–61.

30. Essman TF, Flynn HW Jr, Smiddy WE et al. Treatment outcomes in a 10–year study of endogenous fungal endophthalmitis, *Ophthalmic Surg Lasers* (1997) **28**:185–94.

31. Glasgow BJ, Engstrom RE Jr, Holland GN et al. Bilateral endogenous *Fusarium* endophthalmitis associated with AIDS, *Arch Ophthalmol* (1996) **114**:873–7.

32. Hunt KE, Glasgow BJ. *Aspergillus* endophthalmitis. An unrecognized endemic disease in orthotopic liver transplantation, *Ophthalmology* (1996) **103**: 757–67.

33. Jampol LM, Sung J, Walker JD et al. Choroidal neovascularization secondary to *Candida albicans* chorioretinitis, *Am J Ophthalmol* (1996) **121**: 643–9.

34. Zarbin MA, Becker E, Witcher J et al. Treatment of presumed fungal endophthalmitis with oral fluconazole, *Ophthalmic Surg Lasers* (1996) **27**: 628–31.

35. Henderson T, Irfan S. Bilateral endogenous *Candida* endophthalmitis and chorioretinitis following toxic megacolon, *Eye* (1996) **10**:755–7.

36. Matsuo T, Nakagawa H, Matsuo N. Endogenous *Aspergillus* endophthalmitis associated with periodontitis, *Ophthalmologica* (1995) **209**:109–11.

37. Graham DA, Kinyoun JL, George DP. Endogenous *Aspergillus* endophthalmitis after lung transplantation, *Am J Ophthalmol* (1995) **119**:107–9.

38. Custis PH, Haller JA, de Juan E Jr. An unusual case of cryptococcal endophthalmitis, *Retina* (1995) **15**:300–4.

39. Yohai RA, Bullock JD, Aziz AA et al. Survival factors in rhino-orbital-cerebral mucormycosis, *Surv Ophthalmol* (1994) **39**:3–22.

40. Pavan PR, Margo CE. Endogenous endophthalmitis caused by *Bipolaris hawaiiensis* in acquired immunodeficiency syndrome, *Am J Ophthalmol* (1993) **116**: 644–5.

41. Nakazawa S, Mori T, Hibiya I et al. Analysis of 84 cases with fungemia, *Kansenshogaku Zasshi* (1992) **66**:612–19.

42. Crump JR, Elner SG, Elner VM et al. Cryptococcal endophthalmitis: case report and review, *Clin Infect Dis* (1992) **14**:1069–73.

43. Greenwald BD, Tunkel AR, Morgan KM et al. Candidal endophthalmitis after lithotripsy of renal calculi, *South Med J* (1992) **85**:773–4.

44. McGuire TW, Bullock JD, Bullock JD Jr et al. Fungal endophthalmitis. An experimental study with a review of 17 human ocular cases, *Arch Ophthalmol* (1991); **109**: 1289–96.

45. Pfeifer JD, Grand MG, Thomas MA et al. Endogenous *Pseudallescheria boydii* endophthalmitis. Clinicopathologic findings in two cases, *Arch Ophthalmol* (1991) **109**:1714–17. [Erratum appears in *Arch Ophthalmol* (1992) **110**:449.

46. Denning DW, Armstrong RW, Fishman M et al. Endophthalmitis in a patient with disseminated cryptococcosis and AIDS who was treated with itraconazole, *Rev Infect Dis* (1991) **13**:1126–30.

47. Safnek JR, Hogg GR, Napier LB. Endophthalmitis due to *Blastomyces dermatitidis*, *Ophthalmology* (1990) **97**:212–16.

48. Clinch TE, Duker JS, Eagle RC Jr et al. Infantile

endogenous *Candida* endophthalmitis presenting as a cataract, *Surv Ophthalmol* (1989) **34**:107–12.

49. Khurana AK, Mathur SK, Ahluwalia BK et al. An unusual case of endogenous *Aspergillus* endophthalmitis, *Acta Ophthalmol (Copenh)* (1989) **67**:315–18.

50. Kurosawa A, Pollock SC, Collins MP et al. *Sporothrix schenckii* endophthalmitis in a patient with human immunodeficiency virus infection, *Arch Ophthalmol* (1988) **106**:376–80.

51. Silva MR, Mendes RP, Lastoria JC et al. Paracoccidioidomycosis: study of 6 cases with ocular involvement, *Mycopathologia* (1988) **102**:87–96.

52. Hiss PW, Shields JA, Augsburger JJ. Solitary retinovitreal abscess as the initial manifestation of cryptococcosis, *Ophthalmology* (1988) **95**:162–5.

53. Weiss JN, Hutchins RK, Balogh K. Simultaneous *Aspergillus* endophthalmitis and cytomegalovirus retinitis after kidney transplantation, *Retina* (1988) **83**:193–8.

54. Henderly DE, Liggett PE, Rao NA. Cryptococcal chorioretinitis and endophthalmitis, *Retina* (1987) **7**:75–9.

55. Lance SE, Friberg TR, Kowalski RP. *Aspergillus flavus* endophthalmitis and retinitis in an intravenous drug abuser, *Ophthalmology* (1988) **95**: 947–9.

56. Swan SK, Wagner RA, Myers JP et al. Mycotic endophthalmitis caused by *Penicillium* sp. after parenteral drug abuse, *Am J Ophthalmol* (1985) **100**:408–10.

57. Furia M, Parent de Curzon H, Campinchi R. Favorable development of bilateral *Candida albicans* endophthalmitis. Value of early vitrectomy, *J Fr Ophtalmol* (1984) **7**:689–5 [in French].

58. Baley JE, Kliegman RM, Annable WL et al. *Torulopsis glabrata* sepsis appearing as necrotizing enterocolitis and endophthalmitis, *Am J Dis Child* (1984) **138**:965–6.

59. Wilmarth SS, May DR, Roth AM et al. *Aspergillus* endophthalmitis in an intravenous drug abuser, *Ann Ophthalmol* (1983) **15**:470–2, 74–6.

60. Weis RF, Everett ED, Sprouse R et al. Endogenous cryptococcal endophthalmitis, *South Med J* (1981) **74**:482–3.

61. Shields JA, Wright DM, Augsburger JJ et al. Cryptococcal chorioretinitis, *Am J Ophthalmol* (1980) **89**:210–17.

62. Palmer EA. Endogenous *Candida* endophthalmitis in infants, *Am J Ophthalmol* (1980) **89**:388–95.

63. Peyman GA, Raichand M, Bennett TO. Management of endophthalmitis with pars plana vitrectomy, *Br J Ophthalmol* (1980) **64**:472–5.

64. Aguilar GL, Blumenkranz MS, Egbert PR et al. *Candida* endophthalmitis after intravenous drug abuse, *Arch Ophthalmol* (1979) **97**:96–100.

65. Snip RC, Michels RG. Pars plana vitrectomy in the management of endogenous *Candida* endophthalmitis, *Am J Ophthalmol* (1976) **82**:699–704.

66. Naidoff MA, Green WR. Endogenous *Aspergillus* endophthalmitis occurring after kidney transplant, *Am J Ophthalmol* (1975) **79**:502–9.

67. Edwards JE Jr, Foos RY, Montgomerie JZ et al. Ocular manifestations of *Candida* septicemia: review of seventy-six cases of hematogenous *Candida* endophthalmitis, *Medicine* (1974) **53**: 47–75.

68. Griffin JR, Pettit TH, Fishman LS. Blood-borne *Candida* endophthalmitis, *Arch Ophthalmol* (1973) **89**:450–6.

69. Wålinder PE, Kock E. Endogenous fungus endophthalmitis. *Acta Ophthalmol (Copenh)* 1971; **49**: 263–72.

70. Tarkkanen A, Tommila V, Valle O et al. Endogenous fungus endophthalmitis due to *Candida albicans*, *Br J Ophthalmol* (1967) **51**:188–92.

71. Tanaka M, Kobayashi Y, Takebayashi H et al. Analysis of predisposing clinical and laboratory findings for the development of endogenous fungal endophthalmitis. A retrospective 12–year study of 79 eyes of 46 patients, *Retina* (2001) **21**:203–9.

72. Spencer WH, Chan CC, Shen de F et al. Detection of *Histoplasma capsulatum* DNA in lesions of chronic ocular histoplasmosis syndrome, *Arch Ophthalmol* (2003) **121**:1551–5.

73. Kiratli H, Uzun O, Kiraz N et al. *Scedosporium apiospermum* chorioretinitis, *Acta Ophthalmol Scand* (2001) **79**:540–2.

74. Anteby I, Kramer M, Rahav G et al. Necrotizing choroiditis-retinitis as presenting symptom of disseminated aspergillosis after lung transplantation, *Eur J Ophthalmol* (1997) **7**:294–6.

75. Yau TH, Rivera-Velazquez PM, Mark AS et al. Unilateral optic neuritis caused by *Histoplasma capsulatum* in a patient with the acquired immunodeficiency syndrome, *Am J Ophthalmol* (1996) **121**: 324–6.

76. Morinelli EN, Dugel PU, Riffenburgh R et al. Infectious multifocal choroiditis in patients with acquired immune deficiency syndrome, *Ophthalmology* (1993) **100**:1014–21.

77. Specht CS, Mitchell KT, Bauman AE et al. Ocular histoplasmosis with retinitis in a patient with acquired immune deficiency syndrome, *Ophthalmology* (1991) **98**:1356–9.

78. Dantas AM, Yamane R, Camara AG. South American blastomycosis: ophthalmic and oculomotor nerve lesions, *Am J Trop Med Hyg* (1990) **43**:386–8.

79. Golden SE, Morgan CM, Bartley DL et al. Disseminated coccidioidomycosis with chorioretinitis in early infancy, *Pediatr Infect Dis* (1986) **5**:272–4.

80. Macher A, Rodrigues MM, Kaplan W et al. Disseminated bilateral chorioretinitis due to *Histoplasma capsulatum* in a patient with the acquired immunodeficiency syndrome, *Ophthalmology* (1985) **92**:1159–64.

81. Scholz R, Green WR, Kutys R et al. *Histoplasma capsulatum* in the eye, *Ophthalmology* (1984) **91**:1100–4.

82. Schwarz J, Salfelder K, Viloria JE. *Histoplasma capsulatum* in vessels of the choroid, *Ann Ophthalmol* (1977) **9**:633–6.

83. Chapman-Smith JS. Cryptococcal chorioretinitis: a case report, *Br J Ophthalmol* (1977) **61**:411–13.

84. Font RL, Jakobiec FA. Granulomatous necrotizing retinochoroiditis caused by *Sporotrichum schenckii*. Report of a case including immunofluorescence and electron microscopical studies, *Arch Ophthalmol* (1976) **94**:1513–19.

85. Craig EL, Suie T. *Histoplasma capsulatum* in human ocular tissue, *Arch Ophthalmol* (1974) **91**:285–9.

86. Klintworth GK, Hollingsworth AS, Lusman PA et al. Granulomatous choroiditis in a case of disseminated histoplasmosis. Histologic demonstration of *Histoplasma capsulatum* in choroidal lesions, *Arch Ophthalmol* (1973) **90**:45–8.

87. Cameron ME, Harrison A. Ocular cryptococcosis in Australia, with a report of two further cases, *Med J Aust* (1970) **1**:935–8.

88. Chacko E, Flitcroft I, Condon PJ. Meningococcal septicemia presenting as bilateral endophthalmitis, *J Cataract Refract Surg* (2004) (in press).

89. Frelich VS, Murray DL, Goei S et al. *Neisseria meningitidis* endophthalmitis: use of polymerase chain reaction to support an etiologic diagnosis, *Pediatr Infect Dis J* (2003) **22**:288–90.

90. Kerkhoff FT, van der Zee A, Bergmans AM et al. Polymerase chain reaction detection of *Neisseria meningitidis* in the intraocular fluid of a patient with endogenous endophthalmitis but without associated meningitis, *Ophthalmology* (2003) **110**:2134–6.

91. Jackson TL, Eykyn SJ, Graham EM et al. Endogenous bacterial endophthalmitis: a 17-year prospective series and review of 267 reported cases, *Surv Ophthalmol* (2003) **48**:403–23.

92. Greenwald MJ, Wohl LG, Sell CH. Metastatic bacterial endophthalmitis: a contemporary reappraisal, *Surv Ophthalmol* (1986) **31**:81–101.

93. Lohmann CP, Gabel VP, Heep M et al. *Listeria monocytogenes*-induced endogenous endophthalmitis in an otherwise healthy individual: rapid PCR-diagnosis as the basis for effective treatment, *Eur J Ophthalmol* (1999) **9**:53–7.

94. Wong JS, Chan TK, Lee HM et al. Endogenous bacterial endophthalmitis: an east Asian experience and a reappraisal of a severe ocular affliction, *Ophthalmology* (2000) **107**:1483–91.

95. Rogers SJ, Johnson BL. Endogenous *Nocardia* endophthalmitis: report of a case in a patient treated for lymphocytic lymphoma, *Ann Ophthalmol* (1977) **9**:1123–31.

96. Margo CE, Mames RN, Guy JR. Endogenous *Klebsiella* endophthalmitis. Report of two cases and review of the literature, *Ophthalmology* (1994) **101**:1298–301.

97. Shammas HF. Endogenous *E. coli* endophthalmitis, *Surv Ophthalmol* (1977) **21**: 429–35.

98. Benjamin DK Jr, Poole C, Steinbach WJ et al. Neonatal candidemia and end-organ damage: a critical appraisal of the literature using meta-analytic techniques, *Pediatrics* (2003) **112**: 634–40.

99. Kestelyn P, Taelman H, Bogaerts J. Ophthalmic manifestations of infections with *Cryptococcus neoformans* in patients with the acquired immune deficiency syndrome, *Am J Ophthalmol* (1993) **116**:721–7.

100. Martino P, Gastaldi R, Raccah R et al. Clinical patterns of *Fusarium* infections in immunocompromised patients, *J Infect* (1994) **28** (Suppl 1): 7–15.

101. Ferrer C, Montero J, Alio JL et al. Rapid molecular diagnosis of post-traumatic keratitis and endophthalmitis caused by *Alternaria infectoria*, *J Clin Microbiol* (2003) **41**:3358–60.

102. Ferrer C, Munoz G, Alio JL et al. Polymerase chain reaction diagnosis in fungal keratitis caused by *Alternaria alternata*, *Am J Ophthalmol* (2002) **133**:398–9.

103. Ferrer C, Colom F, Frases S et al. Detection and identification of fungal pathogens by PCR and by ITS2 and 5.8S ribosomal DNA typing in ocular infections, *J Clin Microbiol* (2001) **39**:2873–9.

104. Schulman JA, Peyman GA. Intravitreal corticosteroids as an adjunct in the treatment of bacterial and fungal endophthalmitis: a review, *Retina* (1992) **12**:336–40.

105. Coats ML, Peyman GA. Intravitreal corticosteroids in the treatment of exogenous fungal endophthalmitis, *Retina* (1992) **12**:46–51.

106. Smiddy WE. Treatment outcomes of endogenous fungal endophthalmitis, *Curr Opin Ophthalmol* (1998) **9**:66–70.

107. Samiy N, D'Amico DJ. Endogenous fungal endophthalmitis, *Int Ophthalmol Clin* (1996) **36**:147–62.

108. Schiedler V, Scott IU, Flynn HW Jr et al. Culture-proven endogenous endophthalmitis: clinical features and visual acuity outcomes, *Am J Ophthalmol* (2004) **137**:725–31.

10

Differential diagnosis of endophthalmitis

A number of conditions that either cause or mimic intraocular inflammation may mislead the examiner into making the wrong diagnosis. In this chapter, we will present a broad outline of categories that cause inflammation and discuss some of these entities. Specifically, infectious inflammation, immune-related inflammation, and the masquerade syndrome will be discussed. Posterior uveitis refers to inflammation of the choroid, which extends to the adjacent retina, causing a retinochoroiditis. The cause may be a bacteremia, fungemia, protozoa, or parasite that evolves into endophthalmitis. More commonly, there is a nonpurulent chronic granulomatous reaction. The most common causes of retinochoroiditis in Europe and the USA are *Toxoplasma gondii* infection and larvae migrans from *Toxocara canis* infection. These and other infections associated with retinochoroiditis are discussed below.

Infectious uveitis and chorioretinitis

Bacteria

Brucellosis

Brucellosis arises from drinking unpasteurized milk, due to *Brucella abortus* from the cow or *Brucella melitensis* from the goat. Initially there is an acute phase of generalized fever and systemic disease with leukopenia and a relative lymphocytosis with a slightly enlarged liver and/or spleen. This period is followed by a subacute phase with intermittent bouts of low-grade fever when the ocular manifestations can appear with reduced

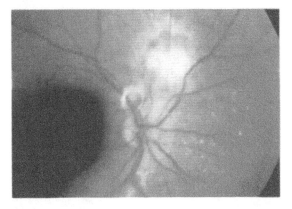

Figure 10.1

Acute chorioretinitis caused by *Brucella melitensis*.

visual acuity from a chorioretinitis. Chronic granulomatous uveitis can also be present with secondary glaucoma. Ocular manifestations are reported as less severe after *B. abortus* than after *B. melitensis* infection, although the former causes more severe systemic symptoms.

Typically, the retinal lesion has distinct margins with a hemorrhage around it (Figure 10.1) and will contain live bacilli that require antibiotic treatment by the systemic route. Chemotherapy traditionally given involves doxycycline 100 mg b.i.d. and streptomycin 1 g daily given intramuscularly; however, this regimen is not always effective and the later appearance of retinochoroiditis can be treated with oral ofloxacin 800 mg daily and oral rifampicin 900 mg daily. Serial fundus examinations should be performed weekly during treatment; progressive improvement should occur over 6 weeks. The choroidal lesion becomes

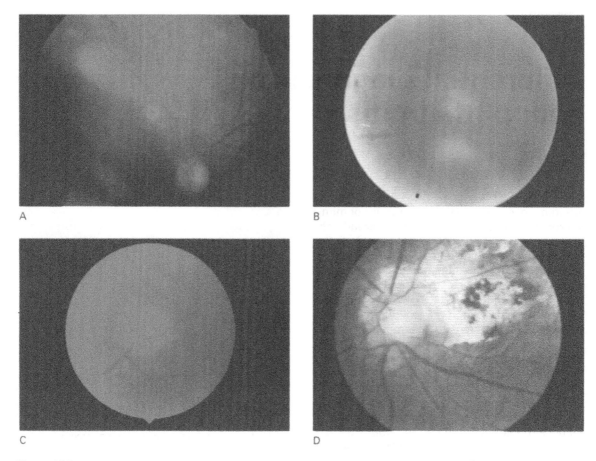

Figure 10.2

(A) Choroidal tubercle on antitubercular therapy. (B) Raised lesions of active tubercular chorioretinitis. (C) Tubercular chorioretinitis after 3 weeks of treatment with antitubercular drugs. (D) Healed lesions with chorioretinal scars 1 year later.

scarred and the retinal lesion disappears; if this does not happen, the advice of an infectious disease physician is needed for additional antibiotics. A serological agglutination test in the third week of illness will confirm the diagnosis with a titer of 1:800 or greater which can normalize after a further 6 weeks.

Tuberculosis

Tuberculosis is caused by *Mycobacterium tuberculosis*, an acid- and alcohol-fast bacillus, with increased incidence in the immunocompromised

population. This organism has an affinity for highly oxygenated tissues such as the lungs. Ocular reaction can be the result of both direct infection, such as choroiditis, and a hypersensitivity reaction to tuberculoprotein manifesting as phlyctenulosis and Eales' disease.

Tuberculosis can affect any part of the uveal tract. The most common appearance is choroiditis (Figure 10.2) which occurs in patients with pulmonary disease, who may even be asymptomatic but have a shadow on a chest X-ray.[1] Such choroiditis also occurs in miliary and chronic disease. Miliary tubercles can be seen especially in tubercular meningitis, and used to be common

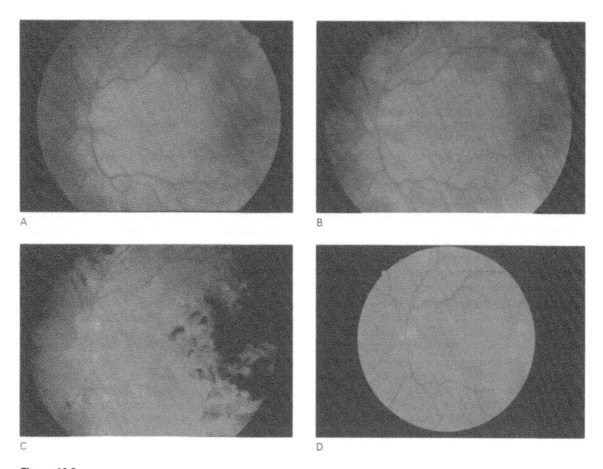

Figure 10.3

Acute posterior multifocal placoid pigment epitheliopathy (APMPPE) caused by *Mycobacterium tuberculosis*. (A) Acute lesions are visible. (B) Lesions after 3 weeks of antitubercular drug therapy. (C) Healed lesions are shown 3 years posttreatment. (D) Acute APMPPE caused by *Mycobacterium tuberculosis* in another patient.

at a late stage in children; these tubercles appear as round, pale yellow spots and vary in number from 3 to 70. Miliary tubercles consist of giant cells around live bacilli. Before chemotherapy, their presence was a prelude to death but recovery is now common with triple antitubercular therapy for a minimum of 6 months. Chronic tuberculosis can occur as a diffuse or disseminated choroiditis with extensive development of granulomatous tissue; it appears only rarely as a solitary mass resembling a neoplasm.

Biswas et al reported five cases of intraocular tuberculosis.[2] Clinical presentation included two patients with subretinal abscesses and one each with granulomatous anterior uveitis with scleral perforation, an exudative mass in the anterior chamber, and a choroidal mass with panuveitis. Three eyes eventually required enucleation, when there was granulomatous inflammation with caseation necrosis, but two showed a significant response to antitubercular therapy.

Pulmonary tuberculosis can also be associated with acute posterior multifocal placoid pigment epitheliopathy (APMPPE). This diagnosis is best established when the acute clinical lesion is associated with culture-confirmed pulmonary disease, and responds to antitubercular therapy.[3] Such cases are illustrated in Figure 10.3.

Endophthalmitis can also be induced by atypical mycobacteria without the association of the acquired immunodeficiency syndrome (AIDS).[4] In one case, there was progressive inflammation that was uncontrolled with corticosteroids and nontubercular antibiotic therapy. A diagnostic vitrectomy for microbiology was negative. The eye became blind with secondary glaucoma and was eviscerated. Histology showed granulomatous inflammation without caseation. A polymerase chain reaction (PCR) test demonstrated mycobacterial gene sequences for atypical types. This type of PCR test is useful because it can be performed on paraffin-fixed or formalin-embedded material.

Tubercular panophthalmitis was more common in the days before antimycobacterial therapy but it was rare even at that time. Ocular inflammation is occasionally seen today in the immunocompetent population, especially in persons from the Indian subcontinent, but is a special problem in patients with AIDS. Both granulomatous and nongranulomatous inflammations are seen and any ocular structure may be involved. Posterior involvement includes retinochoroiditis, choroidal nodules, vitritis, and APMPPE.

Diagnosis is implied by a positive skin tuberculin test, although previous exposure to bacille Calmette–Guérin (BCG) vaccination may also cause a positive reaction. The intensity of the skin reaction and history help to differentiate these entities. Anergy should also be suspected when a negative test result is obtained in an immunocompromised patient. A control antigen specimen such as *Candida* should be used in such cases in order to demonstrate anergy. Sputum cultures and gastric washings can be useful to demonstrate acid-alcohol-fast bacilli. Because true positive diagnoses of tuberculosis resulting from purified protein derivative (PPD) tuberculin screening of uveitis patients are rare, PPD tests are not recommended for routine evaluation of uveitis patients. However, PPD testing is of value in uveitis patients with focal granulomatous lesions and those in whom the use of oral corticosteroids is contemplated.

Treatment of uveitis caused by tuberculosis requires systemic resolution. The regimen initially includes isoniazid and rifampicin (Rifampin). A third agent such as pyrazinamide, ciprofloxacin, or streptomycin is included early in therapy or in endemic areas. Corticosteroids may be required as an adjunct therapy. Various protocols are available for multidrug-resistant strains but the patient should be referred to an infectious disease specialist for treatment.

Leprosy

Leprosy, which is caused by *Mycobacterium leprae,* has the following properties:

- The bacterium is a weekly acid-fast bacillus (AFB) which is an obligate intracellular organism that is noncultivable in artificial media.
- *M. leprae* grows in Schwann cells and other nerve structures.
- The bacterium gives distinctive immunologic reactivity.

The bacteriologic (BI) and morphologic (MI) indices provide information on the bacterial load and viability which is useful for following a response to chemotherapy. The BI is based on the enumeration of AFB in slit-skin smears based on a log scale from 1+ (1–10 bacilli per 100 microscope fields) to 6+ (>1000 bacilli per field). The MI is based on the experience that viable bacilli stain in a uniform manner with even intact cell walls and that fragmented, beaded, or irregularly stained bacilli are dead.

M. leprae does not stain with the full Ziehl–Neelsen stain used for *M. tuberculosis hominis* as it is weakly acid-fast but **not** alcohol-fast. This bacterium requires staining with the modified Ziehl–Neelsen stain, using hot carbol fuschin for 20 minutes, but decolorizing with 5% acetic acid (vinegar) alone. A counterstain is used, such as malachite green, against which the red-staining bacilli can be seen. Focusing on the bacilli with a good image is often difficult because of the thick tissue section.

Clinical forms of leprosy (Ridley-Jopling scale) are as follows.

Lepromatous leprosy is characterized by a long period of incubation and latency. In the early stages, the lesions are diffuse and erythematous with a weak brown pigmentation; they cover extensive areas of the body surface symmetrically. With progression, the skin becomes more infiltrated and sometimes frank symmetrical plaques and nodules appear, which can become multiple to cover the trunk and arms. Neurologic involvement begins with loss of sensitivity followed by enlargement of nerve trunks with muscular atrophy and deformities of the hands and feet.

Lepromatous granulomas contain undifferentiated macrophages that may be full of vacuoles: the foamy cells typical of lepromatous leprosy. Stains for *M. leprae* reveal extremely high numbers of bacilli present in the macrophages of active lepromatous lesions.

Borderline lepromatous lesions are similar to lepromatous leprosy but the borders of the plaques are more sharply defined. Bilateral symmetry is not present and the center of the lesions has a normal appearance. Histology shows undifferentiated macrophages but without foamy cells and with a much smaller number of bacilli.

Borderline leprosy is very characteristic. There are numerous erythematous plaques and nodules of varying sizes that can cover almost the entire surface of the body. Moderate anesthesia is present. Histology reveals a combination of undifferentiated macrophages and various numbers of epithelioid and giant cells. Large numbers of weakly acid-fast bacilli are present; lymphocytes are diffusely distributed.

Borderline tuberculoid leprosy is characterized by macules or plaques in greater numbers than in tuberculoid leprosy but still with well-defined borders and anesthesia or hypothesia. Inflammation of nerves is variable. Histologically, the lesions show some epithelioid differentiation and Langerhans giant cells, similar to tuberculoid leprosy, but the granuloma is less organized and more diffuse. The main difference is the presence of small numbers of weakly acid-fast bacilli.

Tuberculoid leprosy affects both skin and nerves. Skin lesions are single or few and consist of infiltrated plaques with well-defined borders and a sunken center. These lesions are anesthetic, dry, and are accompanied by dissociated anesthesia at other sites. Thickening of nerve trunks is a prominent feature. Tuberculoid granulomas have well-defined characteristics, although it may not be possible to demonstrate bacilli. These granulomas contain epithelioid cells surrounded by an abundant infiltrate of lymphocytes. The granuloma extends from the basal layer of the epidermis to the lower dermis. Nerves passing through these granulomas are obliterated.

Indeterminate leprosy consists of a single or several hypopigmented lesions that are anesthetic. Small numbers of bacilli can be seen on biopsy within a superficial nerve. The inflammatory reaction is nonspecific with a lymphohistiocytic infiltration around blood vessels.

Erythema nodosum leprosum is an exacerbation reaction of lepromatous leprosy, mimicking erythema nodosum clinically during treatment but differing histologically. The scars may ulcerate.

Ocular involvement

Uveitis can accompany leprosy with lepromatous leprosy causing more severe disease than the tuberculoid variety. Systemic treatment is required.

Immunopathology of leprosy

No exotoxins or endotoxins are produced by *M. leprae*. In lepromatous leprosy, there are millions of bacilli per gram of tissue with a high level of antibodies produced but with absent cell-mediated immunity (CMI). The opposite situation occurs with tuberculoid leprosy when the CMI gives a strong reaction but without an antibody response. The phenomenon of CD4 Th1 lymphocyte stimulation (for producing CMI) with CD4 Th2 lymphocyte suppression (for reducing antibody production) and vice versa, mediated through the feedback cytokine system, has been reviewed in Chapter 2 and leprosy is no exception to the general mechanisms. However, why lepromatous leprosy should develop in one patient and tuberculoid leprosy in another is not understood but is thought to involve the role of T suppressor cells in the particular individual. The expression of clinical disease and its type then depend on the immunologic reaction mounted in the individual to the organism.

Therapy of leprosy

Dapsone was introduced in the 1940s and used successfully in many, but not all, patients for several decades until it became apparent that widespread resistance had developed. In 1982, a World Health Organization (WHO) study group recommended that all patients with active leprosy should receive multiple drug treatment with different regimens according to their clinical-immunologic state (the Ridley-Jopling scale). Multibacillary patients (lepromatous leprosy, borderline lepromatous lesions, and borderline leprosy) were given rifampicin 600 mg and clofazimine 300 mg as monthly supervised medication along with dapsone 100 mg and clofazimine 50 mg as daily unsupervised medication. Patients were treated for 2 years and followed for 5 years. Paucibacillary patients (tuberculoid leprosy and borderline tuberculoid leprosy) were given rifampicin 600 mg monthly with daily unsupervised dapsone 100 mg. Therapy was given for 6 months and patients were followed for 2 years. These regimens have been implemented widely with good results; they are effective clinically and bacteriologically without undue toxicity but are still not available to many patients in the developing world.

Whipple's disease

Whipple's disease is a rare systemic disorder with malaise, fever, migrating arthralgias, fatigue, abdominal discomfort, diarrhea, and weight loss. Ocular signs include uveitis, vitritis, and retinal vasculitis. Small bowel biopsy shows characteristic, diastase-resistant, PAS-positive macrophages in the mucosal lamina propria. The etiologic agent has been identified as a Gram-positive actinomycete called *Tropheryma whipplii*. There is some evidence of a predisposing immunodeficiency.[5,6]

This condition, including its ocular features, may be treated successfully with antibiotics; however, relapse is common. The use of antibiotics with good penetration of the blood–brain barrier is important to minimize central nervous system (CNS) complications. Combination therapy is therefore recommended, e.g. 2 weeks of treatment with parenterally administered streptomycin and benzylpenicillin followed by sulfamethoxazole (800 mg) and trimethoprim (160 mg) orally b.i.d. for 1 year.

Cat-scratch disease

Bartonella (Rochalimaea) henselae, the possible etiologic agent of cat-scratch disease, was identified by PCR in a patient with Parinaud's oculog-

Table 10.1 Clinical stages of syphilis

Stage	Characteristics
Primary	Chancre
Secondary	Skin rash (palms, soles), fever, weight loss, arthralgia, uveitis, floaters. Positive reagin test such as VDRL and a specific test such as FTA-ABS or TPHA. Acute iritis roseate or iris roseola, vascularized papules, iritis nodosa, choroiditis, papillitis, vitritis, gummata
Tertiary	General paralysis of the insane, tabes dorsalis, meningovasculitis

FTA-ABS, fluorescent treponemal absorption; TPHA, *Treponema pallidum* hemagglutination assay; VDRL, Venereal Disease Research Laboratories.

landular syndrome in whom culture was unhelpful and specific stains for AFB and fungi of a conjunctival biopsy were negative.[7]

Cat-scratch disease can be associated with persistent vitritis, leading to vitrectomy. Analysis of such a vitrectomy specimen has shown inflammatory cells and necrotic debris but no organism. PCR of the vitreous sample is possible with a novel hemi-nested protocol to demonstrate the presence of *Bartonella henselae* DNA. Treatment with doxycycline led to improvement in the intraocular inflammation but resulted in a poor visual outcome.[8]

Syphilis

Syphilis can mimic many different disorders and is appropriately termed the great masquerader. The causative organism is *Treponema pallidum* of the Spirochete family and is either transmitted congenitally or by a sexual route. The incidence of syphilis has increased since the advent of the human immunodeficiency virus (HIV) and particularly in the last 3 years. The clinical stages of syphilis are listed in Table 10.1.

Systemic manifestations

Chancre, among the first signs of primary syphilis, is an ulcer that appears 10 days to 3 months after exposure to the organism and resolves within a few weeks. This painless lesion is usually found on the penis, vulva, vagina, or rectum, corresponding to the area exposed to a partner's lesion. The chancre disappears within a few weeks whether or not a person is treated.

One-third of untreated people will progress to chronic stages. Secondary syphilis is characterized by a skin rash that appears 3–6 weeks after the disappearance of a chancre. These lesions may appear as dark sores and appear anywhere on the body, although the palms and soles of the feet are always involved. Other symptoms of this stage include mild fever, fatigue, headache, and sore throat, as well as patchy hair loss, and swollen lymph glands throughout the body. These symptoms are transient and may appear intermittently over 1–2 years.

Untreated syphilis may lapse into the latent stage. However, up to one-third of patients with secondary syphilis will progress to tertiary syphilis involving the heart, eyes, brain, nervous system, and almost any other part of the body. This stage may last for years and result in mental illness (general paralysis of the insane [GPI]), blindness, neurologic disorders including tabes dorsalis, heart disease, aortitis, and death. Syphilitic organisms may invade the CNS during the early stages of infection, and 3–7% of untreated patients develop neurosyphilis.[9] Although some patients with neurosyphilis may never develop any symptoms, others may display signs of chronic lymphocytic meningitis, seizures, and stroke. Neurosyphilis may be more difficult to treat and its course may be different in people with HIV infection.

Ocular manifestations

Syphilis can present with retinochoroiditis in the secondary stage that can be associated with syphilitic meningitis. Syphilitic neuroretinitis presents as papillitis, with peripapillary flame-shaped hemorrhages, periarteriolar sheathing, and stellate macular exudates. At this stage, the characteristic macular-papular rash of secondary syphilis with 'snail-track' mouth ulcers may appear or the patient may be asymptomatic apart from a loss of visual acuity. Residual changes include optic atrophy. Necrotizing retinitis may occur associated with panuveitis and retinal vasculitis. Retinitis can become more extensive

and bilateral in patients with AIDS. Progressive changes can become similar to those seen in acute retinal necrosis.[10]

Treatment must be given for 2 weeks with high-dose intravenous penicillin G (3 mega-units, every 4 hours in patients with normal renal function) or a high dose of intramuscular depository penicillin G with oral probenicid. It is essential that the patient's serology be repeated to follow an expected reduction in titer of the nonspecific reagin test. If this reduction has not begun after 6 weeks, then the penicillin course must be repeated and the patient closely followed in a specialty clinic. No reduction in titer is expected with the specific serologic tests.

The failure of the standard 2-week course to treat the patient adequately is not uncommon and if the patient absconds from follow-up, then progression to the tertiary stage of neurosyphilis can occur. Besides the classical presentation of tabes dorsalis (shooting pains in the legs), this stage can present as 'pseudoretinitis pigmentosa' with a progressive decrease in visual acuity and nyctalopia. Findings include a diffuse, granular appearance of the retinal pigment epithelium throughout both fundi with choroidal atrophy.[11]

Systemic findings in neurosyphilis include Argyll Robertson pupils, small, irregular, and reactive to the near response but not to light; and reduced or absent reflexes. Patients may also present with abstruse signs of meningovascular disease with cranial nerve palsies or generalized vascular disease with periarteritis and endarteritis, while a gumma can occur anywhere.

Congenital syphilis is associated with a pigmentary retinopathy that may be segmental or generalized and is morphologically difficult to distinguish from retinitis pigmentosa.[12] Acquired syphilis most commonly produces a patchy and diffuse neuroretinitis with areas of hemorrhage. In some instances, intense patches of chorioretinal infiltrates are seen next to pigmented scarring.

Diagnostic serology includes nontreponemal cardiolipin reagin tests such as the Venereal Disease Research Laboratories (VDRL) and rapid plasma reagin (RPR) tests, which are useful to judge the activity of the disease, although false-positive results can occur. In addition, there are specific antibody tests such as the fluorescent treponemal absorption (FTA-ABS) and micro-hemagglutination-*Treponema pallidum* (MHA-TP) tests. In the case of positive serology without symptoms, asymptomatic neurosyphilis must be ruled out by a lumbar puncture and cerebrospinal fluid (CSF) collected for a reagin and specific test. The reagin test RPR is positive with high titers in active disease and its levels reflect the efficacy of treatment. This finding is in contrast to the specific tests, which remain elevated for life, but the reagin test will return to normal with effective penicillin therapy.

Treatment of syphilitic uveitis involves aqueous crystalline penicillin G (12–24 million units intravenously per day for 10 days) followed by benthazine penicillin G 2.4 million units intramuscularly weekly for 3 weeks.

Lyme disease

Although ocular manifestations are a rare feature of the tick-borne Lyme disease, the spirochete (Borrelia burgdorferi) invades the eye early and remains dormant, accounting for both early and late ocular manifestations. A nonspecific follicular conjunctivitis occurs in approximately 10% of patients with early Lyme disease, while often keratitis occurs within a few months of onset and is characterized by nummular, interstitial opacities. Inflammatory events include orbital myositis, episcleritis, uveitis, vitritis, and retinal vasculitis. In some cases with negative serology, a vitreous tap is required for diagnosis. Neuroophthalmic manifestations include bilateral mydriasis, neuroretinitis, pigmentary retinopathy, involvement of multiple cranial nerves, optic atrophy, and disc edema. Seventh cranial nerve paresis can lead to neurotrophic keratitis. In endemic areas, Lyme disease may be responsible for approximately 25% of new-onset Bell's palsy cases.

Diagnosis is based on a history of exposure within an endemic area, positive serology, and response to treatment.[13] Antibodies may be measured by indirect ELISA and Western blot. PCR has been used successfully for specimens from the vitreous and CSF.[14] Serum RPR or VDRL tests are nonreactive in Lyme borreliosis, but false-positive FTA-ABS tests can occur.

Spirochetes have been identified in the vitreous of a seronegative patient with vitritis and choroiditis and cultured from an iris biopsy in a treated patient. Therapy with doxycycline or amoxicillin is effective in the earliest stages but serious late complications require high doses of intravenous penicillin or ceftriaxone.

Viruses

West Nile fever

The West Nile fever virus spectrum includes headache, stiff neck, myalgia, arthralgia, visual loss (blurred vision) with floaters, and fever with a maculo-papular rash. This virus can be associated with an anterior uveitis, iridocyclitis, vitritis, non-necrotizing creamy yellow circular chorioretinal lesions, and peripheral visual field loss.[15–18] Mild disc edema may be seen. The anterior uveitis responds to topical steroids. The retinal lesions appear hypofluorescent centrally and hyperfluorescent around the edges. Laboratory diagnosis is made by an IgM serologic test. West Nile virus usually causes mild symptoms but occasionally causes neurologic illness with severe morbidity or a fatal outcome.

Acute retinal necrosis syndrome

Acute retinal necrosis (ARN) syndrome, which has been described in both immunocompetent and immunosuppressed individuals, has clinical features which differ according to immune status. Herpes zoster and herpes simplex virus (HSV) have been implicated in immunocompetent patients. ARN tends to follow shingles in older patients and HSV infection in younger patients. ARN is characterized by rapid onset of painful loss of vision with areas of necrotizing retinitis, often peripheral, which enlarge and coalesce. There are vasculitis, macular edema, and acute optic neuritis present. Prompt treatment with intravenous acyclovir at 500–800 mg/m^2 every 8 hours for 7–14 days is effective in halting progression of the infection and may prevent involvement of the other eye. The outcome, however, is reported to be poor. While cytomegalovirus (CMV) occasionally causes retinitis in preterm infants and those on immunosuppressive drugs without HIV infection, this retinitis does not usually progress to ARN. For CMV, see the AIDS section later in the chapter.

PCR (Chapter 3) can be useful for identifying the cause of retinitis based on analysis of a vitreous specimen. In one study, CMV, varicella zoster virus (VZV), or HSV DNA was detected in vitreous samples from 24 patients.[19] CMV DNA was detected in vitreous biopsy specimens from 11 eyes of 10 patients. Nine of the 10 patients with CMV and AIDS developed retinitis over time. VZV was detected in vitreous biopsy specimens from eight patients and HSV from six patients. PCR-based assays on vitreous specimens are useful for diagnostic evaluation of patients with infectious retinitis.

Cidofovir therapy

Cidofovir has been used intravenously for the treatment of CMV retinitis, the most common cause of viral retinitis in AIDS, affecting 25% of patients. Cidofovir has potent antiviral activity against herpes viruses, CMV, and adenovirus which is not dependent on phosphorylation by a virus-encoded nucleoside kinase similar to acyclovir. Reported side effects include uveitis and hypotony, which can be serious.[20] In the latter report, the patient developed almost complete atrophy of the ciliary body, possibly from cidofovir cyclotoxicity.

Leber's idiopathic stellate neuroretinitis

Leber's idiopathic stellate neuroretinitis presents with a sudden loss of vision following a 'viral-type' illness such as hepatitis, cat-scratch fever, or leptospirosis, and occasionally after other systemic infections including toxocaral disease. This condition may also occur in the early stage of asymptomatic neurosyphilis; therefore, appropriate tests should always be performed. In the first week after the onset of decreased visual acuity, usually only swelling of the optic disc may be seen; however, 1 week later a typical macular star (Figure 10.4) is present that is not a maculopathy but is caused by vascular leakage from the optic nerve head followed by reabsorption of serum when lipid precipitates in a stellate pattern. The swelling of the optic disc may be mild, segmental, or massive. Leber's idiopathic stellate neuroretinitis is not related to demyeli-

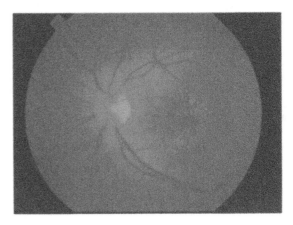

Figure 10.4

Leber's idiopathic stellate neuroretinitis following a systemic virus infection (non-A, non-B hepatitis).

nating diseases but a differential diagnosis for the disc swelling may include leakage from the parafoveal capillaries with diabetes mellitus and hypertension.

There is no specific therapy for this condition. The disc swelling begins to decrease after 2 weeks and resolves within 10 weeks. The macular star begins to decrease after 1 month but requires as long as 1 year for complete resolution. The prognosis for vision is good but there are cases that become exceptions.[21]

Fungi

Candida

Chorioretinitis caused by *Candida albicans* and *Cryptococcus neoformans* has been considered in Chapter 9 (Endogenous endophthalmitis).

Histoplasmosis

Residents in those parts of the world where the soil contains the dimorphic fungus *Histoplasma capsulatum* can suffer from pulmonary disease and posterior uveitis. The uveitis usually follows

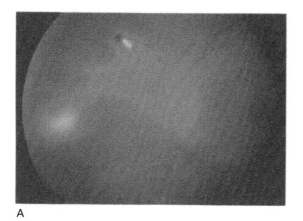
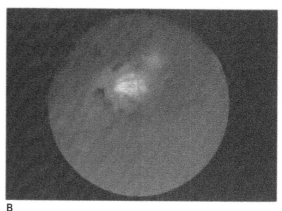

A   B

Figure 10.5

(A and B) Acute chorioretinitis and healed scar following successful therapy for toxoplasmosis. Note that the acute retinal lesion has occurred adjacent to a previous focus of infection.

a benign, asymptomatic course. The histoplasma complement fixation test is positive in 15% of patients; serum must be collected before injecting the histoplasma skin test antigen, which is positive in 90% of cases. This true infection must be distinguished from the pseudoinfection mistakenly labeled 'ocular histoplasmosis syndrome' and diagnosed in patients who have never lived in an area with endemic histoplasma.

Sporotrichosis

Sporothrix schenckii can cause cutaneous and ocular disease (sporotrichosis) in endemic areas, particularly in Brazil,[22] including uveitis. This fungus can be isolated from the aqueous humor. The disease can present as granulomatous uveitis.[23] Other cases are considered in Chapter 9.

Protozoa and helminths

Involvement of ocular tissues by protozoa and helminths is given in Table 10.3.

Toxoplasmosis

Toxoplasmosis, a common cause of intraocular inflammation accounting for 7–15% of all uveitis cases, is caused by *Toxoplasma gondii*, which is an intestinal parasite found in cats. The organism exists in three forms – oocyst, bradyzoite, and tachyzoite – of which the tachyzoite is the active form. Human transmission occurs by consumption of undercooked meats containing bradyzoites and contamination by cat feces. Pregnant women should be especially aware because fetal transmission in the first trimester results in severe CNS, ocular, and systemic complications.

Patients generally report unilateral floaters and visual blurring; the posterior segment tends to be more inflamed than the anterior segment. Examination reveals vitreous opacities and retinal lesions. The retinal lesions occur adjacent to a previous focus of infection and appear as a fuzzy border (Figure 10.5). The affected retinal vasculature shows perivasculitis with diffuse venous sheathing and segmental arterial sheathing. Exudative focal retinitis can occur and the anterior layer of the retina is more involved in proliferation of the organism, although a deeper form may also occur. Toxoplasmal retinitis can also present only with small punctate peripheral lesions called punctate outer toxoplasmosis. Doft and Gass described this entity as having multifocal, gray-white lesions at the level of deep retina and retinal pigment epithelium associated with little or no overlying vitreous reaction.[24]

Table 10.2 Toxoplasmosis treatment options

Drug	Oral therapy	Toxicity
Sulfonamide	4-g loading dose of triple sulfa or sulfadiazine followed by 1 g q.i.d. for 6 weeks	Kidney stones, Stevens–Johnson syndrome
Folinic acid	3 mg daily or IM twice weekly	—
Pyrimethamine	Loading dose of 150 mg followed by 25 mg daily for 6 weeks	Leucopenia, thrombocytopenia
Clindamycin	300 mg q.i.d. for 4–6 weeks	Pseudomembranous colitis

IM, intramuscular.

The recurrent retinochoroiditis usually presents as a yellow inflammatory lesion resulting in an overlying vitreous haze, occurring at the margin of a preexisting choroidal scar. Another presentation is a juxtapapillary lesion at the margin of the optic disc that causes a typical arcuate field defect. Small peripheral retinal lesions may be allowed to run their course but lesions near the macula, optic disc, or maculopapular nerve fiber bundle, or those associated with severe vitritis, should be treated. Therapy is directed both against the dividing organism and the inflammatory host response. The problem is complicated by multiplication of the protozoan within 'tissue cysts' within cells which are impervious to drug penetration, so that recurrence can always be expected. *Toxoplasma* infection is encountered in immunocompromised patients and can be severe in AIDS.

Treatment options for toxoplasmosis include pyrimethamine (Daraprim), sulfonamide, and clindamycin (Table 10.2). Adjunct therapies include folinic acid and steroid therapy. Folinic acid (leucovorin calcium) helps to prevent leukopenia and thrombocytopenia resulting from pyrimethamine therapy. Pyrimethamine and sulfadiazine act synergistically to interfere with folic acid synthesis. These drugs should be commenced early in the course of the disease and continued for 4–6 weeks. Pyrimethamine therapy should be avoided in early pregnancy and monitored closely because of the risk of bone marrow depression. Folinic acid supplements reduce this risk but platelet and white cell counts should be performed weekly.

Clindamycin has also been found to be effective in the treatment of ocular toxoplasmosis[25] and has good ocular tissue absorption properties. However, clindamycin carries the risk of pseudomembranous colitis, although this risk is small when used on an outpatient basis. The role of intravitreal clindamycin with and without steroids needs further evaluation.

Tetracycline and minocycline may also be effective but have not yet been fully evaluated in clinical trials.

Oral corticosteroid therapy is indicated in vision-threatening disease but should not be used without concurrent specific antiprotozoal therapy or in immunocompromised patients.

Ocular *Toxocara* (larva migrans) infection

Toxocara canis is a worm whose natural host is the dog. Man, an accidental host, becomes infected from ingesting the ova from dog-contaminated soil; the larval stage develops, causing visceral and ocular 'larva migrans' although adult worms are not found. These larvae migrate around the body and occasionally deposit themselves in the CNS, including the retina. In the eye, *Toxocara* infection can present as a possible tumor, for which eyes have been eviscerated in the past.

Serologic diagnosis only confirms previous exposure and does not indicate whether the retinal lesion is that of toxocariasis or not. Furthermore, the serologic test may be negative when a

Table 10.3 Involvement of ocular tissues by protozoa and helminths

	Lacrimal sac	Lids	Conjunctiva	Sclera	Cornea	AC	Ciliary body	Iris	Lens	Uvea	Vitreous	Choroid	Retina	Optic nerve	Orbit	Extraocular muscles
Protozoa																
Acanthamoebiasis	[+]	[+]	[+]	(+)	+			[+]		[+]au	+					
Microsporidiosis	[+]	[+]	[+]		+											
Toxoplasmosis						+			(+)	+pu	+	+	+	(+)		
Pneumocystosis												+				
African trypanosomiasis	(+)	(+)	+		(+)			(+)		+au		(+)	+	(+)		
S. American trypanosomiasis	(+)	(+)								+						
Leishmaniasis[a]	(+)	+	(+)		[+]					+au		(+)	(+)	(+)		
Malaria			(+)							+		+	+b	+		
Babesiosis													+	+		
Entamoebiasis	(+)	(+)								+au		+	(+)	+		
Giardiasis		+	+				+	+		+au/pu	+	+	+			
Helminths																
Toxocariasis[c]					(+)	+		(+)		+	+	+	+	+		
'Ocular Larva migrans'[c]		(+)	(+)		(+)	(+)	+	(+)		+	+	(+)	+	+	+	
Paragonimiasis[c]	+	(+)	+			+	+		+	(+)	+	+	(+)	(+)	(+)	+
Schistosomiasis[c]	+	+	+			+					+	+	(+)	+	+	
Alariasis[c]	+						(+)	(+)			+	(+)	(+)			
Ascariasis[c]	+						(+)	(+)				(+)				
Baylisascaris[c]			(+)								+	+	+	+		
Cysticercosis[d,e]			(+)		(+)	+		+	(+)		+	+		(+)	+	
Hydatidosis[f]		+	+			+	+	+		+	+	+	(+)	(+)	+	
Trichinosis		+	+		+	+	+	+		+	+	+	+	+	+	+g
Onchocerciasis[d]		+	+		+	+	+	+		+		+	+	+		
Loiasis	+	+	+			+									+	
Dirofilariasis		+	+			+	+	+		+	+	+				
Brugia filariasis	(+)	(+)	(+)			+	+	+		+au		+			+	
Bancroftian filariasis	+	+	+		(+)	(+)				(+)		(+)			(+)	
Dracunculiasis	+	+	+		(+)	(+)	(+)	(+)	(+)	(+)	(+)	(+)	(+)	(+)	(+)	+
Gnathostomiasis			+	+							+					
Thelaziasis	(+)	(+)	+		(+)	+	+	(+)			+	+	+	(+)		
Angiostrongyliasis			+													
Philophthalmiasis	+	+	+		+	+					+	+	+	+	+	+
Coenurus	(+)	+	+			+					+	+	+	+	+	+
Sparagonosis																

+, Main structure(s) involved. (+), Rare or late effect. [+], Tissue reaction to, but not active infection by, the protozoa or helminth. au, Anterior uveitis. pu, Posterior uveitis.
[a] Depends on type of leishmaniasis. [b] Retinal hemorrhages, retinopathy after chloroquine therapy. [c] Can give signs of diffuse unilateral subacute neuroretinitis (DUSN). [d] Posterior, anterior segments involved – variation depends on geographical location. [e] Cystic stage of Taenia solium. [f] Cystic stage of Echinococcus granulosus. [g] In trichinosis, encysted larvae invade the extraocular muscles preferentially, as well as the orbicularis, to produce a characteristic oedema. (Derived from Seal D et al.[52])

choroidal lesion is present. Serologic diagnosis is thus unreliable and should not be performed. Fine needle biopsy in a reference center, with cytology for tumor cells and a PCR test for *Toxocara* antigen, is the best approach.

If the retinal lesion is peripheral, treatment is conservative or symptomatic; however, lesions close to the macula warrant treatment. Diethylcarbamazine (DEC) is given orally for 3 weeks at 3 mg/kg. The dying larvae may cause symptoms of allergic reaction, for which prednisolone is usually given to suppress such inflammatory reactions in ophthalmic cases. Vitreous traction and localized tractional retinal detachment can be managed by vitrectomy. If blindness develops, it is usually unilateral but bilateral cases are known. Therapy can also be given with albendazole or with a single dose of ivermectin.

Diffuse unilateral subacute neuroretinitis

In the early stages of diffuse unilateral subacute neuroretinitis (DUSN) there is decreased visual acuity and blurred vision often developing over a previous year. The condition presents with vasculitis, multiple foci of outer retinitis, meandering pigmentary retinal changes, papillitis, intraretinal hemorrhages, and later, optic atrophy (Figure 10.6).

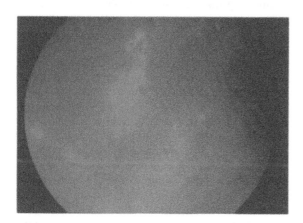

Figure 10.6

Retinal exudates around vessels in visceral larva migrans presenting as diffuse unilateral subacute neuroretinitis (DUSN).

The most common causes of DUSN are the larvae of ascaridoid nematodes, including *Toxocara canis* and the dog hookworm *Ancylostoma caninum*. There are a few reports of trematode infection of the eye including *Paragonimus* sp. (the lung fluke) in endemic areas such as Thailand. Ocular schistosomiasis can also occur. *Alaria* sp., another trematode worm, has infected two Chinese patients in San Francisco.

Drug therapy for nematodes includes thiabendazole and ivermectin; for trematodes, praziquantel and albendazole are used (Chapter 11). Corticosteroid treatment is beneficial for decreasing the associated inflammation. If the nematode is visible in the fundus, one might attempt to coagulate it with a laser. Measuring the aqueous-to-serum antibody ratio to the specific antigen can be useful diagnostically.

Ocular onchocerciasis

Ocular onchocerciasis, or 'river blindness,' results from infection with the filarial parasite *Onchocerca volvulus.* The disease is endemic in areas of Africa and Central and South America where it is a major cause of blindness. The ocular manifestations include keratitis, anterior uveitis, glaucoma, chorioretinitis, and optic neuritis.[25] The inflammatory reaction that occurs is the result of a cell-mediated immune response to the dead microfilariae, which can be seen biomicroscopically at the center of ill-defined opacities which have passed through a sequence of inflammation and scarring. This inflammation is exacerbated by DEC treatment.

For several decades, DEC and sumarin have been used systemically in the treatment of ocular onchocerciasis. Both are effective microfilaricidal drugs with a positive effect on keratitis and uveitis; they are, however, less beneficial in posterior segment disease. The use of DEC may be followed by a severe systemic reaction which is largely prevented by the concomitant use of systemic corticosteroids. An appropriate therapeutic regimen has been provided by Taylor and Dax.[26] DEC was also known to precipitate or exacerbate active optic neuritis in some onchocercal patients as part of a general inflammatory reaction (the Mazzotti reaction).[27]

Ivermectin (12-mg single dose) has also been shown to slowly eliminate microfilariae from the anterior chamber but offers the advantages of minimal ocular inflammation and much less systemic reaction.[28] This agent represents an important advance in the mass therapy of onchocerciasis in endemic areas, by single-dose therapy, for which purpose it has been donated by Merck, Sharpe, and Dohme. A critical feature of its mode of action is that ivermectin acts on the adult female worms to inhibit reproduction, so that no new microfilariae are produced for several months. This drug also kills microfilariae in tissues including the skin and the eye, and has to be given yearly; the eradication program is a continuous one. Ivermectin should not be given to children under 5 years of age, to pregnant women, or to patients with other severe infections such as trypanosomiasis. Ivermectin does not appear to precipitate or exacerbate optic neuritis, at least in the early stages of treatment.[28]

Acute posterior multifocal placoid pigment epitheliopathy

APMPPE was first described by Gass in 1968.[29] APMPPE, which presents with acute or subacute visual blurring, scotomas, or metamorphopsia, is bilateral in approximately 75% of patients. While APMPPE can be self-limiting, there can be an infection such as tuberculosis that requires treatment. In its typical form, APMPPE presents a picture of discrete placoid lesions which in their active phase are cream colored with indistinct margins, blocking a view of the choroid. New lesions can arise within days and there can be fresh lesions concurrently with dwindling ones.[30]

The etiology of APMPPE includes the following infections or noxious stimuli:

- Pulmonary tuberculosis[3]
- Lyme disease
- Adenovirus type 5
- Vaccination for swine influenza
- Sarcoidosis
- Cerebral vasculitis
- Photic damage to the retina
- Lead toxicity
- Idiopathic.

Acquired immunodeficiency syndrome (AIDS)

HIV has been identified in tear fluid, conjunctiva, corneal epithelium, and the retina; however, the principal ophthalmic manifestations of AIDS relate to the occurrence of florid opportunistic infections and to conjunctival and orbital involvement with Kaposi's sarcoma and other neoplasms. Therapy is directed against the relevant organism and is generally more intense and prolonged than is required in immunocompetent individuals.

HIV can cause a characteristic retinitis, resulting from microvasculopathy, of cotton-wool spots, hemorrhages in the nerve fiber layer known as 'flame hemorrhages,' or deeper in the retina as 'blot' or 'sheet' hemorrhages, microaneurysms, macular exudates, and edema with optic neuropathy without other infectious microbes being involved. These signs are illustrated in Figure 10.7A–D. HIV can also cause a characteristic retinopathy (Figure 10.7E).

Treatment is given as part of the systemic therapy of HIV infection and involves dual therapy with an antiretroviral drug inhibiting production of the reverse transcriptase required for replication, namely azidothymidine (AZT) or zidovudine, and a proteinase inhibitor such as dideoxyinosine (ddI) and dideoxycytidine (ddC), preventing virus particle function. This combined approach is prolonging the lifespan of HIV-infected individuals and keeping virus counts in their T cells low so that the infections described below are being seen much less frequently. The therapy causes a lack of HIV reproduction in lymphocytes, although the virus is not eradicated, and a CD4+ Th lymphocyte count rises above 200 per µl, at which level opportunistic infection is prevented by the immune response. Such chemotherapy has to be maintained for the lifespan of the individual.

The *M. tuberculosis* group, including multiple resistant strains of *M. avium-intracellulare*, has been increasingly recognized to cause severe systemic infection which can also manifest as chorioretinitis. The presentation is similar to that given above but endophthalmitis can also occur. The infection can be community-acquired but has also been recognized in hospital-acquired outbreaks in AIDS wards. Systemic antitubercular treatment is required.

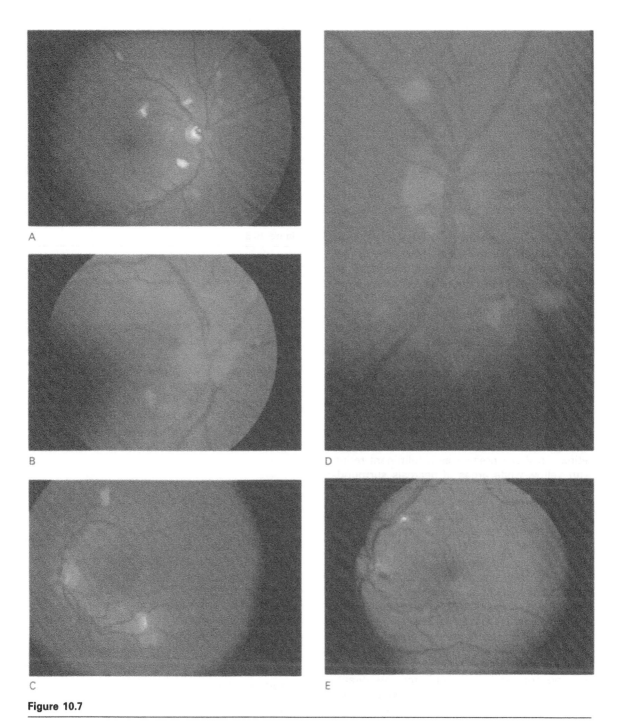

Figure 10.7

(A–D) Flame-shaped hemorrhages and exudates in human immunodeficiency virus infection. (E) Retinopathy of human immunodeficiency virus.

T. pallidum infection can coexist with HIV, with similar modes of transmission. Ocular signs present as described above, but in the presence of HIV infection there can be rapid progression to neurosyphilis. The retinitis that occurs can simulate CMV infection or present as a retinal pigment epitheliitis. Serologic testing in HIV infection can be misleading, particularly with a false-negative cardiolipin reagin test viz. VDRL result.

CMV is the most common of the ocular opportunists and produces a hemorrhagic necrotizing retinitis. During the first 7 years after HIV infection appeared, less than 1% of HIV-infected persons presented with CMV retinopathy as the initial manifestation of AIDS. Today 2% of those with AIDS have CMV retinopathy as the first manifestation. CMV retinitis is found in approximately 20% of terminal AIDS patients and is bilateral in about 17%. The delay from presentation with HIV infection is shorter in bilateral cases. HSV, Epstein–Barr virus, and *Toxoplasma* may occasionally cause a clinically similar retinitis.

Patients with CMV retinitis complain of visual field defects, flashing lights, and symptoms of floaters. If the central retina or optic nerve is involved, the patients report a reduction in visual acuity. CMV causes diffuse, full-thickness retinitis that is sharply demarcated from normal adjacent retina. CMV can present as a fulminant retinitis with yellow-white areas of necrosis surrounded by hemorrhages ('pizza pie' retinitis) (Figure 10.8) or as a 'granular' retinitis in which hemorrhages are not a feature and may be absent. Both types follow a similar clinical course and may coexist in the same eye.

In a study of CMV retinitis in AIDS patients, 58% presented with unilateral disease and 15% of these developed contralateral infection despite treatment with ganciclovir. 'Smoldering retinitis' was a clinical sign seen in 33% of the patients whose retinitis progressed while receiving ganciclovir.[31] Response to therapy is partly related to immune status. At presentation, CMV retinitis does not frequently pose an immediate threat to vision but may do so with the development of retinal detachment, in association with peripapillary disease or with involvement of the central retina. Retinal detachment, an important cause of blindness from CMV retinitis, can be treated successfully by vitrectomy, silicone oil, and endolaser. Elimination of scleral buckling may

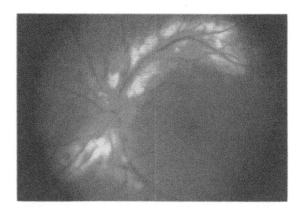

Figure 10.8

Fulminant CMV retinitis with yellow-white areas of necrosis surrounded by hemorrhages ('pizza pie' retinitis) in AIDS.

reduce intraoperative time, patient morbidity, and the risk of an accidental needle stick.

CMV retinitis occurring in AIDS patients implies a high risk for the development of CMV encephalitis (relative risk, 9.5), particularly when the retinitis involves the peripapillary region (relative risk, 13). However, in patients with AIDS without CMV retinitis, CNS symptoms are unlikely to be attributable to CMV encephalitis.[32]

Therapy

Progression of CMV retinitis may be delayed in the short term by intravenous therapy with either ganciclovir or foscarnet. Repeated, local intravitreal therapy is more effective and particularly valuable when there are no signs of disseminated CMV disease. The development of slow-release, intraocular implant systems promises to provide further improvements in management.

Parenteral therapy

The virostatic drugs dihydroxypropoxymethylguanine (DHPG, ganciclovir – similar in structure to acyclovir) and trisodium phosphonoformate (foscarnet) improve or temporarily stabilize retinitis in the majority of patients receiving long-term maintenance therapy. Ganciclovir and foscarnet are equally effective in controling CMV retinitis, but foscarnet is less well tolerated; neither is viricidal. Ganciclovir is myelotoxic while foscarnet causes renal toxicity. Repeated therapy is indicated because of the high relapse rate. Ganciclovir is given by intravenous infusion over 1 hour in a dose of 5 mg/kg every 12 hours.

In a randomized trial of CMV retinitis therapy in AIDS, patients were either immediately treated with intravenous ganciclovir (5 mg/kg b.i.d. for 14 days and then once daily for 14 weeks), or treatment was deferred.[33] Deferred patients whose retinitis progressed were offered ganciclovir. The median time to progression in the deferred treatment group was 13.5 days compared with 49.5 days in the immediate treatment group. Intravenous administration of ganciclovir results in intravitreal concentrations which are subtherapeutic (0.93 ± 0.39 µg/ml) for many CMV isolates, which explains the difficulty of long-term complete suppression of CMV retinitis by this route.

Combined daily therapy with ganciclovir and foscarnet has recently been shown to be beneficial, with prolonged intervals between progressions without increased toxicity. Such therapy may halt the progress of peripheral outer retinal necrosis in AIDS patients. Unfortunately, three of the seven patients in this study had died of other AIDS-related disease before definitive conclusions could be reached, which has also been our experience.

Improved results have been achieved with cidofovir (CDV-HPMPC). Treatment with 5 mg/kg once weekly for 2 weeks, then 5 mg/kg every other week delayed the progression of retinitis in AIDS patients compared with delayed therapy. Proteinuria (23%) and neutropenia (15%) are possibly related to therapy and may lead to discontinuation of the drug.

Intraocular delivery

An effective treatment of CMV retinitis that avoids the risk of systemic toxicity is the intravitreal injection of antiviral agents. Early studies of intravitreal therapy via the pars plana (a region anterior to the retina), with ganciclovir 400 µg, involved induction with two injections per week, followed by maintenance with one weekly injection. In a study by Cochereau-Massin et al with a mean of five intravitreal injections per eye, there was no relapse in 70% of patients at 48 days postinjection.[34]

Intravitreal ganciclovir or foscarnet has been given on a weekly basis with few local ocular complications. An intravitreal dose of ganciclovir (200–400 µg) is as effective as intravenous therapy. A dose of 2 mg in 0.05–0.1 ml provides adequate intravitreal levels (0.25–1.22 µg/ml) for up to 7 days. Levels at 24 hours postinjection have been reported to be 143.4 µg/ml; at 72 hours, the level was 23.4 µg/ml.[35] Intravitreal therapy is a major cost saving in comparison with intravenous therapy.

The intravitreal dose of foscarnet is 2.4 mg in 0.1 ml; 500 µg/0.1 ml of ganciclovir or foscarnet may be given in patients whose eyes contain silicone oil used in retinal surgery.

Intravitreal cidofovir (20 µg/0.1 ml) halted progression of CMV retinitis for 6–10 weeks after a single injection, with a median time to progression of 55 days after the initial injection or 63 days after repeat injections. Patients also received oral probenecid. There was a significant decrease in intraocular pressure from baseline to both 2 and 4 weeks after injection. Cidofovir caused a slight lowering of intraocular pressure and a mild-to-moderate iritis that responded to treatment.

More recently, the development of intraocular, sustained-release devices has provided the opportunity to deliver controlled amounts of drugs for prolonged periods with minimum local toxicity. The median time to progression of CMV retinitis was 226 days following a ganciclovir implant delivering 1 µg/hour compared with 15 days for deferred treatment.

Other opportunistic infections are seen less frequently in AIDS.

Toxoplasma gondii, which causes chorioretinitis less commonly than CNS involvement, may cause the presenting symptom, with blurred vision and floaters or pronounced visual loss from macular, papillomacular bundle, or optic nerve head involvement. The retinochoroiditis is not associated with a preexisting retinochoroidal scar, suggesting that the lesions are a manifestation of acquired rather than congenital disease. The presence of IgM antibodies may support this theory, although antibody levels in AIDS may not reflect the magnitude of disease. Lesions may be single or multifocal, in one or both eyes, or consist of massive areas of retinal necrosis: they may resemble those of CMV retinitis and may occur concurrently in the same eye. In comparison, toxoplasmic lesions tend to be thick and opaque, with smooth borders and a relative lack of hemorrhage. A prominent anterior chamber and vitreous reaction may occur.

Treatment of the toxoplasmic ocular infection with pyrimethamine, clindamycin, and sulfadiazine is effective in more than 75% of patients. Once resolution is observed, maintenance therapy is continued, as relapses occur in the absence of treatment. Corticosteroid treatment is unnecessary and its use has been associated with the development of CMV retinitis.

Pneumocystis carinii causes pneumonia (PCP) in up to 80% of AIDS patients. This protozoal organism can cause choroidopathy in patients with systemic spread from primary lung infections. Multiple yellow placoid fundus lesions are seen.[36,37] Parenteral pentamidine or cotrimoxazole (Septrin) are required for treatment, but pentamidine **should not** be given with foscarnet if there is coexisting CMV infection because of the risk of profound hypocalcemia.

Candida albicans and *Cryptococcus neoformans* can also produce retinal lesions or endophthalmitis, particularly in AIDS patients who are intravenous drug users. Cryptococcosis can present as an iris inflammatory mass and with a differing array of clinical features.[38]

A bilateral epithelial keratopathy caused by *Encephalitozoon* sp. has been described in an HIV-positive patient with cryptococcal meningitis that responded to itraconazole given for the meningitis. In addition, disseminated infection with *Encephalitozoon* sp. has been described recently.[39]

Herpes zoster ophthalmicus, which occurs in a more severe and chronic form in AIDS and may require prolonged systemic penciclovir therapy, can also cause ARN.

Inflammatory uveitis

Sarcoidosis

Sarcoidosis is a multisystem inflammatory disorder primarily affecting the African-American population, typically between 20 and 50 years of age, although any age group may be affected. This chronic, granulomatous inflammatory disorder has an unknown etiology. Although the pulmonary system is affected most frequently, other systems are involved including the liver, CNS, and skin. Ocular involvements are summarized below:

- Lid granuloma
- Conjunctival nodules
- Lacrimal gland infiltration – keratoconjunctivitis sicca
- Iris nodules (Koeppe, Busacca)
- Vascular sheathing
- Neovascularization
- Optic nerve granuloma
- Periphlebitis
- Branch vein occlusion
- Orbital granuloma.

Intraocular inflammation occurs in 25–50% of systemic sarcoidosis patients. Two-thirds of the patients with ocular sarcoidosis have anterior segment inflammation. One-third of the patients with ocular sarcoidosis have posterior segment disease.[40] The posterior segment reveals vitritis and retinal periphlebitis. The latter is distinguished by perivenous sheathing with areas of discrete retinal and choroidal infiltrates around the retinal veins. These nodular granulomas occurring along venules are known as 'candle wax drippings.' Retinal neovascularization, disc edema, and optic nerve granuloma are also seen.

Laboratory diagnostic methods include serum angiotensin-converting enzyme, chest X-ray, gallium scan of the head and neck, and biopsy of suspicious lesions. Unequivocal tests may be repeated as they may become positive with disease progression. Biopsy of the granulomas occurring in the conjunctiva, lacrimal gland, and skin may be considered. Histologic sections will show noncaseating granuloma composed of epithelioid cells, multinucleate giant cells of the Langhans type, and a rim of lymphocytes.

Pars planitis

Pars planitis is a vitreous inflammatory disorder of unknown etiology. Cell-mediated autoimmune responses to type II collagen found in the vitreous may play a role. Sarcoid occurs primarily in young adults, slightly more commonly in men; however, there may be no gender predilection. The differential diagnoses for pars planitis are given below:

- Sarcoidosis
- Lyme disease
- Tuberculosis
- Toxocariasis
- Syphilis
- Demyelinating disease.

Patients with pars planitis present with chronic reduced vision and floaters. The eye is typically white and appears 'quiet.' Mild, nongranulomatous cellular reaction in the anterior chamber may be seen. Vision is limited by cystoid macular edema, posterior subcapsular cataract, band keratopathy, vitreous hemorrhage, glaucoma, disc edema, and perivasculitis. Examination reveals retinal vasculitis with granulomatous inflammation of the peripheral retina and vitreous base. Vitreous snowball opacities consisting of vitreous debris may be seen adjacent to areas of retinal vascular sheathing. These opacities may gravitate inferiorly and form snowbanking of the peripheral retina. Neovascular tufts may arise from these snowbanks.

Diagnosis is suggested in young, healthy patients who present with bilateral, intermediate uveitis with or without pars plana exudation. Although no specific laboratory tests are available, certain tests are performed to rule out other entities which may mimic intermediate uveitis and to guide treatment.

No treatment may be required for patients with visual acuity of 20/40 or better. In patients with visual acuity worse than 20/40 as a result of cystoid macular edema, stepwise increases in corticosteroid administration from topical to periocular to systemic forms may be considered. The following protocol for active inflammation has been proposed:

- Level 1: Periocular corticosteroids and/or oral nonsteroidal antiinflammatory drugs (NSAIDS)
- Level 2: Oral corticosteroid regimens
- Level 3: Pars plana cryopexy
- Level 4: Unilateral disease – vitrectomy
- Severe bilateral disease – vitrectomy or immunosuppression.

Immunologic uveitis

The causes of immunologic uveitis are listed below:

- Type I
  - Hay fever
  - Atopic keratoconjunctivitis
  - Vernal keratoconjunctivitis
- Type II
  - Cicatricial pemphigoid
  - Lens-induced uveitis
- Type III
  - Ankylosing spondylitis
  - Behçet's disease
  - Churg–Strauss syndrome
  - Cogan's syndrome
  - Dermatomyositis and polymyositis
  - Erythema multiforme (Stevens–Johnson syndrome)
  - Inflammatory bowel disease
  - Juvenile rheumatoid arthritis
  - Psoriatic arthritis
  - Reiter's syndrome
  - Relapsing polychondritis
  - Rheumatoid arthritis
  - Polyarteritis nodosa
  - Systemic sclerosis with or without scleroderma
  - Sjögren's syndrome
  - Systemic lupus erythematosus
  - Temporal arteritis or giant cell arteritis
  - Wegener's granulomatosis.

Masquerade syndrome

Masquerade syndrome refers to a number of disorders that simulate chronic uveitis. The term was first used to describe a case of conjunctival carcinoma that presented as chronic conjunctivitis. Because of the nature of the underlying diseases that may have fatal consequences, early diagnosis and prompt treatment are critical.

Intraocular lymphoma (reticulum cell sarcoma)

Intraocular lymphoma is a potentially lethal non-Hodgkin's large-cell lymphoma that is a subset of primary central nervous system (CNS) large-cell lymphoma. It may originate in the eye or brain with rare metastasis outside of the CNS. Although the typical presentation may be vitritis in a patient over 50 years old, it can also mimic a number of other ocular conditions. Patients typically present with floaters and vision loss usually without pain or redness. On examination, discrete, yellow-white lesions located under the sensory retina or the retinal pigment epithelium measuring up to several disc diameters are found. Gill and Jampol reported different presentations of intraocular lymphoma which are listed below:[41]

- Uveitis
- Subretinal pigment epithelium tumors
- Deep retinal white dots from tumor infiltration
- Retinal infiltration causing necrotizing retinitis
- Retinal vasculature infiltration causing vascular obstruction
- Optic nerve invasion.

Up to 80% of patients with intraocular lymphoma will have CNS lymphoma. 'Uveitis' secondary to intraocular lymphoma is refractory to corticosteroids.

Chronic, medically unresponsive uveitis, vitritis, and subretinal infiltrates in an elderly patient with CNS complaints suggest intraocular lymphoma. Multiple vitrectomies may be required before isolating the lymphoma cells that appear as large, pleomorphic cells with mitotic figures and a high nucleus-to-cytoplasm ratio. Transvitreal aspirations may also be performed on some subretinal lesions. The infiltrative lesions appear hypofluorescent early with late staining on fluorescein angiogram. Lumbar puncture, computed tomography, or magnetic resonance imaging may confirm CNS involvement.

Treatment includes corticosteroids that cause a transient decrease of the 'uveitis.' Generally, a combination of ocular irradiation, intrathecal methotrexate, and systemic chemotherapy is required.

Metastatic lesions

The differential diagnoses are listed in Box 10.1. Among these, metastatic lesions should be

---

Box 10.1 Neoplasms masquerading as uveitis

Neoplasms
- Intraocular lymphoma
- Choroidal malignant melanoma
- Metastatic lesions (including carcinoma of breast and kidney)
- Systemic non-Hodgkin's lymphoma
- Retinoblastoma
- Leukemia
- Paraneoplastic syndrome
- Cancer-associated retinopathy
- Bilateral diffuse uveal melanocytic proliferation
- Childhood carcinoma
- Medulloepithelioma
- Juvenile xanthogranuloma

Non-malignant conditions
- Intraocular foreign body
- Retinal detachment
- Myopic degeneration
- Pigment dispersion syndrome
- Retinal degeneration
- Multiple sclerosis
- Intraocular infections
- Drug reactions
- Vaccination

---

considered seriously. Systemic non-Hodgkin's lymphoma (NHL) can metastasize to the eye and mimic chronic inflammation and display hypopyon or hyphema in an uninflamed eye. Primary and metastatic lesions may be identified histologically by location. NHL-CNS cells are located between the retinal pigment epithelium and Bruch's membrane; systemic NHL cells metastatic to the eye are located in the choroid. It is also important to remember that nonmalignant conditions such as retinal detachments can mimic uveitis (Box 10.1).

Vitritis due to mollicutes

Presumed bacteria-like bodies (BLBs), called mollicutes or mycoplasma-like organisms (MLOs), were described in chronic idiopathic vitritis (CIV) 20 years ago by Johnson et al and Wirostko et al.[42–45] They observed ultrastructural properties of BLBs within vitreous leukocyte phagolysosomes. Electron microscopy showed coccal-shaped BLBs 0.5–0.7 μm in size within

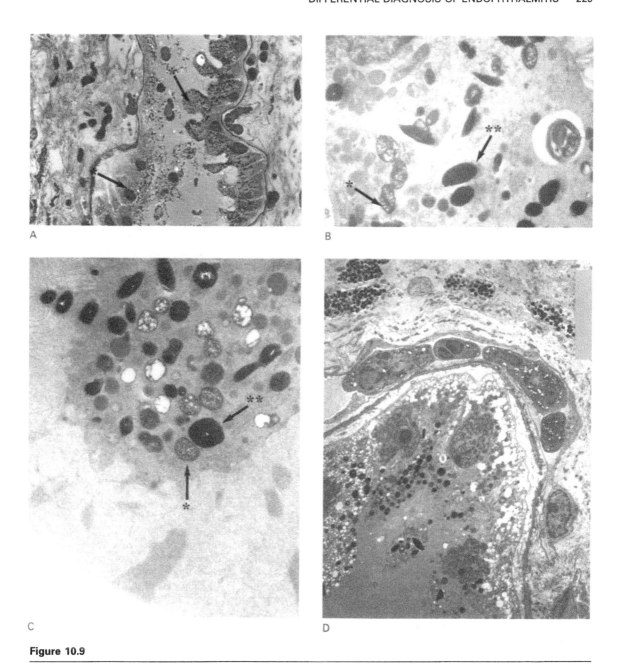

Figure 10.9

(A–C) Electron microscopy of a choroidal and retinal pigment epithelial biopsy showing mollicutes within a phagolysosome; (D) shows leukocytes (PMN cells) in the choriocapillaris. * = mollicute; ** = pigment.

polymorphonuclear (PMN) cell phagolysosomes. These same authors also found parasitization of vitreous leukocytes by these mollicutes in association with Crohn's disease uveitis.[46]

Wirostko et al conducted mouse transmission experiments with vitreous humor from CIV patients containing the 0.5 × 0.7 μm BLBs which they injected into the lower eyelid.[47] After 12 months, 53 mice that received the CIV injection had ocular inflammation which did not occur in any of the controls injected with saline.

There has been debate in *The Lancet* as to whether mollicutes (or mycoplasma-like organisms, MLOs) exist.[48] While the author of the editorial conceded to their possible existence, he did not accept that Wirostko and Johnson had demonstrated that MLOs cause vitritis and uveitis as an infectious disease. Wirostko and Johnson disputed this latter editorial, in particular the role of rifampicin that was dismissed out-of-hand.[49] They had found that rifampicin reduced morbidity of experimental disease due to MLOs and thought that it could be beneficial for treatment of human MLO uveitis.

There has been experience of two patients in whom MLOs were identified by electron microscopy from a biopsy of the choroid and retinal pigment epithelium.[50,51] One patient presented with bilateral retinal pigment epitheliopathy characterized by multiple pigment epithelial detachments and extensive bilateral exudative lesions.[50] Electron microscopy showed the presence of mollicutes in phagolysosomes of the retinal pigment epithelium cells (Figure 10.9). There was a prompt resolution of the clinical features following treatment with rifampicin. Mollicute infection may be a treatable cause of sight-threatening retinal pigment epitheliopathy.

References

1. Helm CJ, Holland GN. Ocular tuberculosis, *Surv Ophthalmol* (1993) **38**:229–41.
2. Biswas J, Madhavan HN, Gopal L et al. Intraocular tuberculosis. Clinicopathologic study of five cases, *Retina* (1995) **15**:461–8.
3. Anderson K, Patel KR, Webb L et al. Acute posterior multifocal placoid pigment epitheliopathy associated with pulmonary tuberculosis, *Br J Ophthalmol* (1996) **80**:186.
4. Grenzebach UH, Busse H, Totsch M et al. Endophthalmitis induced by atypical mycobacterial infection, *Ger J Ophthalmol* (1996) **5**:202–6.
5. Schrenk M, Metz K, Heiligenhaus A et al. Ocular involvement in Whipple disease, *Klin Monatsbl Augenheilkd* (1994) **204**:538–41.
6. Cerf M, Marche C, Ciribilli JM. Whipple disease: a single or multiple origin, *Presse Med* (1995) **24**:119–20, 123–8.
7. Le HH, Palay DA, Anderson B et al. Conjunctival swab to diagnose ocular cat scratch disease, *Am J Ophthalmol* (1994) **118**:249–50.
8. Goldstein DA, Mouritsen L, Friedlander S et al. Acute endogenous endophthalmitis due to *Bartonella henselae*, *Clin Infect Dis* (2001) **33**:718–21.
9. Fact Sheet: Syphilis. July 1998. Office of Communications and Public Liaison, National Institute of Allergy and Infectious Diseases, National Institutes of Health, Bethesda, MD 20892, USA.
10. Wilhelmus K, Lukehart SA. Ocular syphilis. In: Pepose JS, Holland GN, Wilhelmus KR, eds. *Ocular Infection and Immunity* (Mosby Year Book: St Louis, 1996) 1437–66.
11. Lotery AJ, McBride MO, Larkin C et al. Pseudoretinitis pigmentosa due to sub-optimal treatment of neurosyphilis, *Eye* (1996) **10**:759–60.
12. Knox D. Retinal syphilis and tuberculosis. In: Ryan SJ, ed. *Retina*, 3rd edn (Mosby: St Louis, 2002) 1662–74.
13. Lesser RL. Ocular manifestations of Lyme disease, *Am J Med* (1995) **98**(4A): 60S-62S.
14. Karma A, Seppala I, Mikkila H et al. Diagnosis and clinical characteristics of ocular Lyme borreliosis, *Am J Ophthalmol* (1995) **119**:127–35.
15. Adelman RA, Membreno JH, Afshari NA et al. West Nile virus chorioretinitis, *Retina* (2003) **23**:100–1.
16. Anninger WV, Lomeo MD, Dingle J et al. West Nile virus-associated optic neuritis and chorioretinitis, *Am J Ophthalmol* (2003) **136**:1183–5.
17. Bains HS, Jampol LM, Caughron MC et al. Vitritis and chorioretinitis in a patient with West Nile virus infection, *Arch Ophthalmol* (2003) **121**:205–7.
18. Hershberger VS, Augsburger JJ, Hutchins RK et al, Bergmann M. Chorioretinal lesions in nonfatal cases of West Nile virus infection, *Ophthalmology* (2003) **110**:1732–6.
19. Knox CM, Chandler D, Short GA et al. Polymerase chain reaction-based assays of vitreous samples for the diagnosis of viral retinitis. Use in diagnostic dilemmas, *Ophthalmology* (1998) **105**:37–45.
20. Wang L, Damji KF, Chialant D et al. Hypotony after intravenous cidofovir therapy for the treatment of cytomegalovirus retinitis, *Can J Ophthalmol* (2002) **37**:419–22.
21. Dreyer RF, Hopen G, Gass JDM et al. Leber's idiopathic stellate neuroretinitis, *Arch Ophthalmol* (1984) **102**:1140–5.
22. Viera-Dias D, Sena CM, Orefice F et al. Ocular and concomitant cutaneous sporotrichosis, *Mycoses* (1997) **40**:197–201.
23. Cartwright MJ, Promersberger M, Stevens GA. *Sporothrix schenckii* endophthalmitis presenting as granulomatous uveitis, *Br J Ophthalmol* (1993) **77**:61–2.
24. Doft BH, Gass DM. Punctate outer retinal toxoplasmosis, *Arch Ophthalmol* (1985) **103**:1332–6.

25. Klotz SA, Penn CC, Negvesky GJ et al. Fungal and parasitic infections of the eye, *Clin Microbiol Rev* (2000) **13**:662–85.

26. Taylor HR, Dax EM. Ocular onchocerciasis. In: Tabbara KF, Hyndiuk RA, eds. *Infections of the Eye* (Little Brown: Boston, 1986) 653–64.

27. Murdoch I, Abiose A, Babalola O et al. Ivermectin and onchocercal optic neuritis: short-term effects, *Eye* (1994) **8**:456–61.

28. Dadzie KY, Bird AC, Awadzi K et al. Ocular findings in a double-blind study of ivermectin versus diethylcarbamazine versus placebo in the treatment of onchocerciasis, *Br J Ophthalmol* (1987) **71**:78–85.

29. Gass JDM. Acute posterior multifocal placoid pigment epitheliopathy, *Arch Ophthalmol* (1968) **80**:177–85.

30. Jones NP. Acute posterior multifocal placoid pigment epitheliopathy, *Br J Ophthalmol* (1995) **79**:384–9.

31. Gross JG, Bozzette SA, Mathews WC et al. Longitudinal study of cytomegalovirus retinitis in acquired immune deficiency syndrome, *Ophthalmology* (1990) **97**:681–6.

32. Bylsma SS, Achim CL, Wiley CA et al. The predictive value of cytomegalovirus retinitis for cytomegalovirus encephalitis in acquired immunodeficiency syndrome, *Arch Ophthalmol* (1995) **113**:89–95.

33. Spector SA, Weingeist T, Pollard RB et al. A randomized, controlled study of intravenous ganciclovir therapy for cytomegalovirus peripheral retinitis in patients with AIDS, *J Infect Dis* (1993) **168**:557–63.

34. Cochereau-Massin I, Le-Houang P, Lautier-Frau M et al. Cytomegalovirus retinitis in AIDS. Treatment with intravitreal injections of ganciclovir, *Presse Med* (1990) **19**:1313–16.

35. Morlet N, Young S, Naidoo D et al. High-dose intravitreal ganciclovir for CMV retinitis: a shelf life and cost comparison study, *Br J Ophthalmol* (1995) **79**:753–5.

36. Morinelli EN, Dugal PU, Riffenburgh R et al. Infectious multifocal choroiditis in patients with acquired immune deficiency syndrome, *Ophthalmology* (1993) **100**:1014–21.

37. Shami MJ, Freeman W, Friedberg D et al. A multicenter study of pneumocystis choroidopathy, *Am J Ophthalmol* (1991) **112**:15–22.

38. Kestelyn P, Taelman H, Bogaerts J. Ophthalmic manifestations of infections with *Cryptococcus neoformans* in patients with AIDS, *Am J Ophthalmol* (1993) **116**:721–7.

39. Svedhem V, Lebbad M, Hedkvist B et al. Disseminated infection with *Encephalitozoon intestinalis* in AIDS patients: report of 2 cases, *Scand J Infect Dis* (2002) **34**:703–5.

40. Hunter DG, Foster CS. Ocular manifestations of sarcoidosis. In: Albert DM, Jakobiec FA, eds. *Principles and Practice of Ophthalmology* (WB Saunders: Philadelphia, 1994) 443–50.

41. Gill MK, Jampol LM. Variations in the presentation of primary intraocular lymphoma: case reports and a review, *Surv Ophthalmol* (2001) **45**:463–71.

42. Wirostko E, Johnson L, Wirostko B. Chronic orbital inflammatory disease: parasitisation of orbital leucocytes by mollicute-like organisms, *Br J Ophthalmol* (1989) **73**:865–70.

43. Wirostko E, Johnson L, Wirostko W. Chronic intracellular leucocytoclastic bacterial vitritis. A transmission electron microscopic study of the monocytes, *J Submicrosc Cytol Pathol* (1988) **20**: 463–70.

44. Johnson L, Wirostko E, Wirostko B. Chronic idiopathic vitritis. Cytopathogenicity of unusual bacteria for vitreous polymorphonuclear leukocytes, *J Submicrosc Cytol* (1987) **19**:161–6.

45. Johnson LA, Wirostko E. Chronic idiopathic vitritis. Ultrastructural properties of bacteria-like bodies within vitreous leukocyte phagolysosomes, *Am J Clin Pathol* (1986) **86**:19–24.

46. Johnson L, Wirostko E, Wirostko WJ. Crohn's disease uveitis. Parasitization of vitreous leukocytes by mollicute-like organisms, *Am J Clin Pathol* (1989) **91**:259–64.

47. Wirostko E, Johnson L, Wirostko BM. Transmission of chronic idiopathic vitritis in mice by inoculation of human vitreous containing leucocyte phagolysosomal bacteria-like bodies, *Lancet* (1986) **2**:481–3.

48. Editorial. Do human MLO exist? *Lancet* (1990) **335**:1068–9.

49. Wirostko E, Johnson L. Mycoplasma-like organisms, *Lancet* (1990) **336**:246–7.

50. Foulds WS. Uses and limitations of intraocular biopsy, *Eye* (1992) **6**:11–27.

51. Steel DH, Richardson J, Aitken DA. Acute bilateral optic disc neovascularization, *Retina* (1994) **14**:362–9.

52. Seal DV, Bron AJ, Hay J. *Ocular Infection. Management and treatment in practice.* (London: Martin Dunitz, 1998).

11

Pharmacology

The purpose of an antimicrobial drug is to induce damage to the microbe while minimizing injury to the host. Many agents are derived from natural plants and organisms and arrest essential biochemical steps in the proliferation of microorganisms. However, the exact mechanisms of some antibiotics have yet to be discovered. Despite this, a myriad of antibiotics have been discovered including over 10,000 fluoroquinolones since the development of nalidixic acid in 1962.

In evaluating a drug, the minimum inhibitory concentration (MIC) must be determined. The MIC_{90}/MIC_{50} is the concentration of the drug required to inhibit 90%/50% of the isolates. In order to reach this value, the susceptibility of the microorganism and the ability of the drug to reach the target must be considered. Furthermore, inflammation increases vascular permeability and intraocular concentrations of the drugs (Chapter 5).

Antimicrobials are classified as either bacteriostatic or bactericidal. Bacteriostatic drugs such as erythromycin and tetracycline prevent multiplication but depend on host defense mechanisms to kill the organism. Bactericidal drugs such as cephalosporins lead directly to death of the microorganism. Bacteriostatic drugs can become bactericidal if given at high doses; bactericidal drugs can become bacteriostatic if treatment is continued with low doses.

In response, microorganisms have developed genetic and other mechanisms for drug resistance; these include efflux channels which pump out the drugs. Inhibitors of three types of efflux pumps have been identified: two efflux pumps in Gram-positive bacteria, and one in Gram-negative bacteria. Inhibiting these pumps may allow novel approaches to combat drug resistance.

There are also different methods of controling an infection in the future. One method is to decode the microbial genome. Genomic information will reveal new methods for bacteriostatic or bactericidal options. Quorum sensing (a.k.a autoinduction) is the second method and it is a system that allows a bacterium to regulate its own environment. In this system, bacterial gene expression is coupled to population density. Once a threshold is reached, a negative feedback system limits further expression of bacteria. In Gram-positive bacteria, autoinducers belong to the family of N-acylhomoserine lactones (AHL). This may be an inherent control system that exists to limit a bacterial population, which may be exploited as a means of bacteriostasis.

In this chapter, different classes of antimicrobials are discussed that are effective against bacteria and fungi. Most recent developments have been among fluoroquinolones and derivatives of erythromycin, and the triazoles.

ANTIBACTERIAL MEDICATIONS

Fluoroquinolones

Fluoroquinolones (Table 11.1) are antibiotics based on a 7–chloroquinolone molecule identified by Lescher et al in 1962 when they discovered

Table 11.1 Fluoroquinolones	
Generation	Agents
First generation	Norfloxacin
Second generation	Ciprofloxacin, Ofloxacin
Third generation	Levofloxacin, Sparfloxacin, Grepafloxacin*
Third/fourth generation	Moxifloxacin, Gatifloxacin†
Fourth generation	(Trovafloxacin‡)

*Grepafloxacin withdrawn due to QT interval prolongation.
†Systemic use of gatifloxacin may be withdrawn.
‡Trovafloxacin withdrawn due to hepatotoxicity.

nalidixic acid as a byproduct of chloroquine synthesis.[1] Gellert et al subsequently identified the critical enzyme inhibited by this compound and named it DNA gyrase (topoisomerase II).[2] Since then, fluoroquinolone antibiotics have been found to inhibit topoisomerase IV in addition to topoisomerase II. The latter uncoils the DNA superhelix while the former detaches the daughter chromosomes after DNA replication. Unfortunately, nalidixic acid displayed a narrow antibacterial spectrum, short half-life, and high protein binding; its effectiveness was limited.

Four 'generations' of fluoroquinolones have been described since their inception, but not all authors agree with the interpretation for moxifloxacin. The ophthalmic literature has placed moxifloxacin in the fourth-generation group but the general medical literature has classified this new quinolone as a third-generation drug.[3,4] The ability to chemically manipulate the nucleus of the fluoroquinolones to produce new compounds with greater antibacterial activity, improved pharmacokinetics, and fewer side effects has led to successive generations of increasingly potent agents. Fluoroquinolones differ in chemical structure and mode of action from beta-lactam antibiotics and aminoglycosides, and therefore may be active against bacteria resistant to such agents. Bacterial resistance to second-generation fluoroquinolones by community-acquired S. pneumoniae was first reported in the mid-1990s.[5] Resistant bacterial keratitis, especially for Gram-positive organisms, has also been reported. In 2001, 52% of 739 coagulase-negative staphylococci (CNS) isolates were resistant to ofloxacin or ciprofloxacin.[6] These agents are very effective against mycobacteria.

The basic mechanisms of bacterial resistance to fluoroquinolones are through:

- Decreased cell wall permeability
- Altered enzymes that block antibiotic complexing
- Use of efflux pumps that remove antibiotic molecules from the cell.[7]

Toxicity has been linked to the C-8 position. The latter generation fluoroquinolone development resulted from the following observations:

- A fluorine in the C-6 position enhances antimicrobial activity

- A bulky side-chain at C-7 binds to DNA gyrase, impedes efflux of the fluoroquinolone out of the bacterial cell, and increases the serum half-life and potency against Gram-positive organisms.
- A C-8 methoxy group increases potency and decreases toxicity.[8]

Norfloxacin was developed in 1978 and is considered a first-generation fluoroquinolone. Ofloxacin (Ocuflox, Allergan, Inc.) and ciprofloxacin (Ciloxan, Alcon Laboratories, Inc.) are second-generation drugs with improved Gram-negative activity introduced in the 1980s. These drugs showed enhanced activity (1000-fold) against aerobic Gram-negative bacteria and were also active against aerobic Gram-positive bacteria including streptococci and staphylococci.[9] Trovafloxacin and levofloxacin have improved Gram-positive activity and are considered third-generation drugs of this class. They were designed to increase activity against Gram-positive organisms, especially the pneumococci, without losing their broad Gram-negative coverage. Graves et al found Gram-positive bacteria to be 98% sensitive to levofloxacin whereas ofloxacin and ciprofloxacin, respectively, demonstrated 78% and 61% susceptibility.[10] Moxifloxacin and gatifloxacin have shown a better effect against antibiotic-resistant staphylococci and streptococci, as well as having more potency against Gram-positive bacteria and an improved anaerobic coverage, but are less effective against Pseudomonas aeruginosa.[6]

Among fluoroquinolones, ciprofloxacin provides the best coverage against Ps. aeruginosa. However, some resistance has been reported against some Gram-positive organisms.[11] Gatifloxacin, levofloxacin, and ciprofloxacin appear to be uniformly active against other Gram-negative organisms. Gatifloxacin appears to be similar to levofloxacin for Gram-positive and atypical pathogens and, therefore, may prove to be an alternative treatment for community-acquired pneumonia. At this time, resistance to levofloxacin does not appear to be prevalent. Moxifloxacin demonstrated two to four times increased potency against pneumococci as compared with gatifloxacin and levofloxacin, respectively.[6,9,12] However, there is concern about QT interval prolongation, which does not occur with levofloxacin. Finally, Mather et al found that

Table 11.2 Antiarrhythmic agents contraindicated for use with fluoroquinolones

Class	Agents
Class IA	Quinidine, procainamide, disopyramide
Class III	Ibutilide, dofetilide, sotalol, amiodarone, bretylium

moxifloxacin provided in vitro coverage for both Gram-positive and Gram-negative bacteria that are resistant to second- and third-generation fluoroquinolones.[12,13] In general, moxifloxacin exhibited better potency than gatifloxacin against Gram-positive bacteria but was less effective against *Ps. aeruginosa*.[6]

The antiarrhythmic agents which are contra-indicated with fluoroquinolone use are shown in Table 11.2.

Side effects of fluoroquinolones

- Cardiac
  - Prolonged QTc interval in selected patients
  - Avoid in patients with prolonged QTc, un-corrected hypokalemia, and patients on class IA and III antiarrhythmic drugs, both of which prolong repolarization
  - Use with caution in patients with bradycardia, acute myocardial ischemia
  - Additive effect with other drugs that prolong QTc interval – cisapride, erythromycin, antipsychotics, tricyclic antidepressants
  - QTc interval prolongation is dose-dependent
- Gastrointestinal
  - Nausea, diarrhea, vomiting and abdominal pain
  - Liver toxicity (trovafloxacin only?)
  - Toxicity data garnered in clinical trials need to be viewed with some skepticism because healthy volunteers were used in the studies
  - *Pseudomonas* colitis
- Central nervous system
  - Headache, restlessness, insomnia, dizziness, seizures, change in vision, increased intracranial pressure

- Gynecology
  - Vaginitis
- Musculoskeletal
  - Joint and bone deformities found in juvenile animals; therefore, not recommended for pregnant or nursing mothers
  - In children between 9 and 18 years of age, the relative benefit should outweigh the risk. This is not a concern with the ophthalmic products
  - Pain/inflammation/ruptured tendon
- Ophthalmic
  - White corneal precipitate of ciprofloxacin (pH 4.5) noted with topical use.

Exceptions

- QTc prolongation has not been reported with levofloxacin
- Phototoxicity, QTc prolongation, hypoglycemia, and hepatotoxicity were not reported with gatifloxacin
- All fluoroquinolones have the potential to cause phototoxicity, although this side effect has not been shown with levofloxacin and moxifloxacin.

Possible interactions with fluoroquinolones

- Minerals with 2 or 3 positive charges (divalent or trivalent ions) bind fluoroquinolones and reduce the amounts of drugs that are absorbed
- Must be taken at least 2 hours before or after antacids or mineral supplements containing iron, calcium, zinc, or magnesium, which bind the antibiotic and prevents its absorption – sucralfate, didanosine, dDI, and antacids
- Other fluoroquinolones have been shown to increase serum levels of theophylline (Theo-Dur), warfarin (Coumadin), and cyclosporine (Sandimmune; Neoral). However, there have not been any similar reports with trovafloxacin.

Ciprofloxacin

Ciprofloxacin is a monohydrochloride monohydrate salt of 1-cyclopropyl-6-fluoro-1,4-dihydro-4-oxo-7-(1-piperazinyl)-3-quinoline-carboxylic acid.

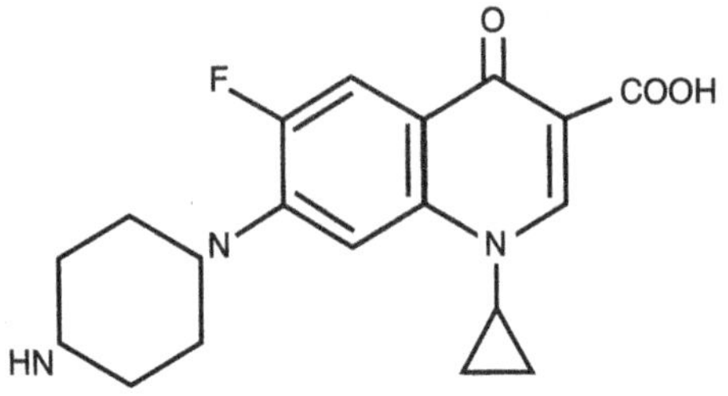

Figure 11.1

Chemical structure of ciprofloxacin.

It differs from other quinolones in that it has a fluorine atom at the 6-position, a piperazine moiety at the 7-position, and a cyclopropyl ring at the 1-position. Ciprofloxacin is a faint to light yellow crystalline powder with a molecular weight of 385.8. Its empirical formula is $C_{17}H_{18}FN_3O_3HCl \cdot H_2O$; its chemical structure is shown in Figure 11.1.

Ciprofloxacin has been shown to be active against most strains of the bacteria listed below both in vitro and in clinical infections.

Gram-positive bacteria
Staphylococcus aureus (including methicillin-susceptible and some methicillin-resistant strains)
Staphylococcus epidermidis
Streptococcus pneumoniae
Streptococcus (viridans group)

Gram-negative bacteria
Haemophilus influenzae
Pseudomonas aeruginosa
Serratia marcescens

Ciprofloxacin has also been shown to be active in vitro against most strains of the following organisms; however, the clinical significance of these data is unknown:

Gram-positive bacteria
Enterococcus faecalis (many strains are only moderately susceptible)
Staphylococcus haemolyticus
Staphylococcus hominis
Staphylococcus saprophyticus
Streptococcus pyogenes

Compared to its cousin (ofloxacin) and forerunner (norfloxacin), ciprofloxacin has:

- Worse MICs against Gram-positive bacteria and chlamydia (ofloxacin)
- Less soluble; therefore produces lower corneal and anterior chamber levels (pH 6.4)
- Norfloxacin has similar but somewhat less effectiveness to ciprofloxacin and is used mostly in urinary tract infections.

Although bacterial resistance was thought to be less of a problem with ciprofloxacin, it may still occur, even with topical ophthalmic use. The first reported resistance to ciprofloxacin involved three cases of keratitis (two cases were *S. epidermidis* with one sensitive to ceftazidime, the other resistant), and one case of *Xanthomonas maltophilia* that was sensitive to ticarcillin.[11]

Indications for and dosages of ciprofloxacin

- Available in 100-mg, 250-mg, 500-mg and 750-mg (ciprofloxacin equivalent) strengths
- Ciprofloxacin HCl oral suspension is available in 5% (5 g ciprofloxacin in 100 ml) and 10% (10 g ciprofloxacin in 100 ml) strengths
- Urinary tract infections, uncomplicated acute urethral cystitis in women, chronic bacterial prostatitis, skin infections, lower respiratory tract infection, urethral and cervical gonococcal infections, acute sinusitis
- Dosage ranges from 500 to 750 mg b.i.d. for 3–14 days, depending on the condition and severity.

Ciloxan (Ciprofloxacin HCl)

Each milliliter of Ciloxan ophthalmic solution contains the following: Active: ciprofloxacin HCl 3.5 mg equivalent to 3 mg base (0.3%). Preservative: benzalkonium chloride 0.006%. Inactive: sodium acetate, acetic acid, mannitol 4.6%, edetate disodium 0.05%, hydrochloric acid and/or sodium hydroxide (to adjust pH), and purified water. The pH is approximately 4.5 and the osmolality is approximately 300 mOsm.

A systemic absorption study (administered in each eye every 2 hours while awake for 2 days followed by every 4 hours while awake for an additional 5 days) reported plasma concentration of ciprofloxacin was less than 5 ng/ml. The mean concentration was usually less than 2.5 ng/ml.

Indications and usage

Corneal ulcers:
Ps. aeruginosa
Serr. marcescens
S. aureus
S. epidermidis
Strep. pneumoniae
Streptococcus (viridans group)

Conjunctivitis:
Haemophilus influenzae
S. aureus
S. epidermidis
Strep. pneumoniae*
*Efficacy for this organism was studied in fewer than 10 infections.

Dosage and administration of ciprofloxacin

Corneal ulcers. Two drops are placed into the affected eye every 15 minutes for the first 6 hours and then two drops into the affected eye every 30 minutes for the remainder of the first day. On the second day, two drops are instilled in the affected eye hourly. On the third through the14th day, two drops are placed in the affected eye every 4 hours. Treatment may be continued after 14 days if corneal reepithelialization has not occurred.

Bacterial conjunctivitis. One or two drops instilled into the conjunctival sac every 2 hours while awake for 2 days and one or two drops every 4 hours while awake for the next 5 days.

Pertinent studies

Vitreous concentrations after oral administration of ciprofloxacin do not reach inhibitory levels for many bacteria associated with endophthalmitis. Typically, intravitreal levels approach 0.19 ± 0.07 µg/ml[14] to 0.29 ± 0.15 µg/ml[15] after a single dose of 750 mg, or 0.51 ± 0.35 µg/ml[16] to 0.56 ± 0.16 µg/ml after two doses. El Baba et al noted that a single 750-mg dose did not reach inhibitory levels for S. aureus and Ps. aeruginosa in vitre-

ous surgery patients.[15] However, MIC$_{90}$ was reached for S. epidermidis, Bacillus spp., and Enterobacteriaceae. On the other hand, Lesk et al noted that after two doses of ciprofloxacin, the vitreous levels exceeded the MIC$_{90}$ of S. epidermidis, Propionibacterium spp., Ps. aeruginosa, Proteus mirabilis, and H. influenzae, as well as the MIC$_{70}$ of S. aureus and Bacillus cereus.[16]

In a rabbit model, Ozturk et al noted that aqueous and vitreous concentrations were increased with topical and oral administration versus topical administration alone in eyes experimentally 'inflamed' with S. aureus.[17] In the topical treatment group, two drops of ciprofloxacin 0.3% were instilled in both eyes every 30 minutes for 4 hours. In the topical-oral treatment group, animals were given two oral 40 mg/kg doses of ciprofloxacin 12 hours apart. In a rabbit and swine model, Alfaro et al noted that surgical trauma increased the amount of ciprofloxacin that penetrated the vitreous exceeding the MIC for common ocular pathogens, except S. aureus and Ps. aeruginosa.[18]

The nontoxic dose of intravitreal ciprofloxacin was determined by Stevens et al to be 100 µg (0.1 mg) in a rabbit model as determined by retinal and corneal toxicity.[19] The authors also suggested that corneal pachymetry was the best method for detecting corneal toxicity that may not be determined by electroretinography (ERG) or light microscopy alone. Pearson et al determined that the half life in rabbits after intravitreal injection of 100 µg ciprofloxacin was 2.2 hours in normal eyes and 1 hour in aphakic, vitrectomized eyes.[20] The majority of the drug appeared to leave by the active retinal pump mechanism via the transretinal route, but clearance was not inhibited by probenecid. Rootman et al found no ocular damage after injection of as much as 3200 µg of ciprofloxacin into the rabbit eye.[21] Histologic study showed mild, transient vacuolation of the nerve fiber layer in all eyes, including the control eyes, 2 hours after injection; at 24 hours no vacuolation was evident except at concentrations of 800 and 3200 µg, at which level plexiform layer damage was evident. This conflicts with the data of Steven et al.[19]

Ofloxacin

Ofloxacin is a fluorinated carboxyquinolone antiinfective for topical ophthalmic use. It is a fluorinated 4-quinolone which differs from other fluorinated 4-quinolones in that there is a six-member (pyridobenzoxazine) ring from positions 1 to 8 of the basic ring structure. Its chemical name is (±)-9-fluoro-2,3-dihydro-3-methyl-1O-(4-methyl-1-piperazinyl)-7-oxo-7H-pyrido[1,2,3-de]-1,4 benzoxazine-6-carboxylic acid. The empirical formula is $C_{18}H_{20}FN_3O_4$; molecular weight is 361.37.

Ocuflox (ofloxacin) solution (0.3%) is un-buffered and formulated with a pH of 6.4 (range 6.0–6.8). It has an osmolality of 300 mOsm/kg, and is preserved with benzalkonium chloride.

Indications for and dosages of ofloxacin

Indications

Bacterial conjunctivitis
- Gram-positive bacteria
  - S. aureus
  - S. epidermidis
  - Strep. pneumoniae
- Gram-negative bacteria
  - Enterobacter cloacae
  - H. influenzae
  - Proteus mirabilis
  - Ps. aeruginosa

Corneal ulcers
- Gram-positive bacteria
  - S. aureus
  - S. epidermidis
  - Strep. pneumoniae
- Gram-negative bacteria
  - Ps. aeruginosa
  - Serr. marcescens
- Anaerobic species
  - Propionibacterium acnes

Usage

Bacterial conjunctivitis
- One to two drops q2–4h for 2 days followed by q.i.d. on days 3–7

Corneal ulcers
- One to two drops q30 minutes for 2 days while awake and q4h while asleep
- One to two drops hourly while awake on days 3–9
- One to two drops q.i.d. while awake until completion.

Pertinent studies

Von Gunten et al suggested that therapeutic levels above the MIC for many bacteria cultured in endophthalmitis could be achieved in the aqueous humor after either topical or oral administration.[22] The authors' data showed that the aqueous humor concentration (mean ± SD) was 0.53 ± 0.35 mg/l with topical ofloxacin (one drop every 3 hours, until 90 minutes preoperatively for six total drops) and 0.63 ± 0.29 mg/l (one drop every 30 minutes, until 30 minutes before aqueous humor aspiration). The aqueous humor concentrations 2 hours after a single 200-mg oral dose (0.38 ± 0.15 mg/l) were significantly lower (p = 0.048) than those 12 hours after the same oral dose (0.58 ± 0.24 mg/l). Two hours after an intravenous infusion of 200 mg of ofloxacin, the aqueous humor concentration was 0.33 ± 0.19 mg/l.

Donnenfeld et al also noted that ofloxacin achieved higher anterior chamber levels than ciprofloxacin or norfloxacin after each was administered 90 and 30 minutes before surgery.[23] In this study, topically applied ofloxacin achieved a mean level in the aqueous humor of 0.338 µg/ml compared with 0.072 µg/ml (ciprofloxacin) and 0.0570 µg/ml (norfloxacin). Donnenfeld et al concluded that topically applied ofloxacin, two drops every 30 minutes for 4 hours preceding surgery, achieved therapeutic levels in the cornea and aqueous, with mean levels well above the MIC_{90} for most ocular pathogens in patients undergoing penetrating keratoplasty.[24] However, in the group of patients that received three oral doses of 400 mg preoperatively at 12-hour intervals in addition to topical therapy, vitreous penetration increased sevenfold (2.55 µg/ml).

Ozturk et al found that the addition of oral ofloxacin to topical administration produced increased aqueous and vitreous humor levels in a rabbit model of endophthalmitis.[25] Although the oral doses were higher than those administered in humans, the study demonstrated that in inflamed eyes, the combination of topical and oral ofloxacin provided higher concentrations in both the aqueous and vitreous humor, especially in inflamed eyes.

Cantor et al studied the penetration of ofloxacin and ciprofloxacin after topical and oral administration into the aqueous humor of eyes with filtering blebs.[26] Patients received either drug one drop every 30 minutes for 4 hours or a combined topical plus oral regimen (ciprofloxacin 400 mg and ofloxacin 400 mg); three doses given 2, 12, and 24 hours before surgery. Aqueous levels were about three times higher in the ofloxacin patients and about 10 times higher in the combined oral and topical regimens with ofloxacin (3.84 µg/ml) than ciprofloxacin (0.35 µg/ml). Ofloxacin penetrated better than ciprofloxacin in the aqueous of eyes with filtering blebs, especially when topical and oral administration was combined. Another study has found that human corneal endothelium can be exposed to a dose of 30 µg/ml of ofloxacin for a period of 3 hours without adverse or ultrastructural or physiologic side effects.[27]

A study that reviewed over 9000 cataract surgeries over a 4-year period determined that the use of topical postoperative ofloxacin was significantly more effective than ciprofloxacin in reducing the incidence of endophthalmitis; in addition, this study reported a 'true' incidence figure of 0.25% following phacoemulsification cataract surgery.[28]

Trovafloxacin

Trovafloxacin (Trovan, Pfizer Pharmaceuticals) was approved by the US Food and Drug Administration (FDA) in 1998; however, its use was restricted in 1999 by the FDA after serious reports of liver failure. The use of trovafloxacin is indicated for enhanced activity against anaerobic and Gram-positive bacteria, including *Strep. pneumoniae*. The recommended dosage is 100–200 mg P.O. q.i.d. for 3–14 days.

Pertinent studies

Ng et al demonstrated that a single dose of trovafloxacin achieved maximal vitreous levels after 8 hours in infected eyes, with a penetration ratio of 36%.[29] Vitreous levels were greater than 15 times the MIC of the *S. epidermidis* strain employed. In animals with established endophthalmitis, treated eyes were sterilized after 5 days (p = 0.0495) compared with control eyes, which autosterilized at 14 days. Clinical and histologic examination revealed significant amelioration of anterior segment inflammation in treated eyes,

although severe destruction of posterior segment structures occurred in both groups after 6 days of therapy.

Trovafloxacin administered 24 or 48 hours after inoculation of rabbit eyes with *S. epidermidis* significantly reduced the number of bacteria compared with the untreated controls.[30] The retinal toxicity of intravitreally injected trovafloxacin was evaluated by Gurler et al in rabbit eyes; a dose of 500 µg was determined to be nontoxic.[31]

Levofloxacin

Levofloxacin is the levo or active isomer of ofloxacin, and produces MICs approximately half of the value provided by ofloxacin. Chemically, levofloxacin, a chiral fluorinated carboxyquinolone, is the pure (-)-(S)-enantiomer of the racemic drug substance ofloxacin. The chemical name is (-)-(S)-9-fluoro-2,3-dihydro-3-methyl-10-(4-methyl-1-piperazinyl)-7-oxo-7H-pyrido[1,2,3-de]-1,4-benzoxazine-6-carboxylic acid hemihydrate. Its empirical formula is $C_{18}H_{20}FN_3O_4\cdot\frac{1}{2}H_2O$ and its molecular weight is 370.38. Peak plasma concentrations are usually attained 1–2 hours after oral dosing. The absolute bioavailability of a 500-mg oral dose of levofloxacin is approximately 99%. Steady state is reached after 48 hours. Levofloxacin is excreted largely as unchanged drug in the urine. The mean terminal plasma elimination half-life of levofloxacin ranges from approximately 6 to 8 hours following single or multiple doses of levofloxacin give orally or intravenously.

Quixin (Vistakon Pharmaceuticals, Jacksonville, Florida) or Oftaquix (Santen Oy, Tampere, Finland, EU) is a sterile topical ophthalmic solution containing 0.5% levofloxacin, a potent, broad-spectrum fluoroquinolone. Levofloxacin's higher solubility, at neutral pH, allows Quixin to be formulated at a higher concentration of active drug (0.5%). It is preserved with benzalkonium chloride with a pH of 6.5. It is not buffered and has an osmolality of 300 mOsm/kg.

Levofloxacin demonstrated activity against both Gram-positive and Gram-negative bacteria.[6] In contrast, second-generation fluoroquinolones (ciprofloxacin, ofloxacin) have less Gram-positive activity.[6]

Indications and dosages of levofloxacin

- **Aerobic Gram-positive microorganisms:**
  S. aureus
  S. epidermidis
  S. saprophyticus
  Strep. pyogenes (BHS Lancefield group A)
  Streptococcus (BHS Lancefield group C/F)
  Streptococcus (BHS Lancefield group G)
  Strep. agalactiae, Strep. pneumoniae
  Viridans group streptococci
  Enterococcus faecalis (moderate activity)
- **Aerobic Gram-negative microorganisms:**
  Acinetobacter anitratus
  Acinetobacter baumannii
  Acinetobacter calcoaceticus
  Acinetobacter lwoffii
  Citrobacter diversus
  Citrobacter freundii
  Enterobacter aerogenes
  Enterobacter agglomerans
  Enterobacter sakazakii
  Klebsiella oxytoca
  Morganella morganii
  Proteus vulgaris
  Providencia rettgeri
  Providencia stuartii
  Pseudomonas fluorescens
  Serratia marcescens
- **Anaerobic Gram-positive microorganisms:**
  Clostridium perfringens, Peptostreptococcus

  – Acute bacterial exacerbation of chronic
    bronchitis, community-acquired pneumonia,
    acute maxillary sinusitis, complicated urinary
    tract infection, pyelonephritis, skin infection
  – Supplied as 250- or 500-mg tabs or as
    injections (500 mg every 24 hours for 7–14
    days).

Pertinent studies

Graves et al reported that levofloxacin demonstrated 98% Gram-positive susceptibility compared with 78% and 61% for ofloxacin and ciprofloxacin, respectively.[10] Following one drop of 0.5% levofloxacin to the conjunctival sac, the drug concentration in human tears remained above the MIC concentration for up to 6 hours, and was higher than previously reported tear concentrations for ciprofloxacin, ofloxacin, and norfloxacin, given in Figure 5.10 on p. 94.[32]

Administered topically before cataract surgery, levofloxacin 0.5% achieved concentrations higher than the MIC in the anterior chamber. Compared with ciprofloxacin, the aqueous absorption rate of levofloxacin was four to seven times higher.[33] Fiscella et al showed that oral levofloxacin produces inhibitory concentrations in the intact vitreous cavity of humans after two doses for the majority of ocular pathogens.[34] A second tablet 12 hours later produced intraocular inhibitory concentrations against the majority of the ocular pathogens that a single dose did not achieve.

Yamada et al evaluated transcorneal penetration of topically applied 0.5% levofloxacin into the aqueous humor of 20 cataract patients.[35] The patients received three drops of 0.5% levofloxacin at 15-minute intervals beginning 90 minutes before surgery. Results showed that the mean aqueous humor level of levofloxacin was $1.00 \pm 0.48\,\mu g/ml$, which was higher than the MIC_{90} values against some common pathogens of postoperative endophthalmitis. In addition, Bucci has shown that five doses of topical 0.5% levofloxacin, given every 10 minutes in the 1 hour before surgery, gave aqueous humor levels of $1.1\,\mu g/ml$, compared with $0.19\,\mu g/ml$ for ciprofloxacin; in addition, dosing with one drop every 6 hours for 48 hours before surgery increased these levels for levofloxacin to $1.6\,\mu g/ml$ and for ciprofloxacin to $0.24\,\mu g/ml$.[36]

Yildirim et al evaluated intravitreal levofloxacin as well as a combination of intravitreal levofloxacin and dexamethasone in S. epidermidis endophthalmitis.[37] Twenty-five albino rabbits were infected with an intravitreal inoculum of S. epidermidis. Groups 1 and 2 received treatment 24 hours after the inoculation, and groups 3 and 4 received treatment 48 hours after the inoculation. No treatment was given to the control group. Treatment efficacy was assessed by vitreous culture, clinical examination, and histopathology. Five days after treatment, groups 1 and 2 had significantly lower clinical and histopathologic scores than the control group. The culture results of the treatment groups were sterile.

Gurler et al showed that in therapeutic doses (500 µg or less), intravitreal injection of levofloxacin does not cause retinal toxicity in rabbit eyes; this dose was well above the MIC_{90} values of ocular pathogens that cause endophthalmitis.[38] Peyman et al have determined the intravitreal dose of 625 µg/0.1 ml to be nontoxic to the retina (unpublished data). In the future, intravitreal injection of levofloxacin may become a therapeutic option.

Table 5.2 on p. 84 includes the measured levels of levofloxacin in the anterior chamber following dosing by either the topical or oral routes.

Gatifloxacin

Gatifloxacin (Tequin, Zymar) is a third/fourth-generation fluoroquinolone approved by the US FDA in December 1999. Chemically, it is (±)-1-cyclopropyl-6-fluoro-1,4-dihydro-8-methoxy-7-(3-methyl-1-piperazinyl)-4-oxo-3-quinolinecarboxylic acid sesquihydrate. Its empirical formula is $C_{19}H_{22}FN_3O_4 \cdot 1.5H_2O$ and its molecular weight is 402.42. Gatifloxacin is well absorbed from the gastrointestinal tract after oral administration and can be given without regard to food. The absolute bioavailability of gatifloxacin is 96%. Peak plasma concentrations of gatifloxacin usually occur 1–2 hours after oral dosing. This drug was designed to improve the side effect profile and reduce the potential for developing bacterial resistance. The oral and intravenous routes of administration can be considered interchangeable because the pharmacokinetics of gatifloxacin 1 hour after intravenous administration are similar to those observed for equal doses of gatifloxacin administered orally.

Gatifloxacin has been chemically altered in the following way:

- 8-methoxy group at position 8 mediates the binding of the DNA–DNA gyrase complex to the DNA–topoisomerase complex and decreases the likelihood of high resistance
- Absence of halogenation at position 8 decreases phototoxicity
- Methyl-substituted piperazinyl ring at the R7 position has the potential to decrease the risk associated with nonsteroidal antiinflammatory drug interactions, central nervous system toxicity, and genotoxicity.[39]

Indications

- Community-acquired pneumonia, acute sinusitis, acute bacterial exacerbation of chronic bronchitis, uncomplicated skin and skin structure infections, uncomplicated and complicated urinary tract infections, and pyelonephritis.

Table 11.3 Recommended dosage of Tequin in adult patients with renal impairment

Creatinine clearance	Initial dose (mg)	Subsequent dose*
≤40 ml/min	400	400 mg every day
<40 ml/min	400	200 mg every day
Hemodialysis	400	200 mg every day
Continuous peritoneal dialysis	400	200 mg every day

*Start of subsequent dose on day 2 of dosing.

- Uncomplicated urethral, pharyngeal, and rectal gonorrhea in men. Endocervical, pharyngeal, and rectal gonorrhea in women.

Dosage

- Tequin is available as 200-mg and 400-mg tabs (Table 11.3)
- Tequin injection is available in 20-ml (200-mg) and 40-ml (400-mg) single-use vials as a sterile, preservative-free aqueous solution of gatifloxacin with pH ranging from 3.5 to 5.5. Tequin injection is also available in ready-to-use 100-ml (200-mg), 200-ml (400-mg) bags.
- 400 mg by mouth or intravenous infusion daily for approved patients whose calculated creatinine clearance is ≤40 ml/min (Box 11.1).
- If creatinine clearance level is <40 ml/min or in patients on hemodialysis or continuous peritoneal dialysis, the manufacturer recommends an initial dose of 400 mg with subsequent daily doses of 200 mg.[40]
- The ocular preparation is 0.3% with preservative of benzalkonium chloride at a pH of 6.0.

Pertinent studies

Orally administered gatifloxacin achieves therapeutic levels in the noninflamed human eye, and the activity spectrum appropriately encompasses the bacterial species most frequently involved in the various causes of endophthalmitis.[41] Mean gatifloxacin concentrations in serum ($n = 19$), vitreous ($n = 19$), and aqueous ($n = 10$) were 4.98

Box 11.1 Creatinine clearance

1. The formula for the calculation of creatinine is:

$$CrCl = \frac{U_{Cr} * U_{Vol}}{P_{Cr} * T_{min}}$$

$$Corrected\ CrCl = CrCl * \frac{1.73}{BSA}$$

Reference range for uncorrected creatinine clearance

- Adult male is 90–139 ml/minute
- Adult female is 80–125 ml/minute
- Many medications must be adjusted for renal impairment when the CrCl falls below 50 ml/min.

2. Creatinine clearance (ml/min) = [Weight (kg) ´ (140 – age)] ⎯ [72 ´ serum creatinine (mg/dl)]
Women: 0.85 ´ the value calculated for men.

CrCl, creatinine clearance; BSA, body surface area; Ucr, urine creatinine; Uvol, urine volume; Pcr, plasma creatinine; Tmin, time in minutes.

± 1.14 µg/ml, 1.35 ± 0.36 µg/ml, and 1.09 ± 0.57 µg/ml, respectively. Gatifloxacin penetrates well into the vitreous cavity in the noninflamed eye. Potential uses for oral gatifloxacin may include prophylaxis against endophthalmitis in open-globe injuries, surgical prophylaxis against postoperative endophthalmitis, and adjunctive therapy for the current management of bacterial endophthalmitis.[42] The nontoxic intravitreal dosage of gatifloxacin was found by Peyman et al (unpublished data) to be 400 µg/0.1 ml.

With in vitro tests, *S. aureus* isolates that were resistant to ciprofloxacin and ofloxacin were statistically most susceptible (p = 0.01) to moxifloxacin. CNS that were resistant to ciprofloxacin and ofloxacin were statistically most susceptible (p = 0.02) to moxifloxacin and gatifloxacin. *Streptococcus viridans* was more susceptible (p = 0.02) to moxifloxacin, gatifloxacin, and levofloxacin than ciprofloxacin and ofloxacin. *Strep. pneumoniae* was least susceptible (p = 0.01) to ofloxacin compared with the other fluoroquinolones. Susceptibilities were equivalent (p = 0.11) for all other bacterial groups. In general, moxifloxacin was the most potent fluoroquinolone for Gram-positive bacteria (p = 0.05), while ciprofloxacin, moxifloxacin, gatifloxacin, and levofloxacin demonstrated equivalent potencies to Gram-negative bacteria.[6,13]

Gatifloxacin showed in vitro bactericidal activity against pathogens resistant to third-generation fluoroquinolones. Compared with ofloxacin, there was 100% sensitivity of *S. epidermidis*, *Streptococcus mitis,* and *Strep. viridans* as opposed to 84%, 8%, and 52%, respectively.[43]

Moxifloxacin

Moxifloxacin (Avelox, Vigamox) was approved by the US FDA in December 1999. It is available as the monohydrochloride salt of 1-cyclopropyl-7-[(S,S)-2,8-diazabicyclo[4.3.0]non-8-yl]-6-9 fluoro-8-methoxy-1,4-dihydro-4-oxo-3-quinoline carboxylic acid with a molecular weight of 437.9. Moxifloxacin's empirical formula is $C_{21}H_{24}FN_3O_4 \cdot HCl$. It is metabolized by glucuronide and sulfate conjugation and is not affected by cytochrome 450 enzyme systems. Therefore, dosage adjustments are not recommended for patients with mild hepatic insufficiency, although experience with this group of patients is limited. Approximately 45% of an oral or intravenous dose of moxifloxacin is excreted as unchanged drug (~20% in urine and ~25% in feces).

Moxifloxacin possesses:

- Methoxy group at position 8 and azabicyclo moiety at position 7, which distinguishes it from the other drugs of this class.
- Differs from gatifloxacin in its different amino acid side-chain rendering it less hydrophobic and reducing the ability of the bacteria to pump out the drug.
- The ophthalmic preparation (0.5%) **without** benzalkonium chloride preservative may allow finer healing of the cornea but predisposes it to fungus contamination. The pH is 6.8.

Indications

Acute bacterial exacerbations of chronic bronchitis, acute bacterial sinusitis, and mild-to-moderate community-acquired pneumonia. Ocular use.

Dosage

400 mg by mouth given once daily for 5–10 days.

Pertinent studies

Garcia-Saenz et al[44] measured the human aqueous humor levels which were determined after two oral doses of ciprofloxacin 12 hours apart and single tablets each of 500 mg levofloxacin and 400 mg moxifloxacin. Aqueous humor concentrations approximately 10 hours after administration were 0.5 ± 0.85 µg/ml for ciprofloxacin, 1.50 ± 0.5 µg/ml for levofloxacin, and 2.33 ± 0.85 µg/ml for moxifloxacin. The mean levels of levofloxacin and moxifloxacin (but not ciprofloxacin) were above the MIC_{90}.

Bronner et al evaluated penetration of moxifloxacin into the vitreous of normal rabbit eyes and of eyes of rabbits infected for 24 hours with methicillin-susceptible S. aureus (MSSA) and MRSA.[45] Following a single intravenous dose of 5 or 20 mg/kg, moxifloxacin penetration was rapid and efficient, ranging from 28% to 52%, regardless of the dose. Penetration of the drug was increased significantly after a 20-mg/kg dose in an inflamed eye, with penetration reaching 52% of serum levels. Concentrations determined in the vitreous cavity following a 20-mg/kg administration showed a 3.5-fold decrease of the bacterial density within 5 hours for MSSA (MIC 0.125 µg/ml) and a 1.6-fold decrease for MRSA (MIC 4 µg/ml) strains.

Moxifloxacin ophthalmic solution (0.5%) demonstrated an 81% eradication rate of bacteria from infected eyes in 53 patients treated twice daily for 3 days.[46] Among 544 bacterial conjunctivitis patients, 82% microbial eradication and 83% clinical cure were seen on the ninth day after medication.[47] In four studies, 336 pediatric patients and 392 adults had no safety concerns or adverse events that were significantly different from placebo.[48] The nontoxic intravitreal dose determined by Peyman et al (unpublished data) is 160 µg/0.1 ml.

Further details on pharmacokinetics can be found in Chapter 5.

Cephalosporins

Mechanism of action

Cephalosporins, derived from the fungus *Cephalosporium acremonium*, inhibit cell wall synthesis. They inhibit the final transpeptidation

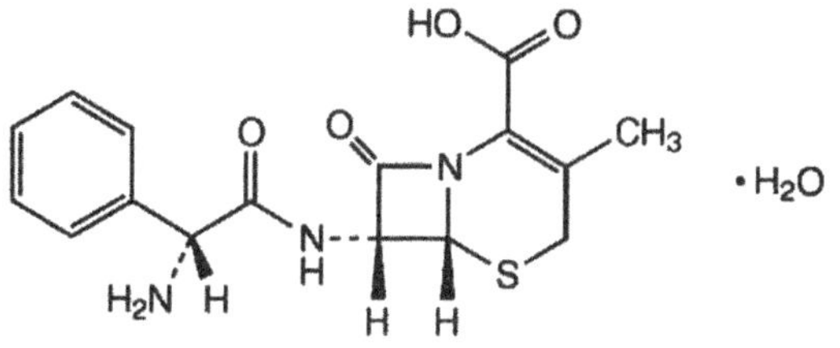

Figure 11.2

Chemical structure of cephalexin.

site of peptidoglycan synthesis by binding to penicillin-binding proteins. Cephalosporins should be used carefully in patients with a history of penicillin allergy because there is a reported 10% cross-reactivity but <1% for anaphylaxis. The mechanism of action is identical to the penicillins.

The chemical structure of a cephalosporin, cephalexin, is illustrated in Figure 11.2. They have a β-lactam ring but are resistant to β-lactamases.

Drugs and spectrum

The first-generation cephalosporins are mainly active against Gram-positive bacteria, including penicillinase- and nonpenicillinase-producing *S. aureus*, *S. epidermidis*, and beta-hemolytic streptococci. Some in vitro activity has been demonstrated against Gram-negative organisms such as *Escherichia coli*, *Klebsiella pneumoniae*, *P. mirabilis*, and *Shigella* spp. Their spectrum includes *Strep. viridans* and *Strep. pneumoniae*, *S. aureus* (not MRSA) and *S. epidermidis*, *Clostridium perfringens*, *Neisseria* spp., *Corynebacterium diphtheriae*, *Klebsiella*, *Shigella*, and *Salmonella* spp. Drugs in this class are listed in Box 11.2.

Box 11.2 First-generation cephalosporins

- Cefadroxil
- Cefazolin
- Cephalexin
- Cephalothin
- Cephradine

Box 11.3 Second-generation cephalosporins

- Cefaclor
- Cefamandole
- Cefmetazole
- Cefotetan
- Cefonicid
- Cefoxitin
- Cefuroxime
- Cefotoxin

The second-generation cephalosporins demonstrate improved Gram-negative coverage at the cost of Gram-positive coverage. These drugs are active against most strains of *H. influenzae*, including ampicillin-resistant isolates. However, some *in vitro* activity against Gram-positive bacteria, especially staphylococci, is lost. Anaerobic coverage is best performed with cefotoxin and cefotetan. *H. influenzae* and *Neisseria* spp. are best covered with cefuroxime. Cefuroxime is active against ampicillin-resistant strains of *H. influenzae*. Drugs in this class are listed in Box 11.3.

Third-generation cephalosporins demonstrate excellent coverage of Gram-negative bacilli with diminished Gram-positive coverage. This class has increased activity against many Gram-negative bacteria, including *Neisseria, Citrobacter, Enterobacter*, and *Pseudomonas* spp. Ceftazidime is excellent against *Pseudomonas* but has poor activity against many Gram-positive cocci and anaerobes. Ceftizoxime has poor activity against penicillin-resistant *Strep. pneumoniae*. Drugs in this class are listed in Box 11.4.

The fourth-generation cephalosporin, cefepime, shows improved Gram-negative coverage against many strains of *Enterobacter, Serratia, C. freundii*, and *Ps. aeruginosa*.

Box 11.4 Third-generation cephalosporins

- Cefixime
- Cefoperazone
- Cefotaxime
- Ceftazidime
- Ceftibutime
- Ceftizoxime
- Ceftriaxone
- Moxalactam

Side effects of cephalosporins

- Gastrointestinal (abdominal cramping, diarrhea, vomiting, seizures in renal failure patients)
- Hematologic (thrombocytopenia).
- Vaginal candidiasis
- Cefotetan, moxalactam, and cefoperazone are associated with hypothrombinemia. This has been attributed to the methyltetrazolethial sidechain that prevents activation of prothrombin.

Pertinent studies

Axelrod et al showed that intravenous ceftriaxone (1 or 2 g) prior to cataract extraction produced inhibitory concentrations in the aqueous humor for many Gram-negative organisms (except *Pseudomonas*) at 2 and 12 hours postoperatively.[49] Levels were also not inhibitory for *S. aureus* or *S. epidermidis*. Sharir et al found that intramuscular injection of 1–2 grams ceftriaxone produced vitreous levels after 4.5 hours of 5.9 µg/ml (range 1.4–19.4) and after 12–13 hours of 11.5 µg/ml.[50] Shockley et al found 2 mg of intravitreal ceftriaxone to be nontoxic; immediately after injection, the vitreous levels were 1345 ± 4.9 µg/ml; by 72 hours, the levels decreased to 17.6 ± 1.4 µg/ml;[51] the mean peak aqueous level was 80.2 ± 12.2 µg/ml at 72 hours.

Aguilar et al noted that vitreous levels above the MIC for *Pseudomonas* spp. were reached in aphakic and vitrectomized eyes within 2 hours of administering intravenous ceftazidime (50 mg/kg).[52] Levels were checked every 8 hours for 72 hours. Shaarawy et al showed that vitrectomy and lensectomy significantly shortened the half-life of ceftazidime after intravitreal injection.[53] Ceftazidime (2.25 mg) was administered intravitreally into control and inflamed rabbit eyes and its levels were assayed at 2, 8, 24, and 48 hours. The half-life was lessened from 13.8 hours in phakic control eyes to 11.8 hours in aphakic eyes to 4.7 hours in aphakic vitrectomized eyes. Schech et al showed that intravenous ceftazidime achieved inhibitory levels for *Pseudomonas* spp. and *Hemophilus* spp. after intravenous administration in traumatized swine eyes.[54] However, gentamicin did not reach MIC in the same eyes, demonstrating that systemic gentamicin is not a viable therapeutic option in traumatized eyes, whereas ceftazidime may be used for prophylaxis. Campochiaro and Green determined that intravitreal injection of ceftazidime 2.25 mg was nontoxic to the primate retina.[55] However, a 10-mg dose caused outer-segment photoreceptor damage in the fovea along with cystic changes and a macular hole.

Other cephalosporins also achieve intraocular concentrations. Jenkins et al showed in human eyes that subconjunctival injection of cefuroxime 25 mg resulted in significant aqueous humor concentrations (20 µg/ml) between 12 and 24 minutes after administration.[56] Forniceal and topical administrations did not achieve adequate aqueous concentrations. Martin et al reported that cefazolin demonstrated inhibitory levels only after repeat dosing.[57] The investigators injected 50 mg/kg of intravenous cefazolin every 8 hours for 48 hours. Vitreous levels progressively increased in inflamed phakic (3, 6.3, 10.6 µg /ml) and aphakic vitrectomized eyes (6.7, 19, 24.9 µg/ml) from 1 hour, 25 hours, and 49 hours, respectively, but were undetectable in noninflamed eyes. The levels obtained at 49 hours were well above MIC for organisms sensitive to cefazolin. Kramann et al injected 1 mg cefotaxime (0.4-ml dose of 0.25% [2.5 mg/ml]) intracamerally in patients undergoing cataract extraction.[58] There were no significant changes in corneal endothelial count or morphology as determined by specular microscopy up to 3 months afterwards.

Details are given in Chapter 5, including the nontoxic effect of 1 mg intracameral (AC) cefuroxime.

Vancomycin

Vancomycin, which inhibits bacterial cell wall synthesis, has excellent Gram-positive coverage and is also used in patients with allergies to penicillin. Its spectrum includes:

- *Strep. pneumoniae, Strep. viridans, Strep. pyogenes, Enterococcus (Strep.) faecalis*
- *S. aureus,* (including MRSA), *S. epidermidis*
- *Bacillus* spp.

Empiric treatment regimens for endophthalmitis now recommend 1 mg of intravitreal vancomycin and amikacin 400 µg (Chapter 8).

Since 1989, a rapid increase in the incidence of infection and colonization with vancomycin-resis-

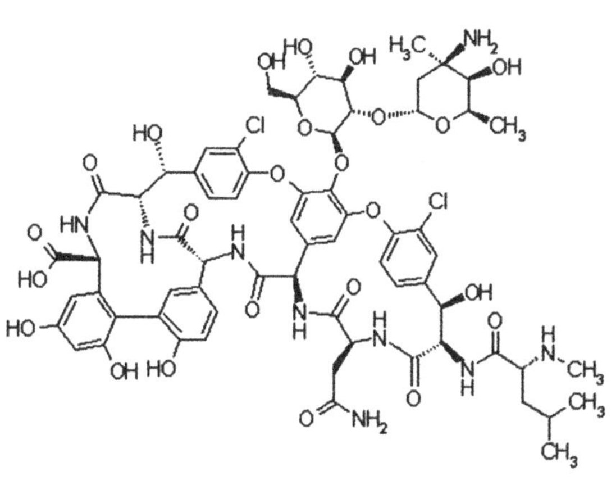

Figure 11.3

Chemical structure of vancomycin.

tant enterococci (VRE) has been reported in US hospitals. The *vanA* gene, which is frequently plasmid-borne and confers high-level resistance to vancomycin, can be transferred in vitro from enterococci to a variety of Gram-positive microorganisms, including *S. aureus*. Because of concerns about drug resistance, the US Centers for Disease Control (CDC) and the American Academy of Ophthalmology recommend that the routine prophylactic use of vancomycin in ocular surgery for topical, intracameral injection or irrigation in cataract surgery be discouraged.[59]

The chemical structure of vancomycin is shown in Figure 11.3.

Side effects

Oral
- Gastrointestinal (bitter taste, nausea, vomiting)
- Chills, drug fever, neutropenia.

Intravenous
- Hypotension
- Flushing
- Red man syndrome (histamine release and rash on face and upper body)
- Chills, drug fever, eosinophilia.

Subconjunctival
• Local irritation.

Co-administration with an aminoglycoside drug has been associated with nephrotoxicity and ototoxicity.

Dosage of vancomycin

• Intravenous: 15 mg/kg q12 hours
• Intravitreal and intracameral: 1 mg/0.1 ml
• Keep serum peaks between 20 and 50 µg /ml
• Keep serum troughs between 5 and 10 µg/m.

Pertinent studies

Meredith et al showed that vancomycin (15 mg/kg every 12 hours × 48 hours) in rabbits produced concentrations in aphakic and phakic vitrectomized eyes after intravenous administration that exceeded the MIC for many Gram-positive ocular pathogens.[60] Ferencz et al reported that in patients with postoperative endophthalmitis, vitreous concentrations were below therapeutic concentrations after intravenous administration but achieved therapeutic levels after intravitreal doses.[61] Haider et al measured intraocular vancomycin levels after intravitreal injections of 1 or 2 mg in cataract patients followed by repeat injections at 48 hours and 72 hours.[62] Aqueous levels varied between 8.4 and 170 µg/ml and vitreous levels varied from 21.2 to 220 µg/ml. Levels were therapeutic for Gram-positive organisms. Souli et al compared intravenous (1 g b.i.d. × 2) and subconjunctival (20 mg) injections of vancomycin and reported that subconjunctival injection is superior for in vivo treatment of Gram-positive bacteria causing eye infections.[63] The subconjunctival group had peak levels at 5 hours of 24.8 ± 3.6 µg/ml versus peak levels of 1.42 ± 0.47 µg/ml at 6 hours for the intravenous group.

Aguilar et al demonstrated in a rabbit model that intravitreal vancomycin had a half-life of approximately 9 hours in aphakic eyes with or without vitrectomy.[64] The half-life was 25.1 hours in phakic rabbit eyes. Inflammation increased the rate of elimination of vancomycin only in the aphakic group. Pflugfelder et al reported that a 2-mg vancomycin dose cleared most slowly in phakic eyes and most rapidly in aphakic vitrectomized eyes without an intact lens capsule.[65] Furthermore, the interaction between vancomycin and gentamicin was noted to be either additive or synergistic, depending on the organism. Park et al, using a rabbit model of pneumococcal endophthalmitis, found that intravitreal dexamethasone reduced the elimination of intravitreal vancomycin while the opposite effect was seen in uninfected eyes.[66]

Hegazy et al demonstrated that nontoxic concentrations of ceftazidime, vancomycin, and ganciclovir injected intravitreally caused toxicity in silicone-filled rabbit eyes.[67] However, 25% of the nontoxic amount did not produce any toxicity in these eyes. The authors speculated that a reduction in the preretinal space may be the reason. Homer et al found vancomycin to be nontoxic in a single intravitreal injection of 1 mg/0.1ml.[68] Therapeutic levels were present for 72 hours in the vitreous and in the aqueous for at least the period between 6 and 48 hours. Injection of MRSA produced a panophthalmitis in nontreated rabbit eyes but a significantly altered course in the treated eyes. However, Piguet et al suggested that even a single dose of amikacin and vancomycin might induce retinal toxicity with permanent damage.[69] The authors described a patient with corneal perforation who developed diffuse retinal edema with intra- and preretinal hemorrhage 12 hours after injection of intravitreal amikacin (1 mg) and vancomycin (1 mg). Visual acuity and ERG were markedly depressed. Oum et al showed that repeated injections of either vancomycin/amikacin or vancomycin/gentamicin may cause toxicity.[70] In rabbit eyes, the authors noted focal areas of retinal toxicity after a second injection 48 hours after initial injection. After a third injection 48 hours later, more advanced toxic reaction was evident with outer segment and retinal pigment epithelial damage. No damage was seen after the initial injection.

Linezolid

Linezolid is a synthetic antibiotic of the oxazolidinone class evaluated recently for its retinal toxicity and aqueous and vitreous penetration.[71,72] This drug has inhibitory action against Gram-positive bacteria including MRSA, VRE, and penicillin-resistant *Strep. pneumoniae*; linezolid also

Box 11.5 Aminoglycosides

- Amikacin
- Gentamicin
- Kanamycin
- Neomycin
- Netilmicin
- Spectinomycin
- Tobramycin

exhibits activity against some anaerobes, including *P. acnes*, *Peptostreptococcus* spp, *Bacteroides fragilis*, *Cl. perfringens*, and *C. difficile*. Buerk et al determined the nontoxic intravitreal dose to be 400 µg/0.2 ml in a rabbit study; its safety was evaluated using fundus examinations, intraoperative pressure measurements, and histopathologic examination.[71] In a noncomparative interventional, prospective case series study in humans, the eyes of patients undergoing pars plana vitrectomy who had not had previous vitrectomy were randomized into two groups; one group of patients was given one dose (one 600-mg linezolid tablet) and the other group two doses (two doses of 600 mg given 12 hours apart). Aqueous, vitreous, and plasma concentrations of linezolid were measured. The mean inhibitory aqueous and vitreous MIC_{90} were achieved against all Gram-positive bacteria, including VRE, MRSA, and streptococcal species after two doses. The MIC_{90} for many Gram-positive pathogens were achieved after only one dose in many patients approximately 4 hours after oral administration.

Aminoglycosides

The topical ophthalmic use of the aminoglycoside (Box 11.5), once a mainstay of ocular topical therapy, is being replaced with topical quinolones. Neomycin (found in Neosporin®) is used often for the treatment of superficial infections such as conjunctivitis. Topical gentamicin or tobramycin in fortified concentrations (10–15 mg/ml) have been used, alternating with cefazolin, for the empiric treatment of bacterial keratitis and inappropriately for endophthalmitis. Subconjunctival administration of gentamicin (20 mg/0.5 ml) is commonly administered postoperatively. Intravitreal administration of gentamicin 100 µg or amikacin 400 µg is used often along with vancomycin in the initial treatment of endophthalmitis. Amikacin has been recommended by many clinicians because of its lower potential for retinal toxicity and its effectiveness against *Mycobacterium* and resistant *Pseudomonas* spp.

The chemical structure of an aminoglycoside is shown in Figure 11.4.

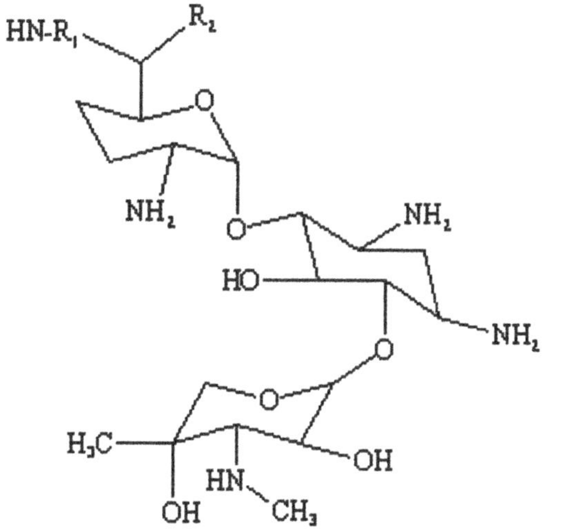

Figure 11.4

Chemical structure of an aminoglycoside.

Gentamicin

Intravenous administration of gentamicin may be recommended along with a drug such as cefazolin for prophylaxis of penetrating injuries. Current pharmacokinetic dosing guidelines and serum monitoring of aminoglycoside levels have reduced the concerns for ototoxicity and nephrotoxicity, especially with short-term administration (less than 1 week). However, the intraocular concentrations of gentamicin after systemic administration are below MIC and MBC levels.

The spectrum of gentamicin includes Gram-negative bacilli (*Ps. aeruginosa, P. mirabilis, Serratia* spp., *Enterobacter* spp., some activity against *S. aureus* and *S. epidermidis*). This drug has a synergistic effect with other medications such as with penicillins or cephalosporins against streptococci.

Tobramycin

Each milliliter of Tobradex contains:

- Tobramycin 0.3% (3 mg)
- Dexamethasone 0.1% (1 mg)
- Benzalkonium preservative
- Inactives: Tuloxapol, edetate disodium, sodium chloride, hydroxymethyl cellulose, sodium sulfate, sulfuric acid, and/or sodium hydroxide.

Each gram of Tobradex ointment contains:

- Tobramycin 0.3% (3 mg)
- Dexamethasone 0.1% (1 mg)
- Chlorobutanol 0.5%
- Inactives: mineral oil, white petrolatum.

Adverse effects of aminoglycosides

- Renal: renal tubular necrosis and renal failure.
- Neuromuscular blockade.
- Cyclosporine, vancomycin, amphotericin B, and radio contrast media increase risk of nephrotoxicity.
- Epithelial toxicity has been reported with the fortified preparations.
- Systemic administration may produce nephrotoxicity and vestibular and auditory toxicity (vestibular – gentamicin, streptomycin; auditory – kanamycin, amikacin, netilmicin, neomycin; both – tobramycin).
- Intravitreal aminoglycosides may be associated with more cases of retinal infarction than originally known.[73,74]

Pertinent studies (also refer to Chapter 5, 'Pharmacokinetics')

Peyman et al reported improved penetration of topical, subconjunctival, and intramuscular injections of gentamicin in the aphakic and phakic rabbit eyes.[75] Surprisingly, combination of routes generally produced higher levels in the noninfected than in the infected eyes. Aqueous levels were generally bactericidal by topical and subconjunctival routes. Levels in the vitreous by the routes of therapy employed in this study were at best inhibitory for the more virulent organisms.

El-Massry et al reported that intravenous administration of neither gentamicin nor amikacin penetrated sufficiently to reach potentially therapeutic concentrations consistently for either *Pseudomonas* spp. or *S. epidermidis* organisms in a rabbit model.[76] The maximum intravitreal concentration achieved for gentamicin was 1.8 ± 0.5 µg/ml. The maximum intravitreal concentration for amikacin was 8.5 ± 3.2 µg/ml. Inflamed eyes demonstrated higher concentrations than those without inflammation.

Peyman et al[77] and Bennett and Peyman[78] reported that intravitreal or intracameral injection of 400 µg or less of gentamicin produced no permanent toxic effects in rabbits. Reports have suggested that only doses up to 200 µg may be safe when given intravitreally. Intravitreal injections greater than 500 µg produced cataracts and retinal degeneration; 500 µg produced therapeutic levels in the vitreous for at least 72 hours. Bennett and Peyman also experimented with tobramycin and showed that intravitreal therapy was required early in the infection (within 7 hours) to treat an experimental *Ps. aeruginosa* endophthalmitis and that systemic and subconjunctival therapy failed to eradicate the infection.[79]

Inadvertent intraocular injections, gentamicin-soaked collagen shields,[80] and 'nontoxic' intravitreal doses of gentamicin[73,81] have produced macular infarction and ocular toxicity, although some patients have recovered useful vision after such incidents. Although amikacin has been demonstrated to have a better safety profile than gentamicin, macular toxicity has also been reported after intravitreal amikacin injection.[82,83]

Conway et al showed the neurotoxic effects of intravitreal gentamicin after injecting 1000–3000 µg of gentamicin intravitreally into monkeys.[84] Macular infarction was demonstrated with fundus examination and fluorescein angiography by 3 days and gradually faded by 21 days. Light and electron microscopic examination of the retina showed no primary vascular lesions; however, damage to the inner retinal layers, mainly the nerve fiber layer, ganglion cell layer, and the inner plexiform and nuclear layer was noted with less severe effects seen in the outer retinal layers and the retinal pigment epithelium. The authors postulated that gentamicin caused a complete shutdown of the regional macular blood flow, perhaps by the mechanism of granulocytic plugging of the capillary bed.

Penicillins

Penicillin is derived from molds of the genus *Penicillium*. The discovery of penicillin in 1926 marked the beginning of the antibiotic era. Penicillin is a bactericidal drug, which prevents cell wall synthesis by binding to the penicillin-binding proteins. This in turn leads to inhibition of peptidoglycan synthesis, an essential component of bacterial cell wall. Systemic uses include dental procedure and rheumatic fever prophylaxis and treatment of otitis media and sinusitis.

The penicillins are classified as:

- **Natural** (susceptible to β-lactamase)
  - Penicillin G, penicillin VK
- **Beta-lactamase resistant**
  - Nafcillin, oxacillin, methicillin, (flu)cloxacillin
- **Enhanced for activity against Gram-negative bacteria** (β-lactamase sensitive)
  - Aminopenicillins
    - Ampicillin, amoxicillin
  - Carboxypenicillins
    - Carbenicillin, ticarcillin
  - Ureidopenicillin
    - Piperacillin, azlocillin, mezlocillin
- **Combination with a betalactamase inhibitor (clavulanic acid)**
  - Unasyn, Augmentin®, Timentin®, Zosyn®.

Depending on the classification, penicillin has excellent activity against:

- *Streptococcus pyogenes* Lancefield group A
- *Streptococcus* group B
- *Streptococcus pneumoniae*
- Anaerobes
- *Staphylococcus aureus*
- *Treponema* and *Neisseria* (resistance was reported more frequently in *Neisseria*).
- Gram-negative bacteria, including *P. aeruginosa*

Susceptible species are inhibited by concentrations as low as 0.02 µg/ml, although resistance has increased dramatically in certain strains of *S. pneumoniae* and penicillinase-producing *S. aureus*.

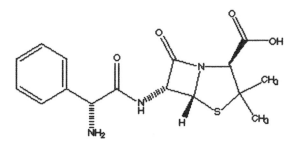

Figure 11.5

Chemical structure of ampicillin.

Many species of Enterobacteriaceae, such as *Proteus* sp. and *E. coli*, remain sensitive to ampicillin (Figure 11.5), while *Klebsiella* sp. is always resistant. Gram-negative bacteria gain plasmids coding for beta-lactamase production that inactivates ampicillin. However, by combining ampicillin, amoxycillin or ticarcillin with clavulanic acid (a beta-lactamase inhibitor), as the combination drugs Augmentin and Timentin, these Gram-negative bacteria are rendered susceptible again.

Side effects

Allergic reactions are probably the most common side effects. In treatment of serious sepsis, 12–24 million units (MU)/day may be administered for 14 days. Central nervous system toxicity in doses of >20 MU/day may become prevalent.

The following hypersensitivity reactions have been reported:

- Skin rashes ranging from maculopapular eruptions to exfoliative dermatitis
- Urticaria
- Reactions resembling serum sickness including chills, fever, edema, arthralgia, prostration
- Fatal anaphylaxis.

Hemolytic anemia, leukopenic anemia, thrombocytopenia, nephropathy, and neuropathy have been reported with high intravenous doses. Patients given continuous intravenous therapy with penicillin G potassium in high dosage (10–100 MU daily) may suffer from severe potassium poisoning, especially in patients with renal compromise. Hyperreflexia, convulsions, and coma are symptoms. Cardiac arrhythmia and cardiac arrest may also occur.

Concurrent administration of bacteriostatic antibiotics (e.g. erythromycin, tetracycline) may diminish the bactericidal effects of penicillins by slowing the rate of bacterial growth. Bactericidal drugs work most effectively against the immature cell wall of rapidly proliferating organisms.

Penicillin blood levels may be prolonged by concurrent administration of probenecid, which blocks the renal tubular secretion of penicillins. Probenecid also blocks the retinal pump mechanism of active removal of penicillins and cephalosporins from the posterior segment of the eye (see Chapter 5).

Ophthalmic use

Topical indication is rare due to limited coverage. Penicillin G is given intravenously 12–24 MU/day × 10 days for neurosyphilis. Although aqueous humor levels may last up to 6 hours after 1 MU in a rabbit model, to achieve equivalent human aqueous levels, doses would be toxic. Vitreous concentrations were reported up to 1 µg/ml in rabbits. Subconjunctival injections of penicillin G 1 MU with epinephrine produced therapeutic aqueous and vitreous levels for approximately 24 hours. Intravitreal doses of 5000 U produced levels similar to those achieved by the subconjunctival route. Because of limited spectrum of activity, a short intravitreal half-life, and difficulty producing posterior segment levels, penicillin is generally not indicated in the treatment of endophthalmitis.

Antistaphylococcal penicillins

Antistaphylococcal penicillins are semisynthetic, acid-stable penicillinase-resistant antibiotics which have coverage against Gram-positive bacteria, especially *S. aureus*. This group includes cloxacillin, dicloxacillin, methicillin, nafcillin, and oxacillin. Methicillin-resistant *S. aureus* (MRSA) are resistant to all antibiotics in this class.

Until the emergence of methicillin-resistant staphylococci, these antibiotics had a much improved spectrum of activity over penicillin for Gram-positive coverage, especially *S. aureus*. Penicillinase-producing strains of *S. aureus* were 15–80 times more susceptible. However, in recent years the advent of MRSA strains has reduced the use of antistaphylococcal penicillins in hospital to superficial lid and oculoplastics procedures; they are widely used in community practice.

The systemic, intravitreal, and subconjunctival administration of these drugs in ocular infections is generally not indicated because of the limited spectrum of activity, relatively limited access, and the availability of broader spectrum antibiotics. The most common use is orally after superficial lid or skin laceration, adult preseptal cellulitis, or some plastics procedures.

Antipseudomonal penicillins (extended-spectrum penicillins)

Antipseudomonal penicillins cover Gram-negative bacilli such as *Klebsiella*, *Proteus*, *Ps. aeruginosa*. These agents are often administered with an aminoglycoside when given systemically because of synergistic activity against *Ps. aeruginosa*. This group includes carbenicillin,[85] ticarcillin,[86] piperacillin,[87] mezlocillin, and azlocillin. The nontoxic intravitreal dose of carbenicillin is 5 mg/0.1 ml;[85] ticarcillin, 3 mg/0.1 ml;[86] and piperacillin, 1.5 mg/ 0.1 ml.[87]

Ophthalmic administration is limited. They are occasionally compounded into an ophthalmic drop for keratitis or may be used in a subconjunctival injection. Compounds are only available in injectable preparations.

Combination penicillins

Ampicillin/amoxicillin

Ampicillin is a semisynthetic penicillinase-sensitive, acid-stable broad-spectrum penicillin that has good Gram-positive and Gram-negative coverage. Amoxicillin has a similar spectrum and is better tolerated. Penicillinase-producing staphylococci and many Gram-negative bacteria including *Ps. aeruginosa* are resistant. However, the addition of clavulanate (ampicillin 500 mg/clavulanate 125 mg as Augmentin®) has improved the spectrum of activity so that this combination is effective against Gram-positive bacteria, including penicillinase-producing *S. aureus*, except MRSA, and resistant strains of *H. influenzae*. Ampicillin has good activity against *Neisseria* spp., *H. influenzae*, *P. mirabilis*, *E. faecalis* and other streptococci.

Ticarcillin/clavulanate (Timentin®) exhibits increased activity against Gram-positive bacteria, including penicillinase-producing *S. aureus* and Gram-negative bacilli. Piperacillin/tazobactam (Zosyn®) is a parenteral beta-lactam/beta-lactamase inhibitor combination which is useful for moderate-to-severe infections caused by staphylococci and anaerobes and some Gram-negative bacteria. Ticarcillin can be effective for *Pseudomonas* with the recommended dose (3 g q6) which is lower than piperacillin alone (18 g/day). Imipenem/cilastatin (Primaxin®) has a wide spectrum of activity including Gram-positive aerobes (*S. aureus* and *S. epidermidis*, penicillinase-producing), and many Gram-negative bacteria, including *Ps. aeruginosa*.

The oral administration of amoxicillin may be helpful in children with preseptal cellulitis. Augmentin® (amoxicillin/clavulanate) may be better because of increased activity against *H. influenzae* (beta-lactamase-producing) and *S. aureus*.

Sulfonamides

The sulfonamides are antagonists of para-aminobenzoic acid (PABA) for bacterial synthesis of folic acid. These agents have a broad spectrum of activity, including Gram-positive and Gram-negative bacteria, *Actinomyces* spp. and *Toxoplasma*. Bacterial resistance is a common problem with topical sulfonamides; other agents have generally replaced them.

The chemical structure of a sulfonamide is shown in Figure 11.6.

The topical preparations of sulfonamides are commonly used for the treatment of blepharitis and conjunctivitis. Sodium sulfacetamide 10% is the most common ophthalmic product available in both ointment and drops. Sodium sulfacetamide 30% has been used in cases of nocardial corneal ulcer. Many sulfacetamide products are also available in combination with steroids (prednisolone acetate or phosphate 0.25–5%) as both ointments and drops.

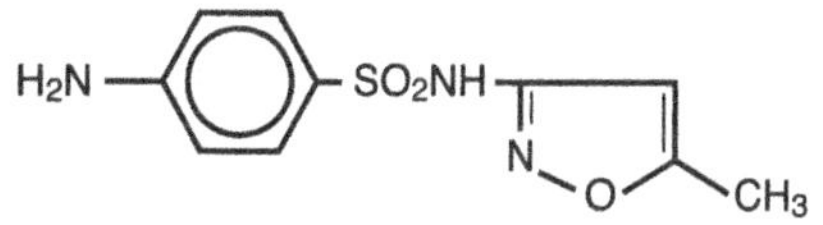

Figure 11.6

Chemical structure of sulfmethoxazole.

Oral administration of triple sulfas (not commercially available) or sulfadiazine (1 g q6h for 4–6 weeks) is used in the treatment of toxoplasmosis.

Side effects of sulfonamides

Hypersensitivity reactions found with the use of sulfonamides include urticaria, rash, erythema nodosum, erythema multiforme (Stevens–Johnson syndrome), and exfoliative dermatitis.

The most common ocular side effect from systemic sulfonamides is a transient, bilateral myopia, possibly with astigmatism.

Clindamycin

Clindamycin is a bacteriostatic agent that is effective against Gram-positive organisms including *B. fragilis*, *P. acnes*, and other penicillin-resistant anaerobic bacteria. Clindamycin has been used in patients who are allergic to penicillin. Clindamycin and gentamicin are an effective combination against most *Bacillus* spp.

The chemical structure of clindamycin is depicted in Figure 11.7.

Systemic clindamycin (300 mg q6h for 4–6 weeks) is used as a single agent or in combination with others in the treatment of toxoplasmosis. Intravitreal injections of up to 1 mg have been used in the treatment of *P. acnes* endophthalmitis and toxoplasmosis. Clindamycin has also been found to be nontoxic in vitrectomy infusion solutions in concentrations up to 10 µg/ml.[88]

Intravitreal administration of up to 1 mg of clindamycin has been used in cases of low-grade postoperative endophthalmitis. Irrigating solution containing clindamycin 10 µg/ml and gentamicin

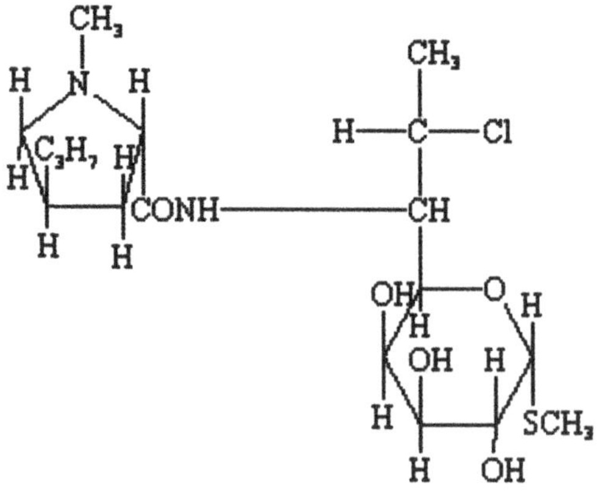

Figure 11.7

Chemical structure of clindamycin.

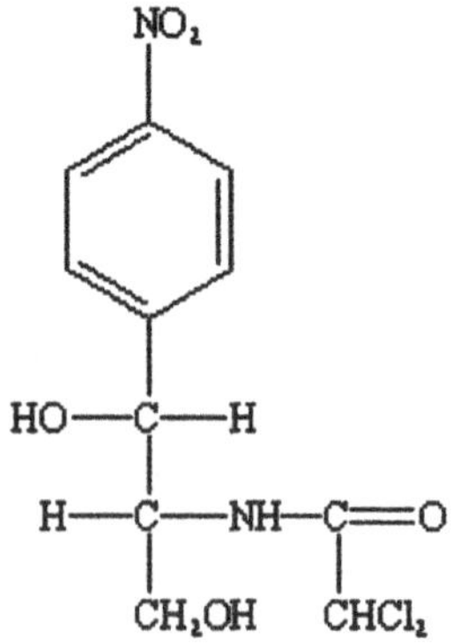

Figure 11.8

Chemical structure of chloramphenicol.

8 µg/ml significantly reduced colony-forming units (cfu) of *S. aureus* in rabbits after vitrectomy.[89] When 1000–2000 cfu of *S. aureus* were injected after vitrectomy, clindamycin and gentamicin in the irrigating solution significantly diminished the intraocular inflammation and the rate of positive bacterial culture. Clindamycin and gentamicin in the irrigating solution were not significantly effective when 4000 cfu bacteria were injected.

Chloramphenicol

Chloramphenicol, a bacteriostatic drug with broad-spectrum activity against Gram-positive and Gram-negative bacteria, except *Ps. aeruginosa*, is also used to treat *Rickettsia* spp., *Mycoplasma* spp., and spirochetes. Chloramphenicol has been used topically for conjunctivitis and keratitis. It works by binding to peptidyl transferase enzyme and inhibiting transfer of the growing peptide chain to an 'acceptor' site aminoacyl-tRNA. The binding is reversible, and thus this drug is bacteriostatic. It is lipid-soluble and thus penetrates well into the corneal stroma from topical application, as well as into the posterior segment of the eye and the cerebral cortex and cerebellum of the brain with systemic use. The chemical structure of chloramphenicol is illustrated in Figure 11.8.

According to Hanna et al, topical application requires repeated applications in order to achieve an aqueous humor concentration of 1 µg/ml, which is the minimum bacteriostatic concentration for many ocular pathogens.[90] George and Hanna showed that the topical route using ointment and the subconjunctival injection route produced bacteriostatic concentrations of chloramphenicol in the aqueous humor lasting for several hours, while the topical powder and intravenous routes yielded relatively low concentrations.[91]

Ophthalmic use has fallen dramatically after reports of aplastic anemia from topical application. Fraunfelder et al reported a 73-year-old woman who died of aplastic anemia less than 2 months after undergoing cataract extraction and beginning topical therapy with chloramphenicol.[92] The authors report that the first signs of pancytopenia began within 1 month of the surgery and that the pattern of the aplastic anemia was associated with an idiosyncratic response to chloramphenicol. Other cases of aplastic anemia, possibly caused by chloramphenicol use, have also been reported in the literature.[93–96]

Walker et al used high-performance liquid chromatography (minimum detection limit, 1 µg/ml) to determine that topical chloramphenicol failed to accumulate in detectable levels in serum.[97] The mean dose of chloramphenicol eye drops used after 1 week of treatment was 8.0 mg, and after 2 weeks, 15.3 mg. The authors asserted that topical chloramphenicol use is not a risk factor for inducing dose-related bone marrow toxicity.[97] In addition, no cases of dose-related aplastic anemia occurred in Scotland before and during the time of the study, with frequent use of chloramphenicol, as would have been expected if topical therapy was implicated as suggested.[92-97] In an international survey including 426 cases of granulocytosis and aplastic anemia and 3118 controls, none of the cases involved the use of chloramphenicol eye drops.[98] These authors also questioned whether topical chloramphenicol use is associated with anemia.

The nontoxic intravitreal dose of chloramphenicol was determined by Koziol and Peyman to be 2 mg.[99]

Macrolides

Erythromycin is a bacteriostatic drug that inhibits protein synthesis at 50S ribosomal subunits but may be bactericidal at high concentrations. Macrolides are effective against Gram-positive cocci such as *Strep. pneumoniae*. Hospital-acquired staphylococci are usually resistant. Gram-positive bacilli (*Cl. perfringens*, *Corynebacterium* spp., and *Listeria* spp.) are sensitive. Erythromycin possesses fair activity against *H. influenzae*, *N. gonorrhoeae*, and *Chlamydia* spp.; it may also be used in patients who are allergic to penicillin. Topical erythromycin ointment is often administered for blepharitis. Systemic administration does not penetrate the eye well. Systemic side effects include gastrointestinal intolerance, nausea, vomiting, and cramping.

Newer oral erythromycin derivatives, clarithromycin (Biaxin®, Klaricid®), and azithromycin (Zithromax®) may be indicated for skin and soft tissue infections because of their extended spectrum, better tolerance, and prolonged activity, requiring less frequent dosing. These agents are promising for *Mycobacterium avium* and other AIDS-related infections. A single 1-g oral dose of azithromycin (Figure 11.9) is approved for chlamydia arthritis. It is also effective for ocular chlamydia as a single 1-g oral dose.

Clarithromycin is particularly useful for treating chronic pseudophakic (saccular) endophthalmitis.[100-102] It is well absorbed to give anterior

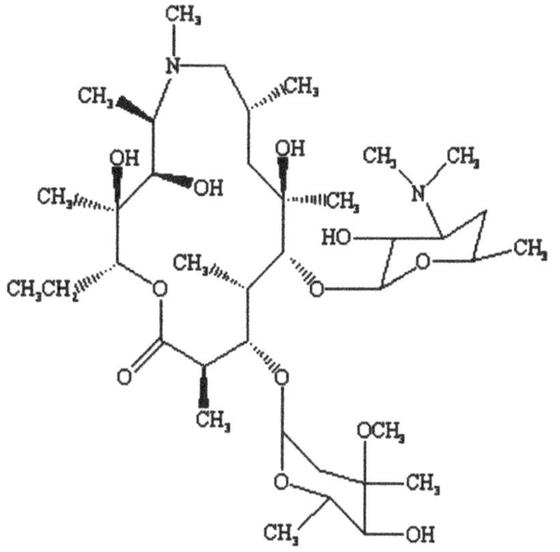

Figure 11. 9

Chemical structure of azithromycin.

chamber levels of 0.13 µg/ml at 4 and 8 hours post-oral dose and of 0.07 µg/ml and 0.06 µg/ml at 10 and 12 hours post-dose from oral doses of 500 mg.[101] In addition, it is concentrated up to 200 times within cells (polymorphonuclear cells and macrophages). In pseudophakic endophthalmitis, the responsible Gram-positive cocci are intracellular and therefore require antibiotic therapy with drugs that penetrate intracellularly (see Chapters 5 and 6). Okhravi et al have shown considerable benefit from the use of oral clarithromycin for treatment of chronic endophthalmitis when a better response was obtained in patients receiving clarithromycin therapy than those who did not.[102] Warheker et al first showed effective use of clarithromycin (500 mg BD) to treat postoperative pseudophakic 'saccular' endophthalmitis, following phacoemulsification surgery and an IOL implant, when the bacterial source was confirmed by PCR on an anterior chamber tap. Further surgery was not needed.[100]

Unal et al investigated ocular toxicity of intravitreal clarithromycin.[103] The authors found the highest nontoxic dose in a rabbit to be 1 mg in 0.1 ml intravitreally; retinal disorganization, necrosis, and cataract occurred with doses of 2 and 4 mg. The half-life was approximately 2 hours, showing that there is active removal of it by the retinal pump mechanism.

ANTIFUNGAL MEDICATIONS

Polyenes

Amphotericin

Amphotericin B acts by binding to a sterol on the cell wall of a sensitive organism, subsequently causing cell membrane permeability and leakage of intracellular components. This drug was derived from the fungus *Streptomyces nodosus* and is both fungistatic and fungicidal. Its wide spectrum of activity includes *Candida, Coccidioides immitis, Histoplasma capsulatum, Cryptococcus neoformans, Blastomyces dermatitidis*, and some *Aspergillus* spp. Notable exceptions include *Trichosporon beigelii, Aspergillus terreus, Pseudallescheria boydii,* and *Malassezia furfur. Fusarium* spp. vary in their susceptibility.

The chemical structure of amphotericin B is illustrated in Figure 11.10.

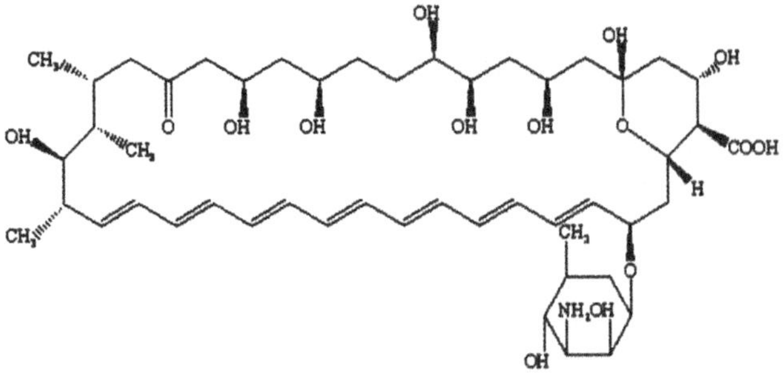

Amphotericin is associated with severe systemic side effects including renal, hematopoietic, and gastrointestinal symptoms. Azotemia, decreased glomerular filtration, loss of urinary concentrating ability, renal loss of sodium and potassium, and renal tubular acidosis and decreased erythropoietin production all occur; normochromic normocytic anemia is a result. Hepatotoxicity, neurotoxicity, allergic reaction, and cardiac arrest can occur with rapid infusion. Thrombophlebitis can also occur during intravenous infusion.

In order to reduce toxicity, three lipid preparations have been created:

- Amphotericin B Colloidal Dispersion (ABCD; Amphocil™, or Amphotec™)
- Amphotericin B Lipid Complex (ABLC; Abelcet™)
- Liposomal Amphotericin B (L-AMB; Ambisome™).

Goldblum et al found that compared with amphotericin B deoxycholate and amphotericin B lipid complex, the liposomal complex of amphotericin B reaches higher drug concentrations in both ocular compartments.[104]

Intravitreal injection of amphotericin B (5 μg/0.1 ml) in conjunction with vitrectomy has been used successfully in humans to treat fungal

Figure 11.10

Chemical structure of amphotericin B.

endophthalmitis.[105,106] However, amphotericin cannot be used in vitrectomy infusion fluid because of its toxicity. In adults, treatment is initiated with 0.25 mg/kg per day intravenously and increased gradually up to 1.0 and 1.5 mg/kg per day, as tolerated. This dosage results in blood levels of 1–2 μg/ml.

Liposomal amphotericin B has been shown to penetrate better into the cornea (2.38 ± 1.47 μg/g) compared with the deoxycholate preparation (0.46 ± 0.2 μg/g) after seven days of intravenous therapy.[107]

Pertinent studies

O'Day et al studied a loading dose approach for the cornea with topical amphotericin in rabbits.[108] Single-drop administration did not produce therapeutic concentrations in the aqueous fluid. Loading dose administration of one drop every 5 minutes for 13 applications was found to penetrate the aqueous fluid and attain therapeutic concentration. In inflamed corneas, a pass-through effect was noted with higher levels initially but rapid fall-off subsequently.

Green et al found that intravenous injection of 1 mg/kg in rabbits revealed no demonstrable levels of amphotericin in normal eyes and in those with chemical keratitis.[109] Aqueous levels of 0.13–0.16 μg /ml were produced from 4 to 24 hours after intravenous injection of 1 mg/kg in eyes with albumin-induced uveitis. Subconjunctival administration of 10 μg of amphotericin B penetrated the aqueous in only trace amounts. Intracameral injection of 20–35 μg was thought to be safe, but aqueous and vitreous levels were not measured. In our experience, this dose was toxic.

Axelrod and Peyman determined that intravitreal injection of 5–10 µg was nontoxic to all intraocular structures.[110] A single intravitreal injection of 5 µg of amphotericin B reversed the course of an experimental *Candida* endophthalmitis when administered up to 5 days after inoculation of the organisms.[111] Perraut et al reported a lack of retinotoxicity following intravitreal amphotericin injection (5 µg) in a 38-year-old woman with culture-positive *C. albicans* endophthalmitis.[112] Orgel and Cohen reported a postoperative case of zygomyctes endophthalmitis after phacoemulsification and posterior intraocular lens insertion that responded to 20 µg of amphotericin B.[113] However, 10 µg was injected into the vitreous cavity and 10 µg between the iris and posterior capsule. The investigators concluded that by keeping the eye bicompartmental, successful treatment with a total dose of 20 µg of amphotericin was possible.

Antifungal agents are not well tolerated systemically; intravitreal administration can be toxic to intraocular tissues. Intravitreal doses of amphotericin B are in the 5–10 µg/0.1 ml range and can cause retinal necrosis if they are given too closely to the retina and in a stream effect.

In a study of the dose-related ocular toxicity of amphotericin B in vitrectomized eyes, Huang et al found that a concentration of up to 5 µg/0.1 ml of the drug was nontoxic to the ocular structure when injected into the anterior part of the vitreous cavity.[114] Intravitreal injection of 2.5 µg of amphotericin B halted experimentally induced fungal endophthalmitis in rabbit eyes, even after 16 days of infection. Combined treatment of vitrectomy and intravitreal injection of amphotericin B not only cured the fungal endophthalmitis but also cleared the ocular media of opacities.

Boldrey described an extrusive vascular occlusion in an eye with *Aspergillus* necrotizing retinitis in an immunocompromised host.[115] Five micrograms of amphotericin B were injected into the center of the vitreous cavity, and an additional 0.75 mg was given subconjunctivally both at surgery and on the second postoperative day, at which time 2 mg of dexamethasone were also given subconjunctivally. Systemic antifungal drugs were not used. Based on this case, the author suggested that early diagnostic vitrectomy and intravitreal amphotericin B can be successful for adequate drug levels.

In recent years, the development of newer antifungal agents has not really improved the outcome of fungal endophthalmitis. Amphotericin B has one of the best spectra of activity and best minimum fungicidal concentration (MFC) of any of the agents currently in clinical use. Reports of synergism between amphotericin B and rifampin have been most promising with certain strains of *Candida* and some of the filamentous fungi such as *Aspergillus, Penicillium*, and *Rhizopus* spp. Christenson et al reported a case of a 16-year-old diabetic patient with *Rhizopus* pneumonia unresponsive to initial treatment with amphotericin B for 7 days.[116] The patient improved clinically when rifampin was added, and histologic examination of lung tissue removed 8 weeks later showed no fungal elements. Christenson subsequently demonstrated synergy between amphotericin B and rifampin against *Rhizopus* spp. with an in vitro study. The activity of amphotericin B in the presence of rifampin (10 or 5 µg/ml) increased fourfold against nine of 10 clinical and one of two environmental *Rhizopus* isolates.

Natamycin

Natamycin (Pimaracin) belongs to the same 'polyene' class of antifungals as amphotericin B and possesses the same mechanism of action in which the fungal cell membrane is altered changing the intracellular osmolarity, leading to cell death. Natamycin possesses a broad spectrum of activity. Unfortunately, the ability of this drug to penetrate the eye is poor.[117]

Natamycin is used topically as a 5% suspension or 1% ophthalmic ointment.[118] Ellison noted that 25 µg of Pimaricin given intravitreally in three dosages spaced 3 days apart in albino rabbits may be effective in inhibiting fungal endophthalmitis; a single dose was ineffective.[119] Although a dose of 50 µg was significantly more effective in inhibiting fungal disease, it also caused significant retinal damage with loss of retinal function and iridoplegia. A dose of 100 µg caused vitreous retraction and degeneration along with retinal detachment.

Ellison and Newmark demonstrated that intracameral doses of natamycin above 250 µg were toxic in infected rabbit eyes but caused no damage in normal eyes.[120] Furthermore, therapeutic

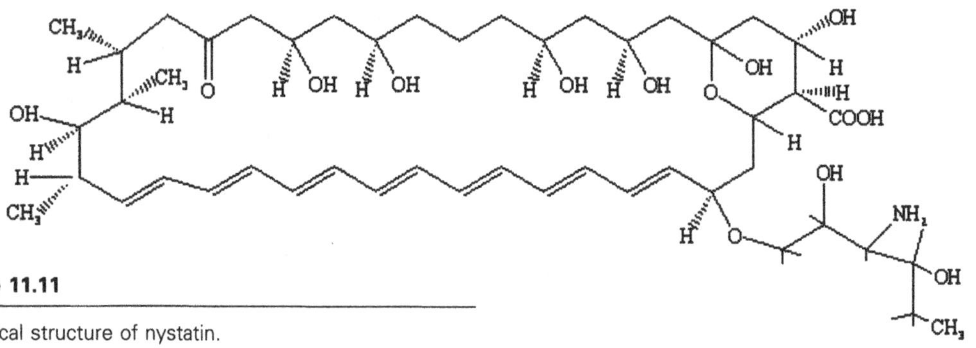

Figure 11.11

Chemical structure of nystatin.

concentrations were maintained for at least 24 hours, demonstrating excretion by the passive route anteriorly. This intracameral dose may be effective in treating a fungal endophthalmitis involving only the anterior segment of the eye.

Nystatin

Nystatin is a fungistatic and fungicidal antibiotic isolated from *Streptomyces noursei* and is also in the 'polyene' group. Its spectrum is mainly yeasts and includes *Candida*, *Cryptococcus*, *Histoplasma*, and *Blastomyces* organisms. The potency of nystatin is expressed in units: 1 µg contains 3.5 U. MICs for sensitive fungi range from 1.5 to 6.5 µg/ml. The mechanism of action of nystatin is similar to that of amphotericin B in which the cell membrane is disrupted by altering intracellular osmolarity. The chemical structure of nystatin is shown in Figure 11.11.

Oral preparations are poorly absorbed and parenteral administration is too toxic to produce adequate systemic levels. Subconjunctival injection of 5000 U appeared to be well tolerated. Intracameral and intravitreal injection of 200 U of nystatin caused transient inflammatory responses. Experimental *Aspergillus* endophthalmitis was treated with an intravitreal injection of 200 U of nystatin. Treatment was successful only if begun 24 hours after inoculation.[121]

Cilofungin

Cilofungin, a semisynthetic lipopeptide antifungal agent, has been found to be very active in vitro against *C. albicans* and *C. tropicalis*; it is moder-

ately active against *Torulopsis glabrata* but is not effective against *C. parapsilosis*, *Cryptococcus* spp., and *Saccharomyces cerevisiae*. Intravitreal injections of cilofungin have been found nontoxic in rabbit eyes in a dose of 320 µg both by ERG and histologic examination.[122]

Flucytosine

Flucytosine (Figure 11.12) (5-fluorocytosine) is an antifungal with a narrow spectrum of activity just for *Candida* spp. Strains of fungi easily acquire resistance to this drug. However, the toxicity of flucytosine is considerably less than that of amphotericin. Flucytosine is administered orally to adults at 100–150 mg/kg per day in four divided doses. Acquired resistance may develop among organisms initially sensitive to this antifungal agent. In addition, flucytosine can be used as an eye drop, although intraocular penetration is poor.[117] Its use is described in Chapter 9.

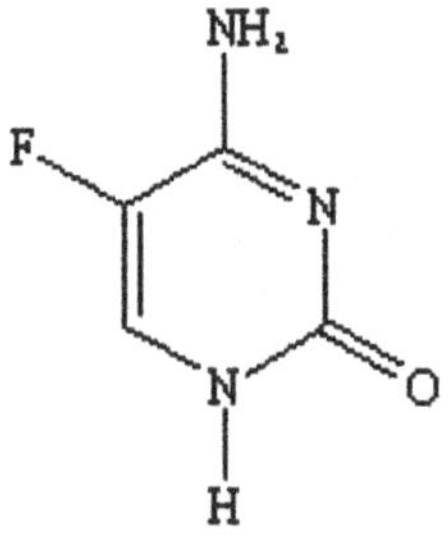

Figure 11.12

Chemical structure of flucytosine.

Table 11.4 Antifungal drugs currently used to treat endophthalmitis*

Drug, features, and advantages	Drawbacks

1. Natamycin (Pimaricin)
  a. Polyene; mol. wt 665.75 Da (28)
  b. Commercially available as topical 5% suspension for ophthalmic use in some countries, where it constitutes first-line therapy for mycotic keratitis
  c. Ophthalmic preparation is well tolerated, stable, and can be sterilized by heat
  d. Relatively high levels reportedly achieved in cornea after topical application
	a. Not commercially available as an ophthalmic preparation in many regions
	b. Effective only when applied topically
	c. Natamycin therapy may not be effective when keratitis is associated with deep stromal lesions
	d. Only about 2% of total drug in corneal tissue is bioavailable
	e. Should *not* be injected into the eye.

2. Amphotericin B
  a. Macrocyclic polyene; mol. wt 924.10 Da
  b. Good in vitro activity against *Aspergillus* spp. and *Candida* spp.; emergence of resistant mutants rare
  c. Can be administered by **topical** (0.15–0.30% solution), **intracameral** (7.5–30 µg/0.1 ml), **intravenous** (0.5–1 mg/kg BW/day) or **intravitreal** (1–5 µg/0.1 ml) routes. Can also be added to **vitrectomy infusion fluid** at a dose of 10 µg/ml
  d. Collagen shields soaked in amphotericin B (0.5%) found useful in experimental mycotic keratitis
  e. Penetrates deep corneal stroma after topical application; bioavailability sufficient for susceptible fungi
  f. Exerts direct fungicidal effect and exhibits immunoadjuvant properties
	a. Intravenous administration frequently associated with renal tubular damage, due to use of deoxycholate as vehicle
	b. Subconjunctival injection causes marked tissue necrosis at the site of injection
	c. Topical application of concentration >5.0 mg/ml may cause ocular irritation (solutions of 1.5–3.0 mg/ml better tolerated)
	d. Not commercially available as topical ophthalmic preparation; needs to be reconstituted from powder or intravenous preparation
	e. Poor intraocular penetration after intravenous administration

3. Miconazole
  a. Synthetic phenylethyl imidazole; mol. wt 416.12 Da
  b. Reported routes of administration include: **topical** (1%), **subconjunctival** (10 mg/0.5 ml), **intravenous** (600–1200 mg/day) and **intravitreal** (10 µg/0.1 ml); topical and subconjunctival administration generally well tolerated
  c. Found to penetrate rabbit corneas after subconjunctival and topical administration; high tissue concentrations achieved
	a. Use of intravenous preparation occasionally associated with toxicity due to the vehicle used
	b. Penetrates poorly to vitreous after intravenous administration with subtherapeutic levels
	c. Anomalous effects after subconjunctival administration in experimental *C. albicans* keratitis
	d. Generally considered useful in *S. apiospermum* ocular infections, but treatment failures have occurred

4. Ketoconazole
  a. Substituted imidazole; mol. wt 531.44 Da
  b. Given by **oral** (200–400 mg/day) or **topical** (1–2% suspension) routes in ophthalmic mycoses
  c. Well absorbed and good tissue distribution after oral administration. Peak serum concentration of 2–3 µg/ml 2–3 hours after 200-mg oral dose
  d. Concentration of 44.0 ± 10.1 µg/g in undebrided, and 1391.5 ± 130.0 µg/g in debrided, rabbit corneas after topical or subconjunctival application of 1% solution
	a. Oral doses >400 mg/day may cause transient rise in concentration of serum transaminases and hepatotoxicity
	b. Acid pH required for absorption
	c. Prolonged administration of high doses may cause impotence, gynecomastia or alopecia or papilledema
	d. No commercially available solution of ketoconazole for topical subconjunctival administration, or intracameral injection
	e. Vitreous penetration from systemic administration is poor

continued overleaf

Synergism has been reported when flucytosine is used in combination with amphotericin B for systemic infections. Codish et al reported the successful treatment of a patient with *Aspergillus* pneumonia with a synergistic combination of amphotericin B and flucytosine.[123] The authors noted that combination therapy decreased the dose of amphotericin B needed for effective therapy.

Table 11.4 Antifungal drugs currently used to treat endophthalmitis* – *continued*

Drug, features, and advantages	Drawbacks

5. Itraconazole
  a. Synthetic dioxolane triazole
  b. Given by **oral** (200–400 mg/day) or **topical** (1% suspension) routes in ophthalmic mycoses
  c. Oral solution and intravenous formulation recently developed; no reports of use in ophthalmic mycoses
  d. Peak serum concentration 0.3 µg/ml after single oral dose of 200 mg; increased to 3.5 µg/ml after 200 mg/day orally for 14 days
  e. Concentration of 200–250 µg/g attained in rabbit corneas after topical application of itraconazole in balanced salt solution, polyvinyl alcohol, boric acid, olive oil
  f. Detectable concentration found to persist in rabbit corneas after subconjunctival administration
	a. Commercially available capsule (100 mg) should be taken with meal; difficult to give in infants and children
	b. May be poorly absorbed after oral administration in certain groups of patients. Caution needed in patients with previous hepatic disease
	c. Absorption after oral dosing affected by antacids and H_2 receptor antagonists; may interact with other drugs
	d. Poor penetration into rabbit ocular tissue, compared with fluconazole and ketoconazole, after oral dosing
	e. Intravitreal injection (>10 µg) causes focal retinal necrosis in rabbits
	f. No commercially available solution of itraconazole for topical, subconjunctival or intracameral injection administration

6. Fluconazole
  a. Synthetic bistriazole; mol. wt 306.3 Da
  b. Soluble in water, hence excreted through kidney; 10–20% protein bound in serum; long half-life
  c. Given by **oral** (50–100 mg/day), **topical** (0.2–2% solution) or **intravenous** routes in ophthalmic mycoses. High bioavailability, low toxicity, good stability
  d. Biodegradable polymeric scleral implant containing fluconazole promising for intravitreal delivery
  e. Commercially available for oral and intravenous use
	a. May interact with cisapride, oral antidiabetic drugs and phenytoin after oral administration
	b. Less active against *Candida glabrata* and *Candida krusei* than against *C. albicans*
	c. May not be effective in treatment of filamentous fungal keratitis

*See also Voriconazole, p. 263.

Faeriefungin

Faeriefungin is a new antibacterial and antifungal agent derived from a strain of *Streptomyces griseus*, a variety of the species autotrophicus. Faeriefungin is a superior antifungal agent with more activity than amphotericin B, nystatin, or natamycin against *Aspergillus fumigatus*, *Microsporum canis*, and *Trichophyton rubrum*. This drug is somewhat less effective against *C. albicans*, with an MIC of 5.5 µg/ml compared with 3.2 µg/ml for natamycin.

Unlike related 'polyene' antibiotics nystatin and amphotericin B, which show no antibacterial activity, faeriefungin exhibits an excellent antibacterial effect against Gram-positive organisms, including MRSA strains. Slightly higher concentrations of faeriefungin are effective against fastidious Gram-negative bacteria such as *N. gonorrhoeae*, *N. meningitidis*, and *Branhamella catarrhalis*, including penicillin-resistant strains. However, other Gram-negative organisms, including *Enterobacter* spp. and *Pseudomonas* spp., are completely resistant to faeriefungin.

Preliminary in vitro toxicity studies of faeriefungin against WB-S cells and human erythrocytes have shown faeriefungin to be 10-fold less toxic than amphotericin B. Dunlap and others reported that intravitreal injection of concentrations of 100 µg or less produced no retinal toxicity.[124] Retinal toxicity was assessed by ERG and light and transmission electron microscopy. Injection of 400 µg resulted in severe retinal toxicity, although indirect ophthalmoscopy was unremarkable. At 200 µg, there was moderate toxicity. Intravitreal injection of concentrations of

100 µg or less produced no neuroretinal toxicity. These data suggest that faeriefungin is a potentially useful drug in the treatment of fungal or bacterial endophthalmitis.

Azoles

Although amphotericin B still remains the drug of choice for most fungal infections, its systemic toxicity limits its usefulness. Azole antifungal drugs and polyenes used to treat endophthalmitis are given in Table 11.4.[125] Azoles have been used as an alternative to amphotericin B. The imidazoles are less toxic than the polyene antibiotics, and are active against dermatophytes, yeasts, fungi, and some bacteria and protozoa. Various imidazole derivatives have been studied for systemic and ocular administration to eradicate fungal endophthalmitis. The chemical structure of an azole is shown in Figure 11.13.

Clotrimazole

Clotrimazole was one of the first agents studied; however, liver microsomal enzyme induction has limited its systemic use but not its topical use in humans. Clotrimazole in a topical 1% arachis oil preparation can be used to treat fungal keratitis.

Miconazole

Miconazole has a broad spectrum of activity and is effective against most organisms and fungi including *Candida*, *Cryptococcus*, and *Coccidi-*oides. At low doses, miconazole is fungistatic, and at higher doses, it is fungicidal. Miconazole demonstrates good vitreous penetration from intravenous administration, and unlike clotrimazole, it can be given intravenously.[126] Miconazole has been used topically as ophthalmic drops in a 10 mg/ml (1%) concentration directly out of the vial or diluted to half strength with saline for fungal keratitis. Stinging and punctuate keratitis from the topical administration of miconazole have been reported. Tests on animals have demonstrated few systemic toxic effects and limited ocular toxicity.[127] Toxic reactions following intravenous administration include thrombophlebitis, chills, nausea, vomiting, rash, and gastrointestinal symptoms; therefore, it has been used mostly as a topical agent and given systemically when amphotericin B or ketoconazole are contraindicated. The chemical structure of miconazole is shown in Figure 11.14.

Tolentino et al proposed that intravitreal use of miconazole in doses not exceeding 40 µg/0.1 ml may be justified in desperate cases of fungal endophthalmitis.[128] Toxicity studies in rabbits and monkeys showed that both miconazole and its vehicle produced toxic damage to the retina and crystalline lens in concentrations of 100 µg or greater. Concentrations of 10–80 µg caused mild-to-moderate retinal necrosis in some rabbit eyes. In monkey eyes, these concentrations did not cause significant histopathologic or ERG changes.

Although miconazole has poor oral absorption, it can be administered orally, with up to 3 g per

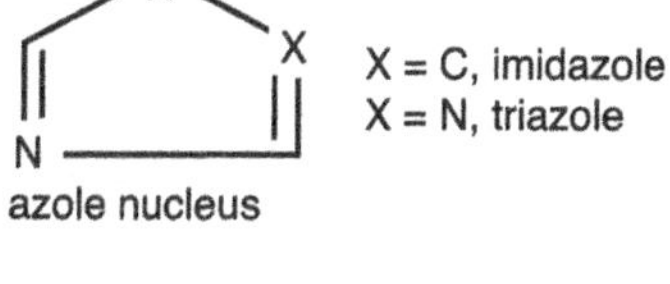

Figure 11.13

Chemical structure of an azole.

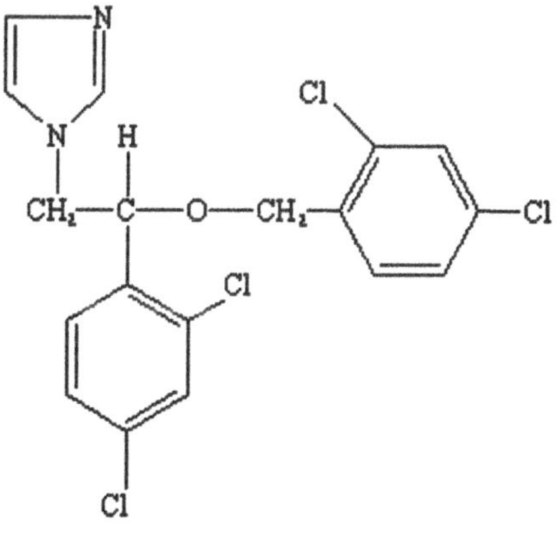

Figure 11.14

Chemical structure of miconazole.

day given to adults in divided doses. The intravenous dose of this drug in adults is usually 600–1200 mg per day administered in three divided doses. The maximal recommended dose is 30 mg/kg per day, but doses ranging from 3 to 6 g per day have been administered for months.[127]

Fowler described an immunosuppressed patient with presumed *Candida* endophthalmitis who failed to respond to intravenous amphotericin B but was successfully treated with a vitrectomy and intravitreal injection of 10 μg of miconazole.[129] Jones described a patient with endophthalmitis from culture-proven *Aspergillus* spp. who was successfully treated with topical and intravenous miconazole.[130]

Blumenkranz and Stevens reported three patients with intraocular fungal infection that progressed despite being treated with intravenous miconazole.[131] Two patients had disseminated coccidioidomycosis and one patient had disseminated candidiasis. Two were being treated with miconazole when the infections developed. The third, with probable *Candida* endophthalmitis, failed to respond to miconazole. All three infections resolved with intravenous administration of amphotericin B.

Foster and Stefanyszyn were unable to demonstrate miconazole in the vitreous of rabbit eyes following intravenous and topical administration.[132] Low levels of the drug were present in the vitreous for 1–2 hours after a 10-mg subconjunctival injection of miconazole. One hour after intravenous administration of 1200 mg of miconazole in a 65-year-old man with endophthalmitis, a vitreous level of 2.77 μg/ml was detected, which is below the effective concentration needed to treat infections with species of *Candida* or *Aspergillus*. Peyman evaluated the toxic effects of intravitreal miconazole but was unable to demonstrate the in vivo efficacy of this drug in managing experimental *C. albicans* endophthalmitis.[133]

Ketoconazole

The chemical structure of ketoconazole is shown in Figure 11.15. Its antifungal activity is similar to that of miconazole, and it is indicated for the treatment of systemic fungal conditions, including candidiasis, histoplasmosis, and blastomycosis. Ketoconazole has fewer side effects in humans

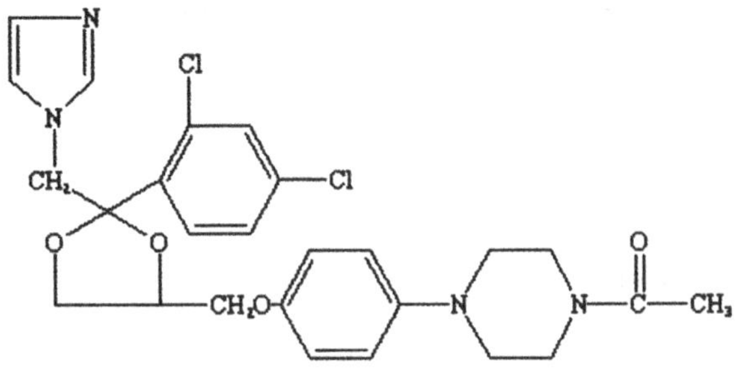

Figure 11.15

Chemical structure of ketoconazole.

than miconazole and, unlike miconazole, it is readily absorbed from the gastrointestinal tract. Vitreous and cerebrospinal fluid penetration from systemic administration is poor. Ketoconazole has been associated with hepatotoxicity and elevated liver function tests after normal oral doses.

The drug is administered orally in a single dose of 200 mg daily in adults;[134] 400 mg per day can be given in severe infections. Children weighing 20 kg or less, 20–40 kg, and over 40 kg are given a single oral dose of 50, 100, and 200 mg, respectively.[135]

In animal experiments, Osato et al demonstrated that oral ketoconazole (80 mg/kg per day) was as effective as parenteral amphotericin B and amphotericin B methyl ester in treating endogenous *C. albicans* in the rabbit eye.[136] Salmon et al successfully treated a patient with metastatic *Candida* endophthalmitis presenting as a unilateral panuveitis in an apparently healthy drug addict.[137] Diagnosis was confirmed with a diagnostic and therapeutic vitrectomy. Treatment with 5-flucytosine (150 mg/day in three divided doses) and ketoconazole (200 μg/kg per day orally) led to resolution.

The use of ketoconazole in human cases of fungal endophthalmitis is somewhat limited and it has usually been given after the intravitreal injection of amphotericin B. Stern et al reviewed 15 patients who developed *C. parapsilosis* infection after intraocular surgery and were treated with intravitreal amphotericin B, ketoconazole (800 mg per day for 12 weeks), and flucytosine.[138] The clinical outcome of the patients could not be correlated specifically with the ketoconazole treatment.

Inflammation may help to increase intraocular levels of ketoconazole. Savani et al measured the penetration of three azole compounds – ketoconazole, itraconazole, and fluconazole – into the ocular tissues and fluids of rabbits in the presence and absence of ocular inflammation.[139] The rank order of penetration into eye tissue was fluconazole > ketoconazole > itraconazole. The presence of inflammation improved penetration of all three compounds into ocular fluids and tissues. Penetration of these azoles into the anterior chamber of uninflamed eyes and into the cerebrospinal fluid was similar.

Mary et al reported a synergistic effect between 5-fluorocytosine and imidazole derivates.[140] The authors tested the eventual synergy between 5-fluorocytosine and imidazole derivatives (miconazole, ketoconazole, fluconazole, itraconazole) against 57 yeast isolates resistant to 5-fluorocytosine. The synergistic effect between 5-fluorocytosine and antifungal imidazoles varied widely with the drug tested; it was more frequent with ketoconazole. Itraconazole and fluconazole present very little synergistic effects in vitro.

The use of ketoconazole in combination with intravitreal amphotericin B deserves further evaluation. There is also some documentation that imidazoles may cause antagonism with amphotericin B, and therefore their concurrent use has not been recommended. Yoshizumi and Banihashemi evaluated the use of intravitreal ketoconazole and found that 540 µg were nontoxic to ocular structures.[141] The authors injected doses varying between 15 µg and 2240 µg dissolved in 0.1 ml of 100% dimethyl sulfoxide (DMSO) intravitreally. Doses of 540 µg or less resulted in no ocular toxicity. Doses of 720 µg revealed ERG abnormalities and photoreceptor degeneration by electron microscopy. Doses of 2240 µg resulted in severe histopathologic and ERG alterations.

Oxiconazole

Oxiconazole is an imidazole derivative that has broad in vitro and in vivo spectra against a wide variety of fungal organisms, including *C. albicans, Cryptococcus neoformans, Aspergillus fumigatus,* and *A. niger.* In vitro studies by Polak demonstrated oxiconazole to be slightly more effective than clotrimazole, econazole, and ormiconazole against *Candida* spp.[142] Oxiconazole is used topically for the treatment of superficial mycoses. Schulman et al reported that dosages up to 100 µg injected intravitreally did not cause any toxic ocular effects in rabbits.[143]

Triazoles

The triazoles are newer azole derivatives that, in contrast to imidazoles (miconazole and ketoconazole), contain a third nitrogen atom on the azole ring. The mechanism of action is similar to that of the imidazoles. The azole compounds appear to inhibit ergosterol biosynthesis and possibly may have some other alternative antifungal properties, of which direct membrane damage on the cell phospholipid membranes, especially at higher dosages, may be one of the most important.

Itraconazole

Itraconazole is active against a wide variety of fungal pathogens, including *Candida, Aspergillus, Coccidioides, Histoplasma,* and *Paracoccidiodes* spp., and *Sporothrix.* It is well absorbed orally, especially when taken after meals in doses of 50–400 mg daily, and is more than 90% protein-bound. Toxicity appears to be low, with some nausea and transient increases in liver enzymes being seen. No effect on steroidogenesis has been noted.

The chemical structure of itraconazole is shown in Figure 11.16.

The ocular toxicity of intravitreal itraconazole was determined in rabbits. Schulman et al showed that intravitreal doses up to 10 µg in 100% DMSO was nontoxic in all eyes.[144] Higher doses caused focal areas of retinal necrosis.

In a rabbit model of *Candida* endophthalmitis, Savani et al reported that itraconazole given early in endogenous *Candida* endophthalmitis was effective despite low drug concentrations.[139] However, the investigators concluded that itraconazole was not effective in fungal endophthalmitis when given 7 days after the infection. In contrast amphotericin B given at the same time interval was found to be efficacious and is still the drug of choice in the animal model.

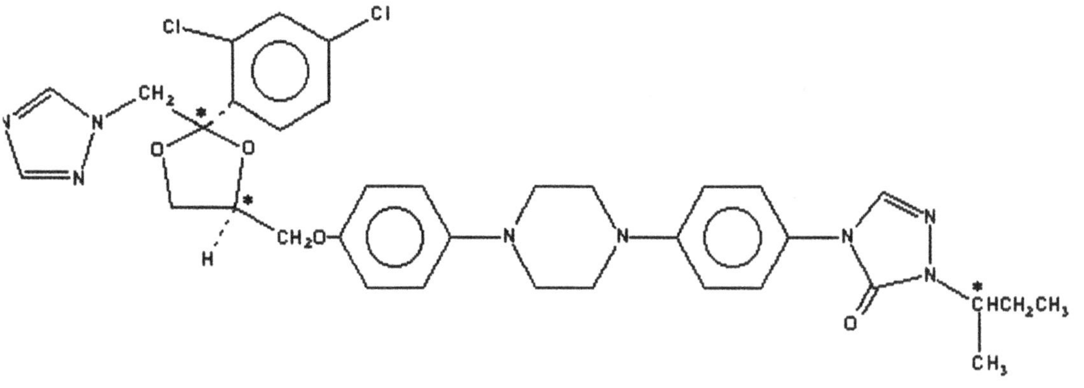

Figure 11.16

Chemical structure of itraconazole.

Table 11.5 Efficacy of the combination of flucytosine and itraconazole against candidiasis and aspergillosis compared with combined flucytosine and amphotericin

5-FC + fluconazole	Synergistic in candidiasis; indifferent in cryptococcosis and aspergillosis
5-FC + itraconazole	Synergistic in candidiasis/aspergillosis; most synergism with a 5-FC-resistant strain of *Candida albicans*
5-FC + amphotericin B	Same synergism as above; indifferent in cryptococcosis
Amphotericin B + itraconazole	Mostly indifferent and weakly antagonistic
Amphotericin B + ketoconazole	More antagonistic than amphotericin B + itraconazole

5-FC, flucytosine.

Polak concluded in an experimental mouse model that the combination of flucytosine and itraconazole was synergistic against candidiasis and aspergillosis, similar in effect to flucytosine and amphotericin B.[145] The results are summarized in Table 11.5. The author noted that further clinical trials should be initiated.

Fluconazole

Fluconazole has activity against *Aspergillus, Candida, Blastomyces, Coccidioides, Crypto-*coccus, and *Histoplasma* spp. Fluconazole may be given by intravenous or oral routes, and appears to have one of the best pharmacokinetic profiles of all available antifungal agents. This drug is water-soluble, weakly protein-bound, and penetrates well into body tissues, including the cerebrospinal fluid. However, there have been some concerns that in vitro and in vivo activities of the drug do not correlate well using the same organisms.

The chemical structure of fluconazole is illustrated in Figure 11.17.

Savani et al noted that in their rabbit model of endogenous candidal endophthalmitis, in spite of high intraocular concentrations, fluconazole did not clear the vitreous and choroid-retina of yeasts when therapy was begun 7 days after infection.[139] The authors concluded that amphotericin B still appears to be the standard of therapy for fungal endophthalmitis in their model.

Schulman et al noted that in rabbit eyes intravitreal fluconazole was nontoxic in doses up to 100 µg/0.1 ml, as measured by biomicroscopy, ophthalmoscopy, and ERG 8 days after the injection.[146] As previously stated, Polak reported that the combination of flucytosine and fluconazole exhibited synergistic activity in a mouse model of candidiasis.[145] However, further clinical trials are warranted to determine the full potential in humans.

Tucker et al reported that the penetration of fluconazole into cerebrospinal fluid was substantial with minimal toxicity.[147] At a dose of 50 mg/day, peak concentrations of 2.5–3.5 µg/ml

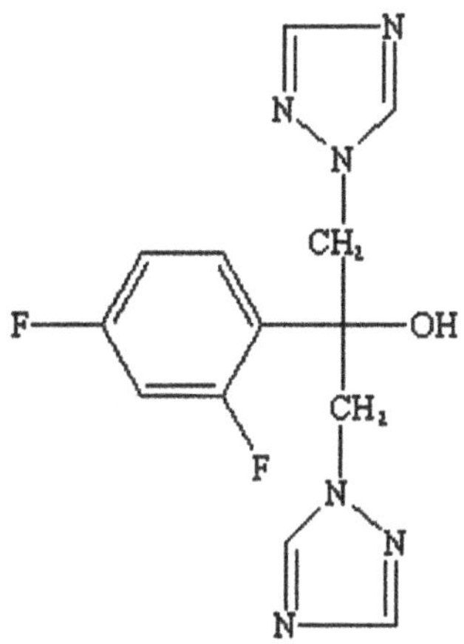

Figure 11.17

Chemical structure of fluconazole.

and 2.0–2.3 µg/ml occurred at 2–6 and 4–8 hours in serum and cerebrospinal fluid, respectively. At 100 mg/day, peak concentrations of 4.5–8.0 µg/ml and 3.4–6.2 µg/ml occurred at 2–4 and 4–12 hours, respectively. The mean ratios of the concentration in cerebrospinal fluid to that in serum were 73.8% at 50 mg/day and 88.7% at 100 mg/day. Minimal toxicity was noted in 34 patient months of therapy (12 months on 50 mg daily; 22 months on 100 mg daily).

Voriconazole

Voriconazole is a triazole that is structurally related to fluconazole. It was developed by Pfizer Pharmaceuticals and its clinical use was approved by the US FDA in May 2002. The trade name of voriconazole is Vfend™.

As with all azole antifungal drugs, voriconazole works principally by inhibition of cytochrome P450 14a-demethylase (P45014DM). This enzyme is in the sterol biosynthesis pathway that leads from lanosterol to ergosterol. Compared with fluconazole, voriconazole inhibits P45014DM to a greater extent but is dose-dependent.

Voriconazole has favorable in vitro activity against a variety of fungi, including Candida spp., Aspergillus spp., C. neoformans, B. dermatitidis, C. immitis, H. capsulatum, Fusarium spp., Paecilomyces lilacinus, and Penicillium marneffei.[148–150] Voriconazole is generally considered to

be a fungistatic agent against Candida spp. and C. neoformans. It may, however, be fungicidal against Aspergillus spp.[151]

Its enhanced activity against fluconazole-resistant Candida krusei, Candida glabrata, and Candida guilliermondii is noteworthy. Some isolates which are resistant to fluconazole and/or itraconazole may possibly exhibit cross-resistance to voriconazole.[152,153] Zygomycetes, such as Mucor spp., and Rhizomucor spp. generate considerably high voriconazole MICs.[154,155]

Voriconazole is active following both oral and intravenous administration. In clinical trials, oral (200 mg twice daily) and intravenous (3–6 mg/kg every 12 hours) doses have produced favorable responses. However, typical doses at individual clinical settings are not yet known. Parenteral administration can be followed by an oral course of voriconazole therapy.[156]

Side effects consist of dose-related, transient visual disturbances, skin rash, and elevated hepatic enzyme levels.

Visual disturbance is an interesting and extensively investigated side effect of voriconazole. It seems to be caused by the blockage of receptor de-excitation by voriconazole. Patients experiencing visual disturbance during voriconazole therapy describe it in various forms: brightness, blurring, light sensitivity, or some changes in color vision. Typically, these visual abnormalities are seen in approximately 30% of patients receiving voriconazole; they begin 30 minutes after the dose and last about 30 minutes.

Clinical use of voriconazole was approved for primary treatment of acute invasive aspergillosis and salvage therapy for rare but serious fungal infections caused by the pathogens Scedosporium apiospermum and Fusarium spp. This drug is only fungistatic against Candida spp. and is not the drug of first choice.

Hariprasad et al determined the vitreous, aqueous, and plasma concentrations of orally administered voriconazole in humans.[156] The authors found that two 400-mg doses given 12 hours apart provide therapeutic aqueous and vitreous levels in the noninflamed eye. They also found that voriconazole has a broad antifungal spectrum, low MIC_{90} levels, and good tolerance and bioavailability. The mean ± SD levels recorded for plasma, vitreous, and aqueous were 2.13 ± 0.93, 0.81 ± 0.31, and 1.13 ± 0.57 µg/ml, respectively.

Garbino et al used voriconazole to treat a case of late-onset postoperative cataract surgery endophthalmitis due to *P. lilacinus* with considerable success.[157] The isolate was resistant to amphotericin (MIC 16 µg/ml), intermediate susceptible to itraconazole (MIC 0.5 µg/ml), and susceptible to voriconazole (MIC 0.25 µg/ml). The patient was treated with voriconazole 400 mg b.i.d. orally for 3 months, after failure of therapy with the other antifungal drugs, with a good clinical response.

References

1. Lescher GY, Froelich ED, Gruett MD et al. 1,8–Naphthyridine derivatives. A new class of chemotherapeutic agents, *J Med Pharm Chem* (1962) **5**:1063–8.
2. Gellert M, Mizuuchi K, O'Dea MH et al. DNA gyrase; an enzyme that introduces superhelical turns into DNA, *Proc Natl Acad Sci USA* (1976) **73**:3872–6.
3. King DE, Malone R, Lilley SH. New classification and update on the quinolone antibiotics, *Am Fam Physician* (2000) **61**:2741–7.
4. Oliphant CM, Green GM. Quinolones: a comprehensive review, *Am Fam Physician* (2002) **65**:455–63.
5. Borek AP, Dressel DC, Hussong J et al. Evolving clinical problems with *Streptococcus pneumoniae*: increasing resistance to antimicrobial agents, and failure of traditional optochin identification in Chicago, Illinois between 1993–1996, *Diagn Microbiol Infect Dis* (1997) **29**:209–14.
6. Kowalski RP, Dhaliwal DK, Karenchak LM et al. Gatifloxacin and moxifloxacin: an *in vitro* susceptibility comparison to levofloxacin, ciprofloxacin and ofloxacin using bacterial keratitis isolates, *Am J Ophthalmol* (2003) **136**:500–5.
7. Drlica K, Malik M. Fluoroquinolones: action and resistance, *Curr Top Med Chem* (2003) **3**:249–82.
8. Saravolatz LD, Leggett J. Gatifloxacin, gemifloxacin, and moxifloxacin: the role of 3 newer fluoroquinolones, *Clin Infect Dis* (2003) **37**:1210–15.
9. Andriole CL, Andriole VT. Are all quinolones created equal? *Medicguide Infect Dis* (2002) **21**:1–5.
10. Graves A, Henry M, O'Brien TP et al. *In vitro* susceptibilities of bacterial ocular isolates of fluoroquinolones, *Cornea* (2001) **20**:301–5. [Erratum appears in *Cornea* (2001) **20**:546.]
11. Snyder ME, Katz HR. Ciprofloxacin-resistant bacterial keratitis, *Am J Ophthalmol* (1992) **114**:336–8.
12. Boswell FJ, Andrews JM, Jevons G et al. Comparison of the *in vitro* activities of several new fluoroquinolones against respiratory pathogens and their abilities to select fluoroquinolone resistance, *J Antimicrob Chemother* (2002) **50**:495–502.
13. Mather R, Karenchak LM, Romanowski EG et al. Fourth generation fluoroquinolones: new weapons in the arsenal of ophthalmic antibiotics, *Am J Ophthalmol* (2002) **133**:463–6.
14. Keren G, Alhalel A, Bartov E et al. The intravitreal penetration of orally administered ciprofloxacin in humans, *Invest Ophthalmol Vis Sci* (1991) **32**:2388–92.
15. El Baba FZ, Trousdale MD, Gauderman WJ et al. Intravitreal penetration of oral ciprofloxacin in humans, *Ophthalmology* (1992) **99**:483–6.
16. Lesk MR, Ammann H, Marcil G et al. The penetration of oral ciprofloxacin in the aqueous humor, vitreous, and subretinal fluid of humans, *Am J Ophthalmol* (1993) **115**:623–8.
17. Ozturk F, Kortunay S, Kurt E et al. Penetration of topical and oral ciprofloxacin into the aqueous and vitreous humor in inflamed eyes, *Retina* (1999) **19**:218–22.
18. Alfaro DV, Hudson SJ, Rafanan MM et al. The effect of trauma on the ocular penetration of intravenous ciprofloxacin, *Am J Ophthalmol* (1996) **122**:678–83.
19. Stevens SX, Fouraker BD, Jensen HG. Intraocular safety of ciprofloxacin, *Arch Ophthalmol* (1991) **109**:1737–43.
20. Pearson PA, Hainsworth DP, Ashton P. Clearance and distribution of ciprofloxacin after intravitreal injection, *Retina* (1993) **13**:326–30.
21. Rootman DS, Savage P, Hasany SM et al. Toxicity and pharmacokinetics of intravitreally injected ciprofloxacin in rabbit eyes, *Can J Ophthalmol* (1992) **27**:277–82.
22. von Gunten S, Lew D, Paccolat F et al. Aqueous humor penetration of ofloxacin given by various routes, *Am J Ophthalmol* (1994) **117**:87–9.
23. Donnenfeld ED, Schrier A, Perry HD et al. Penetration of topically applied ciprofloxacin, norfloxacin, and ofloxacin into the aqueous humor, *Ophthalmology* (1994) **101**:902–5.
24. Donnenfeld ED, Perry HD, Snyder RW et al. Intracorneal, aqueous humor, and vitreous humor penetration of topical and oral ofloxacin, *Arch Ophthalmol* (1997) **115**:173–6.
25. Ozturk F, Kurt E, Inan UU et al. Penetration of topical and oral ofloxacin into the aqueous and vitreous humor of inflamed rabbit eyes, *Int J Pharm* (2000) **204**:91–5.
26. Cantor LB, Donnenfeld E, Katz LJ et al. Penetration of ofloxacin and ciprofloxacin into the aqueous humor of eyes with functioning filtering blebs: a randomized trial, *Arch Ophthalmol* (2001) **119**:1254–7.
27. McDermott ML, Hazlett LD, Barrett R. The effect of ofloxacin on the human corneal endothelium, *Cornea* (1997) **16**:209–14.
28. Jensen MK, Fiscella RG. Comparison of endoph-

thalmitis rates over four years associated with topical ofloxacin vs. ciprofloxacin, *ARVO* (2002) abstract no. 4429.

29. Ng EW, Samiy N, Ruoff KL et al. Treatment of experimental *Staphylococcus epidermidis* endophthalmitis with oral trovafloxacin, *Am J Ophthalmol* (1998) **126**:278–87.

30. Karakucuk S, Mirza E, Sumerkan B et al. Intravitreal trovafloxacin against experimental *Staphylococcus epidermidis* endophthalmitis, *Ophthalmic Res* (2000) **32**:126–31.

31. Gurler B, Ozkul Y, Bitiren M et al. Experimental intravitreal application of trovafloxacin in rabbits, *Ophthalmic Res* (2001) **33**:228–36.

32. Raizman MB, Rubin JM, Graves AL et al. Tear concentrations of levofloxacin following topical administration of a single dose of 0.5% levofloxacin ophthalmic solution in healthy volunteers, *Clin Ther* (2002) **24**:1439–50.

33. Bucci FA. An *in vivo* comparison of the ocular absorption of levofloxacin versus ciprofloxacin prior to phacoemulsification, *ARVO* (2002) abstract no. 1579.

34. Fiscella RG, Nguyen TK, Cwik MJ et al. Aqueous and vitreous penetration of levofloxacin after oral administration, *Ophthalmology* (1999) **106**:2286–90.

35. Yamada M, Mochizuki H, Yamada K et al. Aqueous humor levels of topically applied levofloxacin in human eyes, *Curr Eye Res* (2002) **24**:403–6.

36. Bucci FA Jr. An *in vivo* study comparing the ocular absorption of levofloxacin and ciprofloxacin prior to phacoemulsification, *Am J Ophthalmol* (2004) **137**:308–12.

37. Yildirim O, Oz O, Aslan G et al. The efficacy of intravitreal levofloxacin and intravitreal dexamethasone in experimental *Staphylococcus epidermidis* endophthalmitis, *Ophthalmic Res* (2002) **34**:349–56.

38. Gurler B, Ozkul Y, Bitiren M et al. A study on the toxicity of intravitreal levofloxacin in rabbits, *Curr Eye Res* (2002) **24**:253–62.

39. Breen J, Skuba K, Grasela D. Safety and tolerability of gatifloxacin, an advanced-generation, 8-methoxy fluoroquinolone, *J Respir Dis* (1999) **20** (11 Suppl):S70–S75.

40. Tequin package insert. Bristol-Meyers Squibb Co: Princeton, NJ, 1999.

41. Hariprasad SM, Mieler WF, Holz ER. Vitreous and aqueous penetration of orally administered gatifloxacin in humans, *Arch Ophthalmol* (2003) **121**:345–50.

42. Hariprasad SM, Mieler WF, Holz ER. Vitreous penetration of orally administered gatifloxacin in humans, *Trans Am Ophthalmol Soc* (2002) **100**: 153–9.

43. Zymar package insert. Allergan Inc.: Irvine, CA, 2003.

44. Garcia-Saenz MC, Arias-Puente A, Fresnadillo-Martinez MJ et al. Human aqueous humor levels of oral ciprofloxacin, levofloxacin, and moxifloxacin, *J Cataract Refract Surg* (2001) **27**:1969–74.

45. Bronner S, Jehl F, Peter JD et al. Moxifloxacin efficacy and vitreous penetration in a rabbit model of *Staphylococcus aureus* endophthalmitis and effect on gene expression of leucotoxins and virulence regulator factors, *Antimicrob Agents Chemother* (2003) **47**:1621–9.

46. Sclech BA, Stroman DW, Gower L et al. Eradication of bacteria from infected eyes by a three day BID treatment with moxifloxacin ophthalmic solution 0.5%, *ARVO* (2003) abstract no. 2116.

47. Katz HR, Andrews W, Creager D et al. Moxifloxacin Study Group. Moxifloxacin ophthalmic solution 0.5% hastens cure and eradicates the causative pathogens of bacterial conjunctivitis in pediatric and adult populations, *ARVO* (2003) abstract no. 2114.

48. Silver LH, Burkey R, Montgomery D et al. Safety of ophthalmic moxifloxacin in the treatment of newborns, infants and toddlers, children, and adolescents with bacterial conjunctivitis, *ARVO* (2003) abstract no. 804.

49. Axelrod JL, Newton JC, Sarakhun C et al. Ceftriaxone. A new cephalosporin with aqueous humor levels effective against enterobacteriaceae, *Arch Ophthalmol* (1985) **103**:71–2.

50. Sharir M, Triester G, Kneer J et al. The intravitreal penetration of ceftriaxone in man following systemic administration, *Invest Ophthalmol Vis Sci* (1989) **30**:2179–83.

51. Shockley RK, Jay WM, Friberg TR et al. Intravitreal ceftriaxone in a rabbit model. Dose- and time-dependent toxic effects and pharmacokinetic analysis, *Arch Ophthalmol* (1984) **102**:1236–8.

52. Aguilar HE, Meredith TA, Shaarawy A et al. Vitreous cavity penetration of ceftazidime after intravenous administration, *Retina* (1995) **15**: 154–9.

53. Shaarawy A, Meredith TA, Kincaid M et al. Intraocular injection of ceftazidime. Effects of inflammation and surgery, *Retina* (1995) **15**:433–8.

54. Schech JM, Alfaro DV III, Laughlin RM et al. Intravenous gentamicin and ceftazidime in penetrating ocular trauma: a swine model, *Retina* (1997) **17**:28–32.

55. Campochiaro PA, Green WR. Toxicity of intravitreous ceftazidime in primate retina, *Arch Ophthalmol* (1992) **110**:1625–9.

56. Jenkins CD, Tuft SJ, Sheraidah G et al. Comparative intraocular penetration of topical and injected cefuroxime, *Br J Ophthalmol* (1996) **80**:685–8.

57. Martin DF, Ficker LA, Aguilar HA et al. Vitreous cefazolin levels after intravenous injection. Effects of inflammation, repeated antibiotic doses, and surgery, *Arch Ophthalmol* (1990) **108**:411–14.

58. Kramann C, Pitz S, Schwenn O et al. Effects of intraocular cefotaxime on the human corneal

endothelium, *J Cataract Refract Surg* (2001) **2**:250–5.

59. AAO website: http://www.aao.org/aao/education/library/information/vancomycin.cfm

60. Meredith TA, Aguilar HE, Shaarawy A et al. Vancomycin levels in the vitreous cavity after intravenous administration, *Am J Ophthalmol* (1995) **119**:774–8.

61. Ferencz JR, Assia EI, Diamantstein L et al. Vancomycin concentration in the vitreous after intravenous and intravitreal administration for postoperative endophthalmitis, *Arch Ophthalmol* (1999) **117**:1023–7.

62. Haider SA, Hassett P, Bron AJ. Intraocular vancomycin levels after intravitreal injection in post cataract extraction endophthalmitis, *Retina* (2001) **21**:210–13.

63. Souli M, Kopsinis G, Kavouklis E et al. Vancomycin levels in human aqueous humour after intravenous and subconjunctival administration, *Int J Antimicrob Agents* (2001) **18**:239–43.

64. Aguilar HE, Meredith TA, el-Massry A et al. Vancomycin levels after intravitreal injection. Effects of inflammation and surgery, *Retina* (1995) **15**:428–32.

65. Pflugfelder SC, Hernandez E, Fliesler SJ et al. Intravitreal vancomycin. Retinal toxicity, clearance, and interaction with gentamicin, *Arch Ophthalmol* (1987) **105**: 831–7.

66. Park SS, Vallar RV, Hong CH et al. Intravitreal dexamethasone effect on intravitreal vancomycin elimination in endophthalmitis, *Arch Ophthalmol* (1999) **117**:1058–62.

67. Hegazy HM, Kivilcim M, Peyman GA et al. Evaluation of toxicity of intravitreal ceftazidime, vancomycin, and ganciclovir in a silicone oil-filled eye, *Retina* (1999) **19**:553–7.

68. Homer P, Peyman GA, Koziol J et al. Intravitreal injection of vancomycin in experimental staphylococcal endophthalmitis, *Acta Ophthalmol (Copenh)* (1975) **53**:311–20.

69. Piguet B, Chobaz C, Grounauer PA. Toxic retinopathy caused by intravitreal injection of amikacin and vancomycin, *Klin Monatsbl Augenheilkd* (1996) **208**:358–9.

70. Oum BS, D'Amico DJ, Wong KW. Intravitreal antibiotic therapy with vancomycin and aminoglycoside. An experimental study of combination and repetitive injections, *Arch Ophthalmol* (1989) **107**:1055–60.

71. Buerk BM, Fiscella R, Johnson S et al. Intravitreal toxicity of linezolid in rabbits, *ARVO* abstract (2004), abstract number 4902.

72. Fiscella RG, Lai WW, Buerk B et al. Aqueous and vitreous penetration of linezolid (Zyvox) after oral administration, *Ophthalmology* (2004) **111**:1191–5.

73. Campochiaro PA, Lim JI. Aminoglycoside toxicity in the treatment of endophthalmitis. The Aminoglycoside Toxicity Study Group, *Arch Ophthalmol* (1994) **112**:48–53.

74. Donahue SP, Kowalski RP, Eller AW et al. Empiric treatment of endophthalmitis: are aminoglycosides necessary? *Arch Ophthalmol* (1994) **112**:45–7.

75. Peyman GA, May DR, Homer PI et al. Penetration of gentamicin into the aphakic eye, *Ann Ophthalmol* (1977) **9**:871–80.

76. El-Massry A, Meredith TA, Aguilar HE et al. Aminoglycoside levels in the rabbit vitreous cavity after intravenous administration, *Am J Ophthalmol* (1996) **122**:684–9.

77. Peyman GA, May DR, Ericson ES et al. Intraocular injection of gentamicin: toxic effects and clearance, *Arch Ophthalmol* (1974) **92**:42–7.

78. Bennett TO, Peyman GA. Toxicity of intravitreal aminoglycosides in primates, *Can J Ophthalmol* (1974) **9**:475–8.

79. Bennett TO, Peyman GA. Use of tobramycin in eradicating experimental bacterial endophthalmitis, *Albrecht von Graefes Klin Exp Ophthalmol* (1974) **191**:93–107.

80. Kanter ED, Brucker AJ. Aminoglycoside macular infarction in association with gentamicin-soaked collagen corneal shield, *Arch Ophthalmol* (1995) **113**:1359–60.

81. Conway BP, Campochiaro PA. Macular infarction after endophthalmitis treated with vitrectomy and intravitreal gentamicin, *Arch Ophthalmol* (1986) **104**:367–71.

82. Galloway G, Ramsay A, Jordan K et al. Macular infarction after intravitreal amikacin: mounting evidence against amikacin, *Br J Ophthalmol* (2002) **86**:359–60.

83. Kumar H, Ahuja S, Kumar A. Macular infarction after intravitreal amikacin, *Ann Ophthalmol* (1993) **25**:262–3.

84. Conway BP, Tabatabay CA, Campochiaro PA et al. Gentamicin toxicity in the primate retina, *Arch Ophthalmol* (1989) **107**:107–12.

85. Schenk AG, Peyman GA, Paque JT. The intravitreal use of carbenicillin (Geopen) for treatment of *Pseudomonas* endophthalmitis, *Acta Ophthalmol* (1974) **52**:707–17.

86. Heigle TJ, Peyman GA. Retinal toxicity of intravitreal ticarcillin, *Ophthalmic Surg* (1990) **21**:563–5.

87. Semple HC, Liu JC, Peyman GA. Intravitreal injection of piperacillin, *Ophthalmic Surg* (1989) **20**:588–90.

88. Morgan BS, Larson B, Peyman GA et al. Toxicity of antibiotic combinations for vitrectomy infusion fluid, *Ophthalmic Surg* (1979) **10**:74–7.

89. Liang C, Peyman GA, Sonmez M et al. Experimental prophylaxis of *Staphylococcus aureus* endophthalmitis after vitrectomy: the use of antibiotics in irrigating solution, *Retina* (1999) **19**: 223–9.

90. Hanna C, Massey JY, Hendrickson RO et al. Ocular

penetration of topical chloramphenicol in humans, *Arch Ophthalmol* (1978) **96**:1258–61.

91. George FJ, Hanna C. Ocular penetration of chloramphenicol. Effects of route of administration, *Arch Ophthalmol* (1977) **95**:879–82.

92. Fraunfelder FT, Bagby GC Jr, Kelly DJ. Fatal aplastic anemia following topical administration of ophthalmic chloramphenicol, *Am J Ophthalmol* (1982) **93**:356–60.

93. Rich ML, Ritterhoff RJ, Hoffmann RJ. A fatal case of aplastic anemia following chloramphenicol (chloromycetin) therapy, *Ann Intern Med* (1950) **33**:1459–67.

94. Rosenthal RL, Blackman A. Bone-marrow hypoplasia following the use of chloramphenicol eye drops, *JAMA* (1965) **191**:136–7.

95. Carpenter G. Chloramphenicol eye drops and marrow aplasia, *Lancet* (1975) **2**:326–7.

96. Abrams SM, Degnan TJ, Vinciguerra V. Marrow aplasia following topical application of chloramphenicol eye ointment, *Arch Intern Med* (1980) **140**:576–7.

97. Walker S, Diaper CJ, Bowman R et al. Lack of evidence for systemic toxicity following topical chloramphenicol use, *Eye* (1998) **12** (Pt 5):875–9.

98. Wiholm BE, Kelly JP, Kaufman D et al. Relation of aplastic anaemia to use of chloramphenicol eye drops in two international case-control studies, *BMJ* (1998) **316**: 666.

99. Koziol J, Peyman G. Intraocular chloramphenicol and bacterial endophthalmitis, *Can J Ophthalmol* (1974) **9**:316–21.

100. Warheker PT, Gupta SR, Mansfield DC et al. Successful treatment of saccular endophthalmitis with clarithromycin, *Eye* (1998) **12**:1017–19.

101. Al-Sibai MB, Al-Kaff AS, Raines D et al. Ocular penetration of oral clarithromycin in humans, *J Ocul Pharmacol Ther* (1998) **14**:575–83.

102. Okhravi N, Guest S, Lightman S et al. Assessment of the effect of oral clarithromycin on visual outcome following presumed bacterial endophthalmitis, *Curr Eye Res* (2000) **21**:691–702.

103. Unal M, Peyman GA, Liang C et al. Ocular toxicity of intravitreal clarithromycin, *Retina* (1999) **19**:442–6.

104. Goldblum D, Rohrer K, Frueh BE et al. Ocular distribution of intravenously administered lipid formulations of amphotericin B in a rabbit model, *Antimicrob Agents Chemother* (2002) **46**:3719–23.

105. Peyman GA, Vastine DW, Diamond JG. Vitrectomy in exogenous *Candida* endophthalmitis, *Albrecht von Graefes Arch Klin Exp Ophthalmol* (1975) **197**: 55–9.

106. Peyman GA, Raichand M, Bennett TO. Management of endophthalmitis with pars plana vitrectomy, *Br J Ophthalmol* (1980) **64**:472–5.

107. Goldblum D, Rohrer K, Frueh BE et al. Corneal concentrations following systemic administration of amphotericin B and its lipid preparations in a rabbit model, *Ophthalmic Res* (2004) **36**:172–6.

108. O'Day DM, Head WS, Robinson RD et al. Bioavailability and penetration of topical amphotericin B in the anterior segment of the rabbit eye, *J Ocul Pharmacol* (1986) **2**:371–8.

109. Green WR, Bennett JE, Goos RD. Ocular penetration of amphotericin B: a report of laboratory studies and a case report of postsurgical *Cephalosporium* endophthalmitis, *Arch Ophthalmol* (1965) **73**:769–75.

110. Axelrod AJ, Peyman GA, Apple DJ. Toxicity of intravitreal injection of amphotericin B, *Am J Ophthalmol* (1973) **76**:578–83.

111. Axelrod AJ, Peyman GA. Intravitreal amphotericin B treatment of experimental fungal endophthalmitis, *Am J Ophthalmol* (1973) **76**:584–8.

112. Perraut LE Jr, Perraut LE, Bleiman B et al. Successful treatment of *Candida albicans* endophthalmitis with intravitreal amphotericin B, *Arch Ophthalmol* (1981) **99**:1565–7.

113. Orgel IK, Cohen KL. Postoperative zygomycetes endophthalmitis, *Ophthalmic Surg* (1989) **20**: 584–7.

114. Huang K, Peyman GA, McGetrick J. Vitrectomy in experimental endophthalmitis: Part I. Fungal infection, *Ophthalmic Surg* (1979) **10**:84–6.

115. Boldrey EE. Bilateral endogenous *Aspergillus* endophthalmitis, *Retina* (1981) **1**:171–4.

116. Christenson JC, Shalit I, Welch DF et al. Synergistic action of amphotericin B and rifampin against *Rhizopus* species, *Antimicrob Agents Chemother* (1987) **31**:1775–8.

117. Jones BR. Principles in the management of oculomycosis. XXXI Edward Jackson memorial lecture, *Am J Ophthalmol* (1975) **79**:719–51.

118. Gilman AG, Goodman LS, Gilman A. *Goodman and Gilman's The Pharmacologic Basis of Therapeutics*, 6th edn (MacMillan: New York, 1980) 984.

119. Ellison AC. Intravitreal effects of pimaricin in experimental fungal endophthalmitis, *Am J Ophthalmol* (1976) **81**:157–61.

120. Ellison AC, Newmark E. Effects of subconjunctival pimaricin in experimental keratomycosis, *Am J Ophthalmol* (1973) **75**:790–4.

121. Fine BS, Zimmerman LE. Therapy of experimental intraocular *Aspergillus* infection, *Arch Ophthalmol* (1960) **64**:849–61.

122. Shahsavari M, Peyman GA, Niesman MR. Retinal toxicity and *in vitro* efficacy study of cilofungin (LY121019), *Ophthalmic Surg* (1990) **21**:726–8.

123. Codish SD, Tobias JS, Hannigan M. Combined amphotericin B-flucytosine therapy in *Aspergillus* pneumonia, *JAMA* (1979) **241**:2418–19.

124. Dunlap WA, Karacorlu M, Peyman GA et al. Retinal toxicity of intravitreally injected faeriefungin, *Ophthalmic Surg* (1994) **25**:303–6.

125. Thomas PA. Current perspectives on ophthalmic mycoses, *Clin Microb Rev* (2003) **16**:730–97.

126. Kucers A, Bennett NM. *The Use of Antibiotics: A Comprehensive Review with Clinical Emphasis,* 3rd edn (Lippincott: Philadelphia, 1979) 967.

127. Fitzsimons RB, Nicholls MD, Billson FA et al. Fungal retinitis: a case of *Torulopsis glabrata* infection treated with miconazole, *Br J Ophthalmol* (1980) **64**:672–5.

128. Tolentino FI, Foster CS, Lahav M et al. Toxicity of intravitreous miconazole, *Arch Ophthalmol* (1982) **100**:1504–9.

129. Fowler BJ. Treatment of fungal endophthalmitis with vitrectomy and intraocular injection of miconazole, *J Ocul Ther Surg* (1984) **3**:43–7.

130. Jones DB. Therapy of postsurgical fungal endophthalmitis, *Ophthalmology* (1978) **85**:357–73.

131. Blumenkranz MS, Stevens DA. Therapy of endogenous fungal endophthalmitis: miconazole or amphotericin B for coccidioidal and candidal infection, *Arch Ophthalmol* (1980) **98**:1216–20.

132. Foster CS, Stefanyszyn M. Intraocular penetration of miconazole in rabbits, *Arch Ophthalmol* (1979) **97**:1703–6.

133. Peyman GA. Intravitreal miconazole, *Arch Ophthalmol* (1983) **101**:487.

134. Levine HB. *Ketoconazole in the Management of Fungal Disease* (ADIS Press: New York, 1982) 57.

135. Kastrup EK, Boyd JR. *Facts and Comparisons* (Lippincott: Philadelphia, 1982) 335.

136. Osato MS, Ugland DN, Broberg PH et al. Ketoconazole therapy of endogenous *Candida albicans* endophthalmitis, *Invest Ophthalmol Vis Sci* (1980) **19** (Suppl):113.

137. Salmon JF, Partridge BM, Spalton DJ. *Candida* endophthalmitis in a heroin addict: a case report, *Br J Ophthalmol* (1983) **67**:306–9.

138. Stern WH, Tamura E, Jacobs RA et al. Epidemic postsurgical *Candida parapsilosis* endophthalmitis. Clinical findings and management of 15 consecutive cases, *Ophthalmology* (1985) **92**:1701–9.

139. Savani DV, Perfect JR, Cobo LM et al. Penetration of new azole compounds into the eye and efficacy in experimental *Candida* endophthalmitis, *Antimicrob Agents Chemother* (1987) **31**:6–10.

140. Mary C, Goudard M, Blancard A et al. [Synergic effect of 5–fluorocytosine and imidazole derivatives against yeast strains resistant to 5–fluorocytosine], *Ann Biol Clin (Paris)* (1989) **47**:546–9 [in French].

141. Yoshizumi MO, Banihashemi AR. Experimental intravitreal ketoconazole in DMSO, *Retina* (1988) **8**:210–5.

142. Polak A. Oxiconazole, a new imidazole derivative. Evaluation of antifungal activity in vitro and in vivo, *Arzneimittel-Forschung* (1982) **32**:17–24.

143. Schulman JA, Peyman GA, Dietlein J et al. Toxicity of intravitreal oxiconazole, *Int Ophthalmol* (1989) **13**:201–3.

144. Schulman JA, Peyman GA, Dietlein J et al. Ocular toxicity of experimental intravitreal itraconazole, *Int Ophthalmol* (1991) **15**:21–4.

145. Polak A. Combination therapy of experimental candidiasis, cryptococcosis, aspergillosis and wangiellosis in mice, *Chemotherapy* (1987) **33**: 381–95.

146. Schulman JA, Peyman G, Fiscella R et al. Toxicity of intravitreal injection of fluconazole in the rabbit, *Can J Ophthalmol* (1987) **22**:304–6.

147. Tucker RM, Williams PL, Arathoon EG et al. Pharmacokinetics of fluconazole in cerebrospinal fluid and serum in human coccidioidal meningitis, *Antimicrob Agents Chemother* (1988) **32**:369–73.

148. Arikan S, Lozano-Chiu M, Paetznick V et al. Microdilution susceptibility testing of amphotericin B, itraconazole, and voriconazole against clinical isolates of *Aspergillus* and *Fusarium* species, *J Clin Microbiol* (1999) **37**: 3946–51.

149. Espinel-Ingroff A. *In vitro* activities of the new triazole voriconazole (UK-109,496) against opportunistic filamentous and dimorphic fungi and common and emerging yeast pathogens, *J Clin Microbiol* (1998) **36**:198–202.

150. McGinnis MR, Pasarell L, Sutton DA et al. *In vitro* activity of voriconazole against selected fungi, *Med Mycol* (1998) **36**:239–42.

151. Clancy CJ, Nguyen MH. In vitro efficacy and fungicidal activity of voriconazole against *Aspergillus* and *Fusarium* species, *Eur J Clin Microbiol Infect Dis* (1998) **17**:573–5.

152. Lozano-Chiu M, Arikan S, Paetznick VL et al. Optimizing voriconazole susceptibility testing of *Candida*: effects of incubation time, endpoint rule, species of *Candida*, and level of fluconazole susceptibility, *J Clin Microbiol* (1999) **37**:2755–9.

153. Nguyen MH, Yu CY. Voriconazole against fluconazole-susceptible and resistant *Candida* isolates: *in vitro* efficacy compared with that of itraconazole and ketoconazole, *J Antimicrob Chemother* (1998) **42**:253–6.

154. Johnson EM, Szekely A, Warnock DW. In-vitro activity of voriconazole, itraconazole and amphotericin B against filamentous fungi, *J Antimicrob Chemother* (1998) **42**:741–5.

155. Sheehan DJ, Hitchcock CA, Sibley CM. Current and emerging azole antifungal agents, *Clin Microbiol Rev* (1999) **12**:40–79.

156. Hariprasad SM, Mieler WF, Holz ER et al. Determination of vitreous, aqueous, and plasma concentration of orally administered voriconazole in humans, *Arch Ophthalmol* (2004) **122**:42–7.

157. Garbino J, Ondrusova A, Baligvo E et al. Successful treatment of *Paecilomyces lilacinus* endophthalmitis with voriconazole, *Scand J Infect Dis* (2002) **34**:701–3. [Erratum appears in *Scand J Infect Dis* (2003) **35**:79.]

Index

Numbers in italics refer to *figures* and *tables*.

Printed and bound by CPI Group (UK) Ltd, Croydon, CR0 4YY

23/10/2024

01777691-0006